T0234375

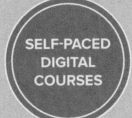
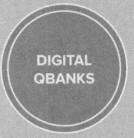
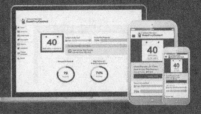
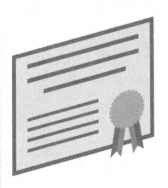
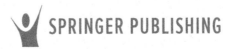

PCCN® CERTIFICATION EXPRESS REVIEW

PCCN® CERTIFICATION EXPRESS REVIEW

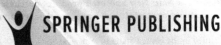

SPRINGER PUBLISHING

Springer Publishing Company, LLC
11 West 42nd Street, New York, NY 10036
www.springerpub.com

Acquisitions Editor: Suzanne Toppy
Clinical Editor: Emily Ferrara, MSN, RN
Compositor: diacriTech

ISBN: 978-0-8261-5957-1
ebook ISBN: 978-0-8261-5958-8
DOI: 10.1891/9780826159588

Printed by BnT

The author and the publisher of this Work have made every effort to use sources believed to be reliable to provide information that is accurate and compatible with the standards generally accepted at the time of publication. Because medical science is continually advancing, our knowledge base continues to expand. Therefore, as new information becomes available, changes in procedures become necessary. We recommend that the reader always consult current research and specific institutional policies before performing any clinical procedure or delivering any medication. The author and publisher shall not be liable for any special, consequential, or exemplary damages resulting, in whole or in part, from the readers' use of, or reliance on, the information contained in this book. The publisher has no responsibility for the persistence or accuracy of URLs for external or third-party Internet websites referred to in this publication and does not guarantee that any content on such websites is, or will remain, accurate or appropriate.

Library of Congress Control Number: 2021923265

Contact sales@springerpub.com to receive discount rates on bulk purchases.

***Publisher's Note*: New and used products purchased from third-party sellers are not guaranteed for quality, authenticity, or access to any included digital components.**

Printed in the United States of America.

CONTENTS

PREFACE

If you have purchased this *Express Review*, you are likely well into your exam prep journey to certification. This book was designed to be a high-speed review—a last-minute gut check before your exam day. We created this review, which is a quick summary of the key topics you'll encounter on the exam, to supplement to your certification preparation studies. We encourage you to use it in conjunction with other study aids to ensure you are as prepared as possible for the exam.

This book, written by certified progressive care nurses, follows the AACN®'s most recent exam content outline, and uses a succinct, bulleted format to highlight what you need to know. This book will help you solidify your retention of information in the month or so leading up to your exam. Special features appear throughout the book to call out important information, including

- **Complications:** Problems that can arise with certain disease states or procedures
- **Nursing Pearls:** Additional patient care insights and strategies for knowledge retention
- **Alerts:** Need-to-know details on how to handle emergency situations
- **Pop Quizzes:** Critical-thinking questions to test your ability to synthesize what you learned (answers in appendix)
- **Medication Tables:** Handy tables at the end of each body system chapter highlighting the indications, mechanisms of action, contraindications, and adverse effects of commonly administered medications
- **List of Abbreviations:** A useful appendix to help guide you through the alphabet soup of clinical terms

We know life is busy. Being able to prepare for your exam efficiently and effectively is paramount, which is why we created this *Express Review*. You have come to the right place as you continue on your path of professional growth and development. The stakes are high, and we want to help you succeed. Best of luck to you on your certification journey. You've got this!

PASS GUARANTEE

If you use this resource to prepare for your exam and you do not pass, you may return it for a refund of your full purchase price. To receive a refund, you must return your product along with a copy of your original receipt and exam score report. Product must be returned and received within 180 days of the original purchase date. Excludes tax, shipping, and handling. One offer per person and address. Refunds will be issued within eight weeks from acceptance and approval. This offer is valid for U.S. residents only. Void where prohibited. To begin the process, please contact customer service at CS@springerpub.com.

1

ABOUT THE EXAMINATION

OVERVIEW

Congratulations on taking one step closer to becoming a progressive care certified nurse (PCCN). The PCCN® examination is written and administered by the AACN and accredited by the NCCA. This exam is designed for RNs and APRNs who practice in progressive care units or provide direct care for acutely ill patients.

PCCN CERTIFICATION REQUIREMENTS

To be eligible to sit for the PCCN exam, test takers must meet the following requirements:
- Have a current, unencumbered nursing license as either an RN or APRN in the United States.
- Meet the requirements of either of the following:
  - Minimum of 2 years of direct care of acutely ill patients, totaling 1,750 clinical hr, with 875 of those hr obtained in the year before application.
  - Have 5 years and at least of 2,000 clinical hr of direct care of acutely ill patients, with 144 of those hr in the most recent year before application.
- Be prepared to provide the name and contact information for a direct supervisor or coworker who can verify clinical hr fulfillment.

ABOUT THE EXAMINATION

- The PCCN examination is a 2.5-hr exam with 125 multiple choice questions.
- Of the 125 multiple choice questions, 100 are scored, and 25 are sample test questions to be used on future exams.
- Passing point/cutoff score:
  - A passing point/cutoff score is predetermined by the exam development committee who carefully reviews each exam question to determine the basic level of knowledge or skill that is expected.
  - The passing point/cutoff score is based on the panel's established difficulty ratings for each exam question.
  - Test takers who meet or exceed this passing point/cutoff score will become PCCN certified.
- Test plan: Test covers two main topics: Clinical Judgment and Professional Caring/Ethical Practice.
  - Clinical Judgment accounts for 80% of the questions and covers each body system, and its related diagnostic tests and nursing interventions. Questions are further broken down by body system and include the following topics:
    - Cardiovascular (27%)
    - Pulmonary (17%)
    - Endocrine/Hematology/Neurology/Gastrointestinal/Renal (20%)
    - Musculoskeletal/Multisystem/Psychosocial (16%)
  - Professional Caring/Ethical Practice accounts for 20% of the questions and includes the following topics:
    - Advocacy/Moral Agency
    - Caring Practices

(continued)

ABOUT THE EXAMINATION *(continued)*

- ○ Response to Diversity
- ○ Facilitation of Learning
- ○ Collaboration
- ○ Systems Thinking
- ○ Clinical Inquiry

HOW TO APPLY

- To apply to take the PCCN examination or for additional information, visit the AACN website at www.aacn.org/certification/get-certified or download the PCCN Exam Handbook from the AACN's website.
- The examination cost for AACN members is $195, and the cost for nonmembers is $300.
- After applying, there is a 90-day window for scheduling and taking the exam at a PSI testing center.

HOW TO RECERTIFY

- After successfully passing the PCCN examination, certification is active for 3 years.
- Online renewal is available to active PCCN certifications 4 months before the scheduled renewal date.
- Nurses who want to recertify must have completed at least 432 hr actively working clinically in acute or critical care. At least 144 of those hr need to be in the year leading up to recertification.
- Certification holders may renew through the following:
  - *CERP*: Complete 100 CERP points in the following:
    - ○ *Category A*: Clinical Judgment/Clinical Inquiry (60–80 points)
    - ○ *Category B*: Advocacy and Moral Agency, Caring Practices, Response to Diversity, Facilitation of Learning (10–30 points)
    - ○ *Category C*: Collaboration, Systems Thinking (10–30 points)
  - *Examination*: Take the PCCN certification exam.
  - *Inactive status*: Nurses can change their status to inactive if they do not meet the criteria for renewal. Inactive status extends the time frame by 3 years to meet the eligibility requirements for recertification. Nurses may not use the PCCN credential while inactive.
- For more information on certification renewal, visit www.aacn.org/certhandbooks.

AACN CONTACT INFORMATION

For more information, visit the AACN website at www.aacn.org/certification/get-certified/pccn-adult. The AACN can also be reached as follows:

- Main Office: (800) 809-2273 available Monday to Friday 7:30 a.m. to 5:30 p.m. PT
- Customer Care: (800) 899-2226 available Monday to Friday 7:30 a.m. to 4:30 p.m. PT
- Mailing Address:
  American Association of Critical-Care Nurses
  27071 Aliso Creek Road
  Aliso Viejo, CA 92656-3399

RESOURCES

American Association of Critical-Care Nurses. (2021, May). *PCCN exam handbook: Acute/critical care nursing certification adult*. https://www.aacn.org/~/media/aacn-website/certification/get-certified/handbooks/pccnexamhandbook.pdf

American Association of Critical-Care Nurses. (n.d.). *Initial eligibility requirements & fees*. https://www.aacn.org/certification/get-certified/pccn-adult

American Association of Critical-Care Nurses. (n.d.). *Renewal eligibility requirements & fees*. https://www.aacn.org/certification/certification-renewal/pccn-adult?tab=Renewal%20by%20Synergy%20CERPs

CARDIOVASCULAR SYSTEM

ACUTE CORONARY SYNDROME

Overview

- ACS describes a group of conditions resulting from a sudden obstruction of the coronary arteries.
- ACS can manifest in three ways:
  - NSTEMI
  - STEMI
  - Unstable angina
- Treatments range from medical management to invasive procedures inducing cardiac catheterization or CABG.
- With timely recognition, ACS can be effectively treated and managed.

Signs and Symptoms

- Patients experiencing ACS may present with any of the following symptoms, with some symptoms varying depending on the manifestation of ACS (Table 2.1):
  - Anxiety, fear, or feelings of imminent demise
  - Decreased pallor
  - Diaphoresis
  - Dyspnea
  - Extra heart sounds (S3, S4, and/or holosystolic murmurs)
  - Fatigue and weakness
  - Initial hypertension and tachycardia, which progresses to hypotension
  - JVD
  - Mental status changes
  - Nausea and vomiting
  - Severe chest pain, heaviness or pressure unrelieved by rest, position changes, and/or medication
  - Palpitations
  - Presyncope or syncope
  - Radiating pain to the chest, neck, jaw, arms, back, and/or epigastrium

COMPLICATIONS

A sudden coronary artery obstruction, if unrecognized and/or untreated, can cause decreased blood flow to the heart and, subsequently, decreased oxygenation of the heart. This can lead to cell injury, dysrhythmia, infarction, left ventricular failure, pericarditis, thromboembolism, tissue injury, and can cause sudden death of the person. Immediate recognition and intervention of obstructions are necessary to prevent deteriorating conditions that can progress to cardiac arrest and death.

NURSING PEARL

The difference between stable and unstable angina can be identified by symptom presentation. Stable angina involves chest pain that is precipitated by activity and relieved by rest and nitroglycerin. In contrast, unstable angina occurs at rest with no precipitating physical activity.

ALERT!

Risk factors associated with ACS include age, diabetes, dyslipidemia, gender, genetics/family history, high fat diet, hypertension, obesity, sedentary lifestyle, and tobacco use. Nurses should recognize the potential development of ACS in high-risk patients.

Table 2.1 Acute Coronary Syndrome Categories

Unstable Angina	NSTEMI	STEMI	Symptoms
✓			Chest pain may be relieved by nitroglycerin
✓	✓	✓	Chest pain may occur at rest
✓	✓	✓	Chest pain has increased frequency and severity
✓	✓	✓	Chest pain lasts >20 minutes
		✓	Unrelenting chest pain
		✓	Patient has dyspnea, pallor, diaphoresis, or cool clammy skin
		✓	Patient has vagal symptoms (bradycardia, nausea, and vomiting)

Diagnosis

Labs
- BNP
- Cardiac enzymes
  - CK may be elevated >308 U/L for men and >192 U/L for women.
  - CK-MB may be elevated >25 IU/L.
  - Troponin may be elevated >0.4 ng/mL.
- C-reactive protein may be elevated >10 mg/L.
- CMP may show elevated or low potassium or calcium. May worsen kidney or liver functions.
- CBC
- Lipid panel may be normal or elevated.

Diagnostic Testing
- 12-lead EKG may show ST elevation (Table 2.2)
- Cardiac catheterization: coronary angiogram and PCI
- Chest x-ray
- Continuous EKG monitoring
- Stress test
- TTE (transthoracic echocardiogram)

 ALERT!

Symptoms and presentation of ACS can vary between gender and in those with diabetes mellitus and/or prior surgical history of CABG or cardiac transplantation. Women are more likely to present with atypical symptoms, such as jaw, neck, or upper back pain with dyspnea and/or fatigue. Patients with a history of diabetes mellitus, CABG, or cardiac transplant may present with silent ischemia, complaining of dyspnea, and fatigue without angina.

Table 2.2 EKG Changes in ACS

EKG Lead Changes	Anatomical Location	Vessel(s) Involved
V1–V2	Septal wall	LAD
V2–V4	Anterior LV	LAD
I, aVL	High lateral wall	Left circumflex
V5–V6	Low lateral LV	LAD
II, III, aVF	Inferior LV	RCA, left circumflex
V8–V9	Posterior wall	Posterior descending, RCA or left circumflex
V3R, V4R	Right ventricular	RCA

Treatment

- Requires timely diagnosis and intervention
- Immediate for suspected ACS:
  - 12-lead EKG and continuous EKG monitoring
  - IV access
  - Oxygen if indicated to maintain an oxygen saturation >90%
    - Compromised airway or rapid patient deterioration: notify provider and prepare for transfer to higher level of care
- Medications (Table 2.8*):
  - ACEI
  - Antiplatelet inhibitors
  - Anticoagulation
  - Aspirin
  - Beta-adrenergic blockers
  - Fibrinolytic therapy (Table 5.1)
  - Morphine (Table A.2)
  - Nitroglycerin
  - Oxygen
- Possible cardiac catheterization or CABG (see Cardiac Catheterization section)

NURSING PEARL

One popular mnemonic, MONA-B, can be used to recall the common medications used when treating ACS patients (morphine, oxygen, nitroglycerin, aspirin, and beta blockers).

Nursing Interventions

- Assess and manage anxiety as needed.
- Draw serial laboratory tests as ordered and monitor results.
- Update patient and/or family on current clinical status, plan of care, and upcoming tests or procedures.
- Perform continuous physiologic monitoring through frequent physical assessment of cardiac, pulmonary, and neurologic systems for signs of worsening condition or complications.
  - Cardiac:
    - Auscultate for extra heart sounds (S3, S4, holosystolic murmurs).
    - Assess for fluid retention/overload.
  - Pulmonary:
    - Auscultate for adventitious lung sounds (crackles, rhonchi, wheezes, rubs, etc.).
    - Assess for the ability to maintain a patent airway.
    - Assess for signs of respiratory distress or compromise.
  - Neurologic:
    - Assess for changes in alertness to person, place, time, and situation.
    - Assess Glasgow Coma Scale (See Chapter 10 for review of Glasgow Coma Scale).
- Monitor vital signs:
  - Maintain oxygenation and perfusion.
  - Position patient with HOB >30°.
  - Titrate appropriate oxygen delivery system to achieve oxygen saturation >90%.
  - Use continuous SpO_2 monitoring.
  - Prepare for transfer to higher level of care if hemodynamically unstable or unable to maintain adequate oxygenation and ventilation.
  - Assess EKG monitoring system for presence of dysrhythmias.
  - Assess for both hypertension and/or hypotension.
- See the Cardiac Catheterization section for information relating to cardiac catheterization treatment and management.

NURSING PEARL

When monitoring vital signs for a patient experiencing ACS, BP and HR may initially be elevated. As cardiac output decreases, the patient may develop acute hypotension. This decreased perfusion can result in acute kidney injury and decreased urine output.

---

* Table 2.8 is located at the end of this chapter.

Patient Education

- Adhere to dietary recommendations as ordered for lipid and sodium control (DASH diet).
- See Cardiac Catheterization section for information on care of femoral access site post cardiac catheterization. Increase physical activity as recommended. If referred by provider, participate in cardiac rehab program.
- Follow up as appropriate with outpatient appointments.
- Follow exercise and weight management recommendations.
- Pursue smoking cessation as advised.
- Take medication as prescribed.

ACUTE INFLAMMATORY DISEASE

Overview

- Acute inflammatory disease of the heart consists of endocarditis, myocarditis, and pericarditis. It can manifest with a wide range of signs and symptoms depending on etiology and type.
  - *Endocarditis:* Inflammation of the inner lining of the heart (endocardium).
  - *Myocarditis:* Inflammation of the middle layer of the heart (myocardium).
  - *Pericarditis:* Inflammation of the outermost layer of the heart (pericardium).
- Treatments range from lifestyle modifications, medications, and invasive procedures.

Signs and Symptoms

- Endocarditis may have vague or nonspecific symptoms involving multiple organ systems:
  - Abdominal pain
  - Chills
  - Clubbing of fingers
  - Fatigue
  - Fever
  - Headache
  - Malaise
  - Myalgia
  - New or changing heart murmur
  - Weakness
- Pericarditis:
  - Dyspnea
  - Pericardial friction rub
  - Severe chest pain
    - ○ Described as sharp and pleuritic
    - ○ May radiate to neck, arms, or left shoulder
    - ○ Worse with deep breath in supine position
- Myocarditis may present with a range of symptoms:
  - Angina
  - Crackles

 ALERT!

The DASH diet is a nutrition and lifestyle modification approach to moderate BP. The DASH diet includes restricting daily sodium intake to 1500 mg in addition to increasing fruit and vegetable intake, decreasing meat intake to one 6 oz. portion or less of lean meat a day, as well as limiting sweets, fats, and alcohol intake.

 POP QUIZ 2.1

A 48-year-old female is admitted to the PCU with ACS. Her EKG in the emergency department showed no ST elevation; however, after completing her admission EKG in the PCU, there are ST elevations in leads II, III, and AVF. She complains of worsening shortness of breath and anxiety. HR is 136, BP is 98/62, oxygen saturation is 89% on 2 L nasal cannula, and oral temperature is 99 °F (37.2 °C). What should the nurse's next action be?

 COMPLICATIONS

- A severe complication of inflammatory cardiac disease, specifically infective endocarditis, is the development of a septic pulmonary embolism. Bacterial vegetations, which develop on or near the heart valves, become dislodged, travel through the vasculature, and disrupt circulation and perfusion like native clots, ruptured plaques, or emboli. These septic emboli can affect any organ system and can result in sudden death.
- Risk factors for developing an acute inflammatory disease of the heart include age, alcohol and/or IV drug use, family history, gender, poor dentition, medical conditions including cancer, diabetes, renal disease, and/or conditions that alter the body's immune system such as HIV/AIDs, severe burns, or trauma.

- Dyspnea
- Fatigue
- Fever
- HF
- JVD
- Lymphadenopathy
- Myalgia
- Nausea and vomiting
- Peripheral edema
- S3 heart sounds
- Syncopal episodes

Diagnosis

Labs

- Blood cultures to identify organisms responsible for infection
- CBC to show elevated WBCs
- Cardiac enzymes: possible troponin elevation in cardiac inflammation
- Possible inflammatory marker elevation in infection or inflammatory process
  - ESR
  - CRP
- Viral titers: possible elevation if viral infection present

 ALERT!

Prior to performing invasive procedures, coagulation values should be drawn and treated if elevated to decrease the risk for additional bleeding in the pericardial space. Excessive bleeding can worsen patient condition, leading to pericardial effusion and/or tamponade.

Diagnostic Testing

- 12-lead EKG
- Cardiac biopsy
- Cardiac catherization
- Chest x-ray
- CT or MRI
- Echocardiogram
- Pericardiocentesis

Treatment

- Medications (Table 2.8)
  - Antiarrhythmics
  - Antibiotic and/or antifungal IV therapy (Table A.1)
  - Autoimmune/immunosuppressive therapy
- IABP (requires transfer to higher level of care)
- Valve replacement

Nursing Interventions

- Administer antibiotic, antifungal, or immunosuppressant therapy as ordered.
- Follow institutional policy for accessing and administering IV medications through PICC line to prevent CLABSIs.
- Monitor vital signs and physical assessment for any changes. Notify provider immediately if condition worsens.
- Position patient to decrease cardiac workload.

 ALERT!

Patients with a suspected or confirmed history of intravenous drug use are at high risk for developing infective endocarditis. Most commonly, these patients present with MSSA or MRSA infections. Both MSSA and MRSA are treated with long-term antibiotics. This may require a PICC line or other long-term IV injection devices. Patients with intravenous drug use history are often reluctant to comply with this course of treatment, which worsens the infection and results in valvular disease and/or HF.

(continued)

Nursing Interventions *(continued)*

- Perform or have patient perform daily oral hygiene.
- Refer patients with history of intravenous drug use to treatment as appropriate.

Patient Education

- Avoid lifestyle actions that place at risk for recurrence of intravenous drug use.
- Avoid others who are ill, especially with upper respiratory infections.
- Consider participating in drug or alcohol rehabilitation program.
- Determine the cause of inflammatory disease (if identifiable).
- Educate on PICC line maintenance and care if receiving IV antibiotic therapy in outpatient or home health setting.
- Perform daily oral hygiene practices and regularly visit the dentist.
- Use antibiotic prophylaxis for dental or other procedures.

 POP QUIZ 2.2

A 67-year-old female is admitted to the PCU after a motor vehicle accident. She was restrained (as evidenced by a positive seatbelt sign), and the airbags were deployed. In the emergency department, she complains of frequent sharp chest pain. She says the pain is worse when she takes a deep breath or lies down. The pain radiates to her shoulders and upper back. EKG shows no ST elevation, and cardiac enzymes are negative. VS are as follows: HR 122, BP 130/81 mmHg, SpO$_2$ 98% on 2 L nasal cannula, T 98.4 °F (36.9 °C). What should the nurse's next action be?

ANEURYSM

Overview

- An aneurysm is an abnormal outpouching or dilation of a vessel wall that can occur in the abdominal aorta, thoracic aorta, or as a cerebral aneurysm.
- While an abdominal and thoracic aortic aneurysm often present with no symptoms, dissection or rupture of the aneurysm presents with sudden and severe excruciating pain in the chest and/or back with hypotension.
- Cerebral aneurysms are also asymptomatic, usually only presenting with symptoms after rupture.
- The mortality rate of ruptured or dissecting aneurysms (regardless of location) is high.
- Treatment requires strict BP management and surgical repair.

 COMPLICATIONS

A life-threatening complication of aortic aneurysm and dissection includes rupture and hemorrhage that can lead to exsanguination, hypovolemia, and death. Rupture of cerebral aneurysm can result in a devastating hemorrhagic stroke, resulting in total loss of voluntary function and cognitive ability and may result in herniation or death. Preventing these complications requires rapid identification, monitoring, and BP management.

Signs and Symptoms

- Aortic and thoracic aneurysm: most commonly asymptomatic and found on routine, unrelated examinations, or imaging; symptoms, if any, include the following:
  - Epigastric pain
  - Dull generalized back or chest pain
  - Pulsatile mass in the periumbilical area
  - Bruits may be present on abdominal auscultation
- Aortic or thoracic aneurysm dissection present with:
  - Dyspnea
  - Mental status changes
  - Sudden severe pain radiating to the back, shoulders, chest, and/or neck often described as tearing, ripping, or sharp
  - Hypotension
  - Signs and symptoms of hemorrhagic or cardiovascular shock

- Cerebral aneurysms: often asymptomatic and usually found in unrelated imaging studies; rupture symptoms:
  - Severe headache that may be accompanied with a brief loss of consciousness
  - Nausea and vomiting
  - Sudden onset headache (described as a thunderclap headache or as "the worst headache of my life")
  - Cerebral aneurysms leading to subarachnoid hemorrhage: possible sentinel leak, also known as a warning leak, presenting 6 to 20 days before the event

Diagnosis

Labs
There are no labs specific to diagnose aneurysm. However, the following may be helpful when determining severity and treatment:
- CBC
- Coagulopathies and clotting
  - D-dimer
  - Fibrinogen
  - INR
  - Interleukin-6
  - PT/PTT

Diagnostic Testing
- 12-lead EKG
- Angiography
- Chest x-ray
- Chest, abdomen, or head CT scan
- Echocardiogram
- MRI
- Ultrasound

 ALERT!

For patients with abdominal aortic aneurysm with or without suspected dissection, strict BP control is essential to prevent dissection growth or rupture. BP control is managed with pain medication, antihypertensives, and continuous bedside monitoring. Instruct patients to immediately report any change in pain or status.

Treatment

- Medications
  - BP control (Table 2.8)
    - ACEIs
    - Beta blockers
    - Calcium channel blockers
    - Nitrates (e.g., nitroglycerine)
  - Opioid analgesics (Table A.2)
- Surgical repair
  - EVAR:
    - Minimally invasive, performed through a femoral access site much like cardiac catheterization
    - Aortic stent deployed around aneurysm site
    - Postoperatively, recovery consistent with cardiac catheterization
    - Criteria for EVAR include the following:
      - 1.0 to 1.5 cm aneurysm neck
      - Neck diameter <3.2 cm
      - Aortic angulation <60°
      - Access to vessels amendable to endograph delivery
  - Endovascular cerebral aneurysm repair:
    - Minimally invasive; performed through femoral access site in interventional radiology
    - Coils placed within the lumen of the aneurysm promoting clot formation and obliteration of the residual dilation or outpouching

(continued)

Treatment *(continued)*

- Open aortic surgical repair:
  - ○ Typically reserved for emergency repair of ruptured abdominal aortic aneurysms involving the renal arteries or for patients who do not meet the anatomical criteria for EVAR
- Open cerebral aneurysm surgical repair:
  - ○ Involves craniotomy under general anesthesia in the operating room
  - ○ Skull removed, then metal clips placed across the neck of aneurysm to prevent blood from entering residual dilation or outpouching

Nursing Interventions

- In patients with known aortic aneurysm:
  - Monitor BP to maintain a goal of SBP of 110 mmHg.
  - Encourage bedrest and a quiet, calm environment.
  - See Cardiac Catheterization section for post procedure care and management. Gather a complete history and detailed physical assessment.
  - If the patient presents with symptoms of a retroperitoneal bleed post cardiac catheterization, immediate surgical consult should be made as retroperitoneal bleed is a surgical emergency.
  - Manage pain and anxiety.
  - Monitor for:
    - ○ New onset of sudden pain in the back, chest, or abdomen
    - ○ Diaphoresis
    - ○ Weakness
    - ○ Vital sign changes (hypotension and/or tachycardia)
  - Monitor vital signs:
    - ○ Assess EKG monitoring system for presence of dysrhythmia or rate change
    - ○ Assess for both hypotension and hypertension
    - ○ Maintain oxygenation and perfusion.
      - ▪ Position patient with HOB >30°
      - ▪ Use appropriate oxygen delivery system to achieve oxygen saturation >90%.
      - ▪ Use continuous SpO$_2$ monitoring.
      - ▪ Titrate up oxygen delivery system or L/min as needed.

ALERT!

If decompensating, alert the provider and call for rapid response team to ensure all available resources are available for intubation and transfer to higher level of care.

NURSING PEARL

Patients experiencing aortic dissection are at risk to develop cardiac tamponade. Remember, the hallmark signs for cardiac tamponade include Beck's triad: hypotension, distended neck veins, and muffled heart sounds.

Patient Education

- Adhere to dietary recommendations as ordered for lipid and sodium control (e.g., DASH diet).
- During suspected or confirmed aortic dissection, patients must be educated on importance of remaining in bed and minimizing exertion.
- Explain the purpose of any medication therapy.
- Follow up as appropriate with outpatient appointments.
- Follow exercise and weight management recommendations.
- Increase physical activity as recommended and, if referred by provider, participate in cardiac rehab program.

POP QUIZ 2.3

A 65-year-old male is admitted to the PCU after a witnessed syncopal episode in the yard while gardening with his wife. The patient fell forward and hit a large rock during the syncopal episode. While in the emergency department, a chest x-ray revealed a right-sided hairline fracture in rib 5, but most notably a dilation in the aorta, which is concerning for an abdominal aortic aneurysm. The physician has ordered a STAT CT and BP goals of SBP 110 mmHg. What additional orders should the nurse request at this time?

CARDIAC CATHETERIZATION

Overview

- Cardiac catheterizations are performed to provide visualization of the vascular system and/or coronary arteries using contrast media and x-rays.
- There are two types of cardiac catheterization:
  - Left heart catheterizations:
    - ○ Angioplasty with or without stenting
    - ○ Coronary angiography
    - ○ Pressure measurements of the chambers
    - ○ Ventriculography
  - Right heart catheterizations:
    - ○ Pressure and flow measurements
- Left heart catheterization angiography can help identify areas and lesions of concern in the coronary arteries. If a concerning lesion is identified, it may be treated with balloon angioplasty or stent placement.
- Not all lesions can be treated with a balloon angioplasty or stent placement. If revascularization is not possible with stenting or balloon angioplasty, then a CABG is indicated.

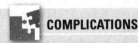

COMPLICATIONS

Complications of cardiac catheterization and/or stent placement include reocclusion of the stent/vessel, dysrhythmia, arterial dissection, pseudoaneurysm, hematoma, retroperitoneal bleed, myocardial infarction, and death.

Signs and Symptoms

A cardiac catheterization is indicated if a patient presents with the following signs, symptoms, or past medical history:

- Dysrhythmia
- Congenital heart disease
- New or worsening symptoms of HF including dyspnea, increasing oxygen requirements, fluid overload, pulmonary edema, or cardiogenic shock.
- Sudden onset of chest pain with or without:
  - Anxiety, fear, or feelings of imminent demise
  - Decreased pallor
  - Diaphoresis
  - Dyspnea
  - Extra heart sounds (S3, S4, and/or holosystolic murmurs)
  - Fatigue and weakness
  - Initial hypertension and tachycardia, which progresses to hypotension
  - JVD
  - Mental status changes
  - Nausea and vomiting
  - Palpitations
  - Presyncope or syncope
  - Radiating pain to the chest, neck, jaw, arms, back, and/or epigastrium
  - ST changes
  - Severe chest pain, heaviness, or pressure unrelieved by rest, position changes, and/or medication

Diagnosis

Labs

- Lab drawn prior to beginning a cardiac catheterization procedure
- BMP

(continued)

Labs (continued)

- Creatinine
  - Iodine contrast media can be nephrotoxic to kidneys and result in increased creatinine and kidney function post procedure.
  - If creatinine is mildly elevated from baseline and the patient does not have a history of kidney disease, hydrate with IV fluids prior to procedure.
- Magnesium
  - Hyper- or hypomagnesemia can produce lethal dysrhythmias while in the cardiac catheterization procedure.
  - Low magnesium should be supplemented pre procedure.
- Potassium
  - Hyper- or hypokalemia can produce lethal dysrhythmias while in the cardiac catheterization procedure.
  - Low magnesium should be supplemented pre procedure.
  - High potassium should be treated as necessary based on patient condition.
- Coagulopathies
  - INR: will be evaluated for patients taking Coumadin
  - PT
  - PTT: baseline evaluation, as heparin given intraoperatively and will increase coagulation times
- CBC
  - Hematocrit
  - Hemoglobin
  - Platelets: indicates potential clotting issues
  - WBCs: indicates whether infection is present
- Type and screen

Diagnostic Testing
- 12-lead EKG
- Continuous EKG monitoring
- Positive Allen test for radial approach
- TTE

 ALERT!

Patients receiving iodine contrast are at risk for developing an acute kidney injury due to the nephrotoxic properties of contrast. Patients receiving iodine contrast for catheterization procedure should be well hydrated pre and post procedure. Additionally, baseline renal function should be assessed to monitor for the development of acute kidney injury post procedure.

Treatment

- Before the procedure, patients should receive the following:
  - Aspirin as ordered pre procedure
  - IV access
  - IV fluid replacement as ordered
  - Potassium or magnesium supplementation if needed based on potassium or magnesium labs
  - Vitamin K as needed based on INR (Table 5.6)
- If coronary angiogram demonstrates evidence of blockage of the coronary arteries, patients may receive the following:
  - Balloon angioplasty
  - Bare metal stent
  - Drug-eluting stent
- Post procedure, patients should receive the following:
  - Clopidogrel or prasugrel if PCI performed (Table 2.8)
  - Strict bed rest procedures until femoral sheath is removed and hemostasis is achieved
  - Complications of stent placements include:
    - Coronary artery perforation
    - Device embolization
    - Longitudinal stent deformity
  - Post-procedure, 12-lead EKG
- Assess for bleeding or hematoma around cardiac catheterization insertion site (usually the femoral or radial arteries)

Nursing Interventions

- Assess and manage anxiety.
- Assess vital signs for hemodynamic and oxygenation changes.
  - Assess for evidence of reperfusion dysrhythmias or HR change.
  - Assess for both hypertension and/or hypotension.
  - Maintain oxygenation and perfusion.
    - Position patient with HOB flat per institutional policy following sheath removal.
    - Use appropriate oxygen delivery system to achieve oxygen saturation >90%.
    - Use continuous SpO$_2$ monitoring.
    - Titrate up oxygen delivery system as needed.
    - Prepare for rapid sequence intubation if airway is lost or patient progresses to respiratory failure and/or cardiac arrest.
- Draw serial laboratory tests as ordered and monitor results.
- Describe what to expect during procedure.
- Prep patient pre procedure.
  - Clipping hair
  - Cleaning site
- Discuss bedrest orders post procedure.
- Explain sedation.
  - Typically, patients receive a combination of versed and fentanyl.
- Perform continuous physiologic monitoring through frequent physical assessment of the following systems:
  - Cardiac
    - Auscultate for extra heart sounds (S3, S4, holosystolic murmurs).
    - Assess for fluid retention/overload.
    - Palpate peripheral pulses.
  - Pulmonary
    - Auscultate for adventitious lung sounds (crackles, rhonchi, wheezes, rubs, etc.).
    - Assess for ability to maintain airway.
    - Assess for signs of respiratory distress or compromise.
  - Neurologic
    - Any neurologic change should be identified and the provider should be notified immediately.
    - If neurologic changes consistent with stroke are present, follow the alert procedure for your institution (notify attending, call a code stroke or rapid response) to obtain a STAT head CT. See Chapter 10 for additional information on signs and symptoms of stroke.
- Monitor for symptoms of
  - internal and external manifestations of bleeding or hemorrhage. These may present as:
  - Bleeding or oozing around the puncture or catheter insertion site.
    - Arterial bleeds can progress to lethal situations rapidly if appropriate action is not taken. If an arterial access site begins to ooze or bleed, immediately apply firm manual pressure to the site. Do not remove manual pressure until hemostasis is achieved or appropriate pressure device is applied.
    - Apply supplemental oxygen as needed.
    - If hemodynamically unstable, notify provider and prepare to place patient in reverse Trendelenburg and administer IV fluid bolus. If hemodynamic changes unresponsive to position change and IV fluid bolus, prepare to administer vasopressors.
    - Keep head of the bed flat.
    - Provide extra support if the patient must cough.
  - Hematoma and/or ecchymosis around the catheter insertion site.

(continued)

Nursing Interventions *(continued)*

- ○ A small degree of ecchymosis is expected after cardiac catheter site insertion; however, if bruising appears to be expanding and the skin becomes firm, raised, and painful to the touch, this is a hematoma.
- ○ A hematoma is evidence of bleeding under the surface of the skin and can be just as lethal as bleeding outside of the puncture site. Interventions for hematoma is the same as external bleeding or oozing:
  - ■ Immediately apply firm manual pressure to the site. Do not remove manual pressure until hemostasis is achieved or appropriate pressure device is applied.
  - ■ Apply supplemental oxygen as needed.
  - ■ If hemodynamically unstable, notify provider and prepare to place patient in reverse Trendelenburg and administer IV fluid bolus. If hemodynamic changes unresponsive to position change and IV fluid bolus, prepare to administer vasopressors and possible surgical consult.
  - ■ Keep HOB flat.
  - ■ Provide extra support at the insertion site with manual pressure if the patient must cough.
- • Retroperitoneal bleeding
  - ○ Presentation may be vague and nonspecific; however, if symptoms present, they may include the following:
    - ■ Abdominal pain
    - ■ Back pain
    - ■ Dizziness
    - ■ Flank bruising (also known as Grey-Turner sign)
    - ■ Hypotension or shock
    - ■ Pallor
    - ■ Syncope
  - ○ If the patient presents with symptoms of a retroperitoneal bleed post cardiac catheterization, immediate surgical consult should be made as retroperitoneal bleed is a surgical emergency.

 NURSING PEARL

During catheter removal and pressure application to the site to achieve hemostasis, patients may experience a vasovagal response. During this vasovagal response, the patient may complain of feeling nauseous and hot. They may also become diaphoretic, hypotensive, and bradycardic. Atropine and fluid bolus may be indicated for this symptomatic bradycardia.

Patient Education

- • Adhere to dietary recommendations as ordered for lipid and sodium control. Follow the DASH diet.
- • Maintain care of femoral access site:
  - • Post procedure:
    - ○ HOB must remain flat for 2 to 6 hr (depending on institutional policy).
    - ○ Advanced activity as allowed per institutional policy and femoral access site integrity.
    - ○ Reinforce femoral access site if you need to cough or bear down.
    - ○ Do not lift or carry anything >10 lbs.
    - ○ Do not bend over at the hip.
    - ○ Do not pick any scabs that may form.
    - ○ Do not scrub femoral access site.
  - • Notify the nurse or proceed to the emergency department for any of the following:
    - ○ Cold, numbness, tingling pain, or burning in the extremity distal to the femoral insertion site
    - ○ Change in color to the extremity

 POP QUIZ 2.4

A 52-year-old female returns to the PCU post cardiac catheterization. She was found to have a 99% blockage in the left circumflex, an 85% blockage in the right anterior descending artery, and 85% blockage in the left anterior descending artery. Vital signs are as follows: HR 109, BP 110/85 mmHg, RR 16, SpO_2 96% on 2L of oxygen via nasal cannula, and T 97.2 °F (36.2 °C). She received 100 mcg of fentanyl and 2 mg of midazolam for sedation. She did not receive any stenting or balloon angioplasty during the procedure. What should the nurse expect as the next step for the patient in treating her blockages?

○ Intense pain at the femoral access site
○ Increased bruising or swelling at the femoral access site
○ For frank bleeding from femoral access site: lay down flat, hold pressure, and immediately call for help
- Follow up as appropriate with outpatient appointments.
- Follow exercise and weight management recommendations.
- Increase physical activity as recommended.
  - If referred by provider, participate in cardiac rehab program.
- Perform self-assessments of the femoral access site for any new swelling, changes in bruising, bleeding, or oozing.
- Pursue smoking cessation as advised.
- Take medication as prescribed.

CARDIAC TAMPONADE

Overview

- Cardiac tamponade develops when there is fluid or blood accumulation in the pericardial sac surrounding the heart.
  - As fluid and/or blood accumulation increases in the pericardial sac, the heart's pumping ability is constricted.
  - This constriction decreases the cardiac output of the heart and sends patients into shock.
- Most common causes of cardiac tamponade are pericarditis, surgical complications, and trauma.

 COMPLICATIONS

Cardiac tamponade is a medical emergency that requires immediate intervention to prevent shock and death. As cardiac tamponade progresses, patients rapidly develop hypotension and shock. If surgical intervention is not urgently performed, the patient will experience a cardiac arrest and death.

Signs and Symptoms

- Beck's triad:
  - Muffled heart sounds
  - Bulging neck veins
  - Hypotension
- Chest pain
- Dizziness
- Dyspnea
- Mental status changes
- Narrowed pulse pressures
- Palpitations
- Pulsus paradoxus (SBP drop of >10 mmHg on inspiration)
- Syncopal episodes
- Tachycardia

Diagnosis

Labs

Labs not specifically diagnostic for detecting cardiac tamponade; labs provide more information to guide treatment plan:

- BMP
- CBC
- Coagulation labs
  - PT/PTT
  - INR

Diagnostic Testing

- Chest x-ray
- Chest CT scan
- MRI
- Pressure monitoring during cardiac catheterization
- TTE

Treatment

- Needle pericardiocentesis
- Surgical intervention:
  - Pericardial window:
    - Surgical removal of a small part of the pericardial sac, which allows rapid drainage of fluid
    - Can be done in the operating room or at the bedside in an emergency
  - Open thoracotomy: done as a surgical procedure in the operator room
- Vasopressors (Table 2.8)
- Volume replacement

 ALERT!

Coagulation time values (PT, PTT, INR, etc.) alone do not help diagnose cardiac tamponade; however, this information is valuable pre- and postoperatively. Reversal agents may be ordered as needed. Elevated coagulation times place patients at a higher risk for bleeding, making drainage of the pericardium or performing a pericardial window difficult.

Nursing Interventions

- Continuously monitor vital signs.
  - HR
  - BP
  - Oxygen saturation
- If condition deteriorates, prepare for arterial line insertion and/or transfer to a higher level of care.
- If patient undergoes surgical procedure, monitor for signs and symptoms of infection post procedure:
  - Chills
  - Fever
  - Foul-smelling drainage
  - Pus or purulent drainage
  - Redness around surgical site
  - Warmth or pain to touch around incision site
- Maintain continuous physiologic monitoring and assessment:
  - Heart and lung sounds
  - Mental status changes
  - Peripheral pulses
  - Skin color and temperature
  - Assess for worsening:
    - Chest pain
    - Dizziness
    - Dyspnea
    - Palpitations
- Maintain oxygenation and perfusion. Administer oxygen therapy as ordered, increasing oxygen as needed.
- Prepare for possible bedside pericardiocentesis.

 NURSING PEARL

Patients with cardiac tamponade can quickly decompensate. Ensure that emergency supplies are readily available and discuss plan of care with responsible provider.

Patient Education

- Educate on the severity and time-sensitive nature of treating cardiac tamponade.
- Discuss possibility of transfer to ICU and/or OR.
- Discuss surgical treatment options.
- Discuss full plan for course of recovery.

- Educate on what to expect during and after invasive procedure.
- Notify the nurse of new or worsening:
  - Chest pain
  - Dizziness
  - Dyspnea
  - Palpitations
- Review the purpose of bedside EKG monitoring.
- Once cardiac tamponade is resolved, follow up with cardiologist after discharge home.
- Take all prescribed medications.

CARDIOGENIC SHOCK

Overview

- Cardiogenic shock is a type of systemic shock defined as decreasing cardiac output and evidence of tissue hypoxia and end-organ hypoperfusion in the presence of adequate intravascular volume.
- Cardiogenic shock can develop following myocardial infarctions, HF, dysrhythmias, acute valvular dysfunction, ventricular or septal rupture, myocardial or pericardial infections, massive pulmonary embolism, cardiac tamponade, or drug toxicity.
- Cardiogenic shock results in decreased ventricular filling which then causes decreased stroke volume ultimately decreasing cardiac output despite adequate filling pressures.

Signs and Symptoms

- Abnormal heart sounds:
  - Diastolic murmur with aortic insufficiency
  - Muffled heart tones with cardiac tamponade
  - Murmurs if aortic stenosis or mitral regurgitation
  - S3 or S4
- Abnormal lung sounds: rales or crackles associated with pulmonary vascular congestion and/or fluid overload
- Altered mental status
- Cool, clammy, or mottled extremities
- Cyanosis
- Decreased peripheral pulses
- JVD
- Peripheral edema

Diagnosis

Labs

- Blood gases
  - ABG to show hypoxia
  - VBG to show hypoxia
- BMP with magnesium
- BNP
- Cardiac enzymes may be elevated
  - CK
  - CK-MB
  - Troponin

POP QUIZ 2.5

A patient is admitted to the progressive care unit 24 hr after CABG. The patient begins to exhibit sudden shortness of breath, palpitations, and chest pain. The nurse notices that he has JVD, hypotensive, and muffled heart sounds. Given his recent cardiac surgery and clinical presentation, the nurse suspects he may be developing cardiac tamponade. What is the nurse's next action?

COMPLICATIONS

Complications associated with cardiogenic shock include dysrhythmia, cardiac arrest, renal failure, ventricular aneurysm, stroke, pulmonary embolism, and death. Prompt recognition and treatment is necessary to improve outcomes.

(continued)

Labs (continued)

- CBC
- Coagulation studies may be either high or low
  - INR
  - PT
  - PTT
- Lactate may be elevated in shock

Diagnostic Testing

- 12-lead EKG
- Cardiac catheterization/angiogram with PCI if indicated
- Cardiac pressure assessment in the cardiac catheterization lab
- Continuous EKG monitoring
- Chest x-ray
- Cardiac CT

 ALERT!

Serial ABGs and lactate values can help determine if interventions are improving the patient's condition. Increasing lactate levels indicate the status of myocardial and other organ and tissue ischemia or hypoperfusion. This can be treated with fluid, as permitted by cardiac function. Other values in the ABG, such as PCO_2, PaO_2, and HCO_3 can be best treated with mechanical ventilation IABP deployment.

Treatment

- CABG
- Hemodialysis if kidney damage is extensive
- Coronary angiography/PCI
- Medications
  - Anticoagulation/antiplatelets
  - Antiplatelet drugs
  - Antiarrhythmics
  - Diuretics if pulmonary edema is present
  - Fluids
  - Fibrinolytic therapy (transfer to higher level of care)
  - Vasopressors and inotropes
- Ventricular assistive devices
- Ventilator/oxygen support

Nursing Interventions

- Assess airway, breathing, and circulation.
- Assess vital signs and telemetry monitor.
- Maintain continuous physiologic monitoring.
  - Physical assessment:
    - Heart and lung sounds
    - Mental status changes
    - Changes in perfusion as evidence by worsening skin color or cyanosis
    - Peripheral edema
    - Worsening chest pain
  - Vital signs:
    - HR and rhythm assessment
    - Oxygenation and perfusion; appropriate oxygen delivery system and continuous SpO_2 monitoring
    - Dysrhythmias monitoring
    - Hypotension monitoring
- Manage anxiety.
  - Nonpharmacological methods (i.e., guided imaging and deep breathing)
  - Pharmacologic methods as ordered by provider

- Position patient as appropriate.
  - Flat with HOB elevated if prepping for ECMO/IABP deployment and transfer to higher level of care
  - Trendelenburg if severe drop in BP
  - Semi-Fowler's to decrease work of breathing
- Reduce activity to decrease cardiac workload.

Patient Education

- Adhere to full plan for course of recovery.
- Ask questions about clinical condition.
- Discuss what to expect during/after invasive procedures.
- Notify the nurse (if possible) of new or worsening:
  - Chest pain
  - Dizziness
  - Dyspnea
  - Palpitations
- Once cardiac tamponade is resolved, follow up with cardiologist after discharge home.
- Recognize the severity and time-sensitive nature of treating cardiac tamponade.
- Review surgical treatment options.
- Review the purpose of bedside EKG monitoring.
- Take all prescribed medications.

NURSING PEARL

Patients with cardiac tamponade can quickly decompensate. Ensure that emergency supplies are readily available and discuss plan of care with responsible provider.

POP QUIZ 2.6

A patient is admitted in suspected cardiogenic shock. Vital signs are as follows: HR 138, BP 100/64, RR 24, SpO_2 94% on 4L of oxygen via nasal cannula, and T 99 °F (37.2 °C). He has IV fluids running through a 20-gauge peripheral IV in his right hand. He also has an 18-gauge PIV in the left antecubital. The provider places an order for a dobutamine drip. What should the nurse's next action be?

CARDIOMYOPATHY

Overview

- *Cardiomyopathy* classifies a group of disorders that affect the myocardium.
- Cardiomyopathy can be further classified as dilated, hypertrophic, or restrictive based on clinical presentation and diagnostic testing.
  - *Dilated cardiomyopathy:*
    - Most common type of cardiomyopathy
    - Results in diffuse inflammation and muscle breakdown that results in expansion and dilation of the atria and ventricles accompanied by stasis and impaired contractility
    - Can be inherited, autoimmune secondary to infection, related to metabolic disorders, toxins (alcohol or cocaine), connective tissue disorders, or viral myocarditis
  - *Hypertrophic cardiomyopathy:*
    - Results in an asymmetrical enlargement of the left ventricle without ventricular dilation
    - Can cause diastolic dysfunction
    - Most commonly has familial component
    - May be related to neuromuscular disorders, hypoparathyroidism, or hypertension
  - *Restrictive cardiomyopathy:*
    - Least common type
    - Results in ventricular wall stiffness, which impairs pumping ability of the heart
    - May be idiopathic or infiltrative, such as with amyloidosis or sarcoidosis

COMPLICATIONS

Complications of cardiomyopathy include HF, renal or hepatic damage, dysrhythmia, valvular dysfunction, pulmonary hypertension, thromboembolism, cardiac arrest, and/or sudden death. Patients with progressive HF and cardiomyopathy can receive a ventricular assistive device as a bridge to cardiac transplant. Otherwise, patient outcomes are poor and may result in death.

Signs and Symptoms

Signs and symptoms of cardiomyopathies are outlined in Table 2.3.

Diagnosis

Labs

- ABG to determine acid base balance and compensation
- BNP elevated >100 pg/mL
- BMP with magnesium to determine electrolyte balance, renal and liver function
- Cardiac enzyme (CK, CK-MB, and troponin) elevation
- HIV viral loads
  - HIV can result in direct myocardial damage, autoimmune reactions, and cardiac inflammation, which may result in left ventricular dysfunction. Antiretroviral therapy is also known to contribute to additional myocardial damage.
- Iron studies to rule out hemochromatosis
- Thyroid function elevation
  - Long-term untreated hyperthyroidism can cause dilated cardiomyopathy.
- Toxicology screening for cocaine and methamphetamines
  - Illicit drug use can cause cardiomyopathy.

Table 2.3 Signs and Symptoms of Cardiomyopathies

Dilated cardiomyopathy	<ul><li>Anorexia</li><li>Cough</li><li>Crackles</li><li>Decreased peripheral pulses</li><li>Dysrhythmia</li><li>Edema</li><li>Hepatomegaly</li><li>JVD</li><li>Nausea and vomiting</li><li>Narrow pulse pressure</li><li>Palpitations</li><li>PMI and apical pulse lateral displacement</li><li>S3 and S4 heart sounds</li><li>Tricuspid insufficiency</li><li>Vital sign changes</li></ul>
Hypertrophic cardiomyopathy	<ul><li>Angina</li><li>Dysrhythmias (A-fib, SVT, V-tach, V-fib)</li><li>Lateral displacement of apical pulse</li><li>Paroxysmal nocturnal dyspnea</li><li>S4 and systolic murmur</li></ul>
Restrictive cardiomyopathy	<ul><li>Ascites</li><li>Cardiac enlargement</li><li>Edema</li><li>Hepatojugular reflex</li><li>JVD</li><li>Mitral and tricuspid insufficiency</li><li>Pulmonary congestion</li><li>S3 and S4 heart sounds</li></ul>
Findings common to all types	<ul><li>Dyspnea on exertion</li><li>Fatigue</li><li>Orthopnea</li></ul>

Diagnostic Testing

- 12-lead EKG
- Cardiac biopsy
- Continuous EKG monitoring
- Coronary angiogram (right and left-sided)
- Cardiac catheterization
- CT scan
- Chest x-ray
- Genetic testing
- Nuclear stress test
- TEE and/or TTE

Treatment

- Cardiac transplantation (if severe)
- Identification of underlying causes of cardiomyopathy and reverse if possible (e.g., infection)
- ICD
- LVAD
- Medication to optimize afterload and preload using ACEIs, beta blockers, and antiarrhythmics (Table 2.8)
- Pacing if indicated (transfer to higher level of care)
- Sodium restriction

Nursing Interventions

- Assess for signs of decreased cardiac output as evidence by worsening:
  - Chest pain
  - Dyspnea
  - Edema
  - Fatigue
  - JVD
  - Lung crackles
  - Orthopnea
  - Palpitations
  - Skin color changes
  - Skin temperature changes (cool/clammy)
  - Weight gain (assess weight daily)
- Closely monitor vital signs.
  - BP
  - HR, rhythm, and dysrhythmia presence
  - SpO_2
- Maintain oxygen saturation >90%. Titrate oxygen and switch oxygen delivery system as ordered.
- Position patient in semi-Fowler's position to decrease cardiac workload.

Patient Education

- Adhere to a sodium and fluid restriction.
- Continuously update and educate on status and situation.
- Discuss the plan of care and what to expect.

ALERT!

Early identification and treatment of cardiomyopathy is essential to enhance and improve patient outcomes. There is currently no cure to cardiomyopathy. Patients are managed with lifestyle modifications, medication management, and bridge to cardiac transplantation. Nearly 50% of patients diagnosed with dilated cardiomyopathy, progress to HF and a life expectancy of no greater than 5 years. To improve outcomes, diet, exercise, and medication compliance is essential.

NURSING PEARL

Dietary education and modification is essential for appropriate management of cardiomyopathy and associated HF. Consultation with a dietician may be warranted to improve patient and family understanding of necessary dietary changes.

POP QUIZ 2.7

A 35-year-old patient is admitted to the progressive care unit with a diagnosis of idiopathic dilated cardiomyopathy. The nurse notices that he has a pending HIV antibody test. How could the HIV antibody test result impact the patient's diagnosis?

(continued)

Patient Education *(continued)*

- Discuss importance of interventions and diagnostic testing.
- Exercise as advised.
- Follow BP control guidelines.
- Follow antibiotic prophylaxis prior to dental procedures to reduce risk of infective endocarditis as prescribed.
- Take medications as prescribed.

DYSRHYTHMIAS

Overview

- To understand and identify dysrhythmias, a basic understanding of NSR is essential.
- NSR includes the presence of an upright P wave (indicating depolarization of the atria), a QRS complex (indicating ventricular depolarization and atrial repolarization) and an upright T wave (indicating ventricular repolarization):
  - PR intervals should be between 0.12 and 0.2 seconds.
  - QRS intervals should be <0.1 seconds.
  - QT intervals should be <0.38 seconds.
  - There should be one P wave for every QRS complex (Figure 2.1).
- A dysrhythmia is a disturbance of the NSR that can have a wide variety of presentations.
- Recognition of dysrhythmias is key to delivering appropriate intervention and care.
- Often, the cause of dysrhythmias results from accessory pathways, cardiomyopathy, conduction, defects, HF, myocardial infarction, infection, trauma, shock, or valvular disease.
- In the progressive care setting, patients are particularly vulnerable and may develop dysrhythmias due to medications, fluid and electrolyte imbalances, and blood loss, as well as other causes.
- Some dysrhythmias can be lethal, so adequate understanding of the advanced cardiac life support protocol is essential and should be reviewed.
- Dysrhythmias can be classified as atrial dysrhythmias, sinus dysrhythmias, ventricular dysrhythmias, and myocardial conduction system abnormalities.

COMPLICATIONS

Dysrhythmias can cause complications including stroke, HF, cognitive impairments, and cardiac arrest. Rhythm identification is essential to providing appropriate intervention to prevent complications.

Atrial Dysrhythmias

- *Atrial fibrillation*, or A-fib, is an abnormal electrical conduction in the atria that causes quivering of the upper chambers and results in ineffective pumping of the heart (Figure 2.2). RVR, a potential

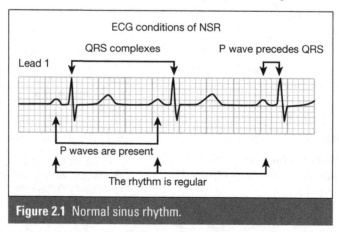

Figure 2.1 Normal sinus rhythm.

Source: From Thaler, M. S. (2019). *The only EKG book you'll ever need* (9th ed.). Wolters Kluwer.

sequela of A-fib, is common during critical illness and can lead to hemodynamic instability. A-fib with RVR can be treated with medications (e.g., metoprolol, amiodarone, and diltiazem) or cardioversion.

- P waves will not be seen on the EKG because the atrial rate is so fast and the action potentials produced are of such low amplitude.
- The QRS rate is variable, and the rhythm is irregular.
- In patients with A-fib with RVR, the ventricles may beat >100 times per minute, resulting in elevated HR.
- The irregularity of the atrial contraction causes decreased filling time of the atria. This results in a smaller volume of oxygenated blood being circulated.
- A-fib may be caused by any of the following: advanced age, congenital heart disease, underlying heart disease, alcohol consumption, hypertension (systemic or pulmonary), endocrine abnormalities, genetic predisposition, cerebral hemorrhage or stroke, mitral or tricuspid valve disease, left ventricular dysfunction, pulmonary embolism, OSA, myocarditis, or pericarditis.

- *Atrial flutter* occurs when the atria beat more rapidly than the ventricles (Figure 2.3). The hallmark sign of this arrythmia is a "saw tooth" like EKG tracing.
  - EKG shows a P rate between 251 and 300 and a PR interval is usually not observable.
  - Irregularity and rate of atrial contraction causes decreased filling time of the atria.
  - This results in a smaller volume of oxygenated blood being circulated.
  - The cause begins with an ectopic beat which depolarizes one segment of the normal conduction pathway.

- *Premature atrial contractions* are contractions of the atria that are triggered by the atrial myocardium but have not originated from the sinoatrial node (Figure 2.4). Early P waves are often caused by hypercalcemia, altered action potentials, hypoxia, or elevated preload.
  - EKG shows early P waves with normal PR interval and one QRS complex for each P wave.
  - Irregularity of rhythm can sometimes decrease filling times and BP.
  - The cause is commonly idiopathic; however, higher incidence of PACs occurs in patients with MI, CHF, HTN, DM, COPD, CAD, hypertrophic cardiomyopathy, left ventricular hypertrophy,

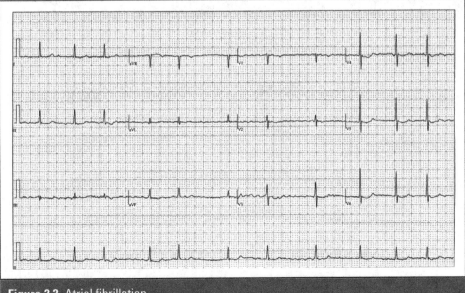

Figure 2.2 Atrial fibrillation.

Source: From Knechtel, M. A. (2021). *EKGs for the nurse practitioner and physician assistant* (3rd ed.). New York: Springer Publishing Company.

(continued)

Atrial Dysrhythmias (continued)

    valvular heart disease, septal defects, or congenital heart disease. Medications like beta-agonists, digoxin, chemotherapy, tricyclic antidepressants, and MAOIs can also induce PACs.

- *Sinus dysrhythmia* is a variation of a NSR with an R–R interval >0.12 seconds (Figure 2.5). This is a normal finding in children and young adults which requires no treatment. Incidence decreases with age.

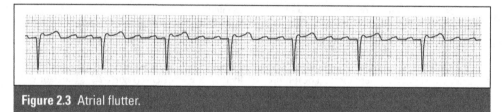

Figure 2.3 Atrial flutter.

Source: From Knechtel, M. A. (2021). *EKGs for the nurse practitioner and physician assistant* (3rd ed.). Springer Publishing Company.

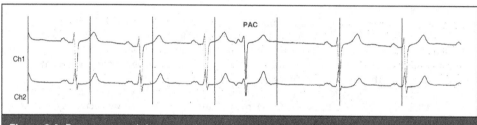

Figure 2.4 Premature atrial contractions.

Source: From Green, J. M., and Chiaramida, A. J. (2015). *12-lead EKG confidence* (3rd ed.). Springer Publishing Company.

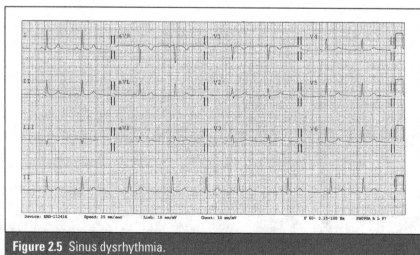

Figure 2.5 Sinus dysrhythmia.

Source: From Knechtel, M. A. (2021). *EKGs for the nurse practitioner and physician assistant* (3rd ed.). Springer Publishing Company.

Ventricular Dysrhythmias

- *Supraventricular tachycardia* is a rapid heartbeat that develops when the electrical impulses in the AV node affect the atria (Figure 2.6). The patient's HR can be anywhere from 150 to 220 beats per minute.
  - EKG shows a narrow QRS complex and rhythm between 150 and 220 beats per minute.
  - SVT results in decreased cardiac output from loss of atrial contribution to ventricular preload for the beat.
- *Ventricular tachycardia* has a wide QRS complex and ventricular beat >100 beats per minute (Figure 2.7). VT can be further classified as monomorphic or polymorphic based on characteristics of the QRS complex. Torsade's de Pointes is an example of polymorphic ventricular tachycardia.
  - EKG has absent or independent P wave with a QRS >0.11 and rate >100 beats per minute.
  - VT results in decreased cardiac output and increased myocardial demand.
  - Can occur commonly in patients with underlying ischemic heart disease, structural heart disease, abnormal electrical conduction, infiltrative cardiomyopathy, electrolyte imbalances, cocaine or methamphetamine use, or digitalis toxicity.
  - Common triggering events for VT include hypokalemia and hypomagnesemia.

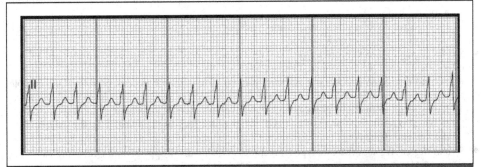

Figure 2.6 Paroxysmal supraventricular tachycardia.

Source: From Roberts, D. (2020). *Mastering the 12-lead EKG* (2nd ed.). Springer Publishing Company.

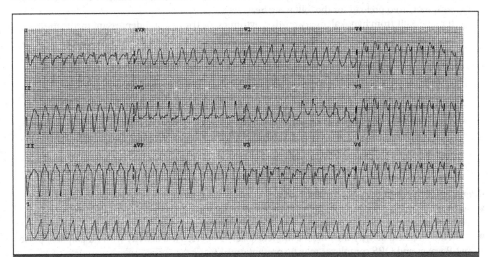

Figure 2.7 Ventricular tachycardia.

Source: From Knechtel, M. A. (2021). *EKGs for the nurse practitioner and physician assistant* (3rd ed.). Springer Publishing Company.

(continued)

Ventricular Dysrhythmias (continued)

- *Ventricular fibrillation* is a quivering or shaking of the ventricles. This results in ventricular standstill and incomplete pumping (Figure 2.8). Ventricle fibrillation is a life-threatening dysrhythmia that requires prompt recognition and treatment to improve outcomes.
  - Ventricular fibrillation has an absent P wave with a QRS rate >300 and is usually not observable.
  - Ventricular fibrillation is a life-threatening dysrhythmia and often causes ventricular standstill.
  - Ventricular fibrillation can occur commonly in patients with underlying structural heart disease, MI, A-fib, electrolyte abnormalities, hypothermia, hypoxia, cardiomyopathies, QT abnormalities, and alcohol use.
  - Common triggering events for ventricular fibrillation include hypo/hyperkalemia and hypomagnesemia.
  - Myocardial conduction system abnormalities include first-degree AV block, second-degree AV block types 1 and 2, and third-degree AV block.
- *First-degree AV block* results when there is an abnormally slow conduction through the AV node, resulting in a prolonged PR interval (Figure 2.9).
  - First-degree AV block has a PR interval >0.2 seconds.
  - Patients with first-degree AV block may not have any symptoms and may only be detected with a routine EKG.
  - First-degree AV block may result from hyperkalemia or hypokalemia, or with the formation of myocardial abscess in endocarditis.
- *Second-degree AV block* (Mobitz type I, or Wenckebach) includes a progressively prolonged PR interval until one QRS is dropped (Figure 2.10).
  - Second-degree AV block has progressive prolongation of the PR interval until one QRS complex is dropped.
  - It may result from electrolyte abnormalities (hypokalemia), digoxin toxicity, or beta blockade.
  - It may also result from preexisting CAD, MI, hypoxia, increased preload, valvular surgery or disease, and diabetes.
- *Second-degree AV block* (Mobitz type II) includes occasionally dropped P and QRS complexes (Figure 2.11).
  - A second-degree AV block (Mobitz type II) has occasionally absent P waves with the loss of a QRS complex for that beat.
  - Second-degree AV block (Mobitz type II) can cause an occasional decrease in cardiac output with increased preload for the following beat.
  - It may result from hypokalemia, anti-dysrhythmics, or tricyclic antidepressant medications, or in patients with preexisting CAD, MI, hypoxia, increased preload, valvular surgery or disease, and diabetes mellitus.
- *Third-degree AV block* (complete heart block) includes P waves and QRS complexes that beat independently of one another (Figure 2.12).
  - P waves and QRS complex both present; however, there is no observable relationship between the P wave and QRS complex.
  - Rate is usually <60 beats per minute.
  - Third-degree AV block may result from hypokalemia, conduction abnormalities in the bundle of His, or MI (inferior wall).
  - Third-degree AV block can cause decreased cardiac output.

Other Lethal Dysrhythmias

- *Asystole* includes a complete absence of electrical activity as evidenced by no palpable pulse, paired with a flat waveform on EKG monitoring (Figure 2.13).
- *Pulseless electrical activity* includes a complete absence of electrical activity with no palpable pulse but P waves and QRS complexes may be present on EKG.

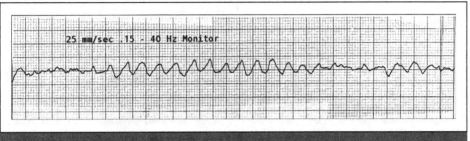

Figure 2.8 Ventricular fibrillation.

Source: From Knechtel, M. A. (2021). *EKGs for the nurse practitioner and physician assistant* (3rd ed.). Springer Publishing Company.

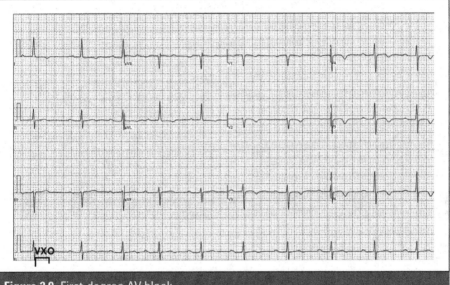

Figure 2.9 First-degree AV block.

Source: From Knechtel, M. A. (2021). *EKGs for the nurse practitioner and physician assistant* (3rd ed.). Springer Publishing Company.

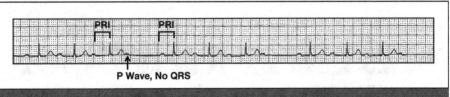

Figure 2.10 Second-degree AV block Mobitz type I.

Source: From Knechtel, M. A. (2021). *EKGs for the nurse practitioner and physician assistant* (3rd ed.). Springer Publishing Company.

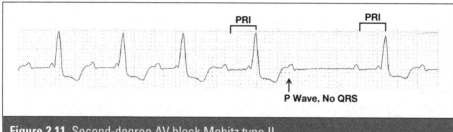

Figure 2.11 Second-degree AV block Mobitz type II.

Source: From Knechtel, M. A. (2021). *EKGs for the nurse practitioner and physician assistant* (3rd ed.). Springer Publishing Company.

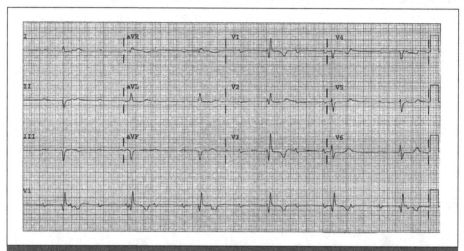

Figure 2.12 Third-degree AV block.

Source: From Knechtel, M. A. (2021). *EKGs for the nurse practitioner and physician assistant* (3rd ed.). Springer Publishing Company.

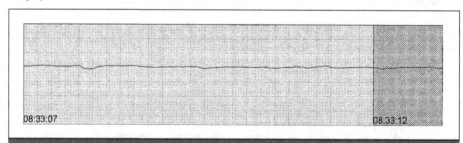

Figure 2.13 Asystole.

Source: From Knechtel, M. A. (2021). *EKGs for the nurse practitioner and physician assistant* (3rd ed.). Springer Publishing Company.

Signs and Symptoms

Any disruption to regular HR and rhythm may result in the following symptoms:
- Anxiety and/or feelings of impending doom
- Dyspnea
- Diaphoresis
- Dyspnea

- Mental status changes and/or syncope resulting from decreased cerebral perfusion
- Nausea and/or vomiting
- Pain in chest, back, or arms
- Pallor
- Palpitations
- Nausea and/or vomiting
- Vital sign changes
  - Decreasing oxygen saturation
  - Hypotension or hypertension
  - Irregular HR and rhythm findings on continuous EKG monitoring
- Weak and/or irregular peripheral pulses

Diagnosis

Labs

There are no labs specific to detect dysrhythmias. However, the following labs may be indicated to treat potential causes of dysrhythmias:
- BMP with magnesium
- Cardiac enzymes:
  - CK
  - CK-MB
  - Troponin

Diagnostic Testing
- 12-lead EKG
- Continuous EKG monitoring
- Coronary angiogram
- Echocardiogram
- Electrophysiology study
- Holter monitor for extended cardiac monitoring
- Stress test

Treatment

Treatment highly dependent on type of dysrhythmia (Table 2.4). Adhere to the advanced cardiac life support protocol if patient acutely decompensating or experiencing cardiac arrest.

 ALERT!

Failure to capture may occur if the pacer voltage is too low. Notify provider and increase voltage as ordered or per institutional protocol until capture is achieved at desired rate (Table 2.6).

Table 2.4 Dysrhythmia Treatments

Dysrhythmia	Treatment	Other Interventions
Atrial		
• Atrial fibrillation	• Amiodarone • Ibutilide • Disopyramide • Flecainide • Procainamide • Propafenone • Quinidine • Sotalol • Dofetilide • Anticoagulation • Calcium channel blockers (e.g., diltiazem) • Digoxin • Dronedarone • Metoprolol	• Ablation • Cardioversion • Pacemaker implantation

(continued)

Table 2.4 Dysrhythmia Treatments *(continued)*

Dysrhythmia	Treatment	Other Interventions
Atrial (continued)		
• Atrial flutter	• Ibutilide • Flecainide • Propafenone • Sotalol • Procainamide • Amiodarone • Beta blockers • Calcium channel blockers • Digoxin	• Ablation • Cardioversion • Pacemaker implantation
• PACs	• Electrolyte replacement (Table 8.4)	• Reverse hypoxia or other identifiable causes of elevated preload
Sinus		
• Sinus dysrhythmia	• No treatment required	• None
Ventricular		
• SVT	• Adenosine	• Vagal maneuvers
• Monomorphic V-tach	• Amiodarone • Epinephrine • Lidocaine	• Cardioversion if pulse present • High-quality CPR and defibrillation if pulse not present • ICD (if recurrent V-tach)
• Polymorphic ventricular tachycardia (also referred to as Torsade's de Pointes)	• Magnesium	• Cardioversion if pulse present • High-quality CPR and defibrillation if pulse not present
• V-fib	• Amiodarone • Epinephrine • Lidocaine	• High-quality CPR • Defibrillation
Myocardial conduction abnormalities		
• First-degree AV block	• None	• Usually involves minimal treatment; identify/correct cause
• Second-degree AV block (Mobitz type I or Wenckebach)	• If hypotensive or experiencing altered LOC: atropine	• Pacemaker
• Second-degree AV block (Mobitz type II)	• None	• Pacemaker

(continued)

Table 2.4 Dysrhythmia Treatments *(continued)*

Dysrhythmia	Treatment	Other Interventions
Myocardial conduction abnormalities (continued)		
• Third-degree AV block (complete heart block)	• Atropine • Dopamine • Epinephrine	• Transcutaneous pacing • Permanent pacemaker
Other lethal dysrhythmias		
• Asystole	• Epinephrine	• High-quality CPR • Obtain advanced airway if not already in place
• Pulseless electrical activity	• Epinephrine	• High-quality CPR • Obtain advanced airway if not already in place

Nursing Interventions

- Administer ordered medications and titrate drips to achieve ordered parameter goals.
- Assess airway, breathing, and circulation.
- Insert at least two large bore peripheral IVs and consider the need for central line placement.
- If a pacemaker is implanted, assess implantation site for:
  - Bleeding
  - Colored or foul-smelling drainage
  - Capturing, sensing, and pacing within ordered parameters (Tables 2.5 and 2.6)
  - Icepack placement over pacemaker implantation site to reduce swelling
  - Erythema
  - Warmth
- Maintain continuous physiologic monitoring and observe for:
  - Changes in diaphoresis
  - Changes in pallor
  - Changes in peripheral pulses
  - Mental status change
- Monitor vital signs for hemodynamic instability.
- Monitor telemetry for rhythm changes or conversion to potentially unstable dysrhythmias.
- Perform 12-lead EKG if rhythm change is observed.
- Provide therapeutic support for patient and family. A chaplain can be called to the bedside to provide additional support if needed.

 NURSING PEARL

Electrolyte replacement in patients with cardiac dysfunction or dysrhythmia is essential. Electrolyte imbalance affects the electrical conduction of the heart and can predispose already at-risk patients for worsening dysrhythmias. Closely monitor these laboratory values and notify providers of abnormal results.

Table 2.5 Pacemaker Characteristics

First Initial—Chamber That Is Paced	Second Initial—Chamber That Is Sensed	Third Initial—Response of Pacer to Intrinsic Activity
• A—atria • V—ventricle • D—dual	• A—atria • V—ventricle • D—dual	• I—inhibits pacer • D—inhibits or triggers pacer • O—neither

Table 2.6 Types of Pacer Failure and Common Causes

Failure to Pace	Failure to Capture	Failure to Sense
• Battery failure	• Battery failure	• Battery failure
• Lead or wire dislodgement	• Lead or wire dislodgement	• Lead or wire dislodgement
• Sensing threshold too low	• Pacer voltage too low	• Sensitivity set too high
	• Ventricular perforation	

Patient Education

- Notify the nurse if following symptoms are present:
  - Difficulty in breathing
  - Dizziness
  - Nausea/vomiting
  - New onset or changes to chest pain
  - Palpitations

HEART FAILURE

Overview

- HF is a disorder in which the ventricles of the heart either do not fill or do not eject blood efficiently, resulting in decreased cardiac output. It develops when there is impaired cardiac pumping (contractility) or filling.
- HF can be classified as either chronic or acute right- or left-sided HF, each with distinguishable symptoms and varying treatment.
- Risk factors for HF include a past medical history of HTN, CAD, MI, diabetes, tobacco use, obesity, elevated cholesterol levels, and advanced age.

Signs and Symptoms

- CHF:
  - Abdominal distention
  - Anorexia
  - Dyspnea
  - Fatigue
  - Peripheral edema
- Acute HF:
  - Dyspnea at rest or on exertion
  - Lightheadedness
  - Orthopnea
  - Palpitations
  - Paroxysmal nocturnal dyspnea
- Left-sided HF
  - Altered mental status/confusion
  - Anxiety
  - Crackles on auscultation
  - Dyspnea (with or without exertion)
  - Extra heart sounds (S3/S4)

 POP QUIZ 2.8

A 38-year-old male is admitted to the progressive care unit after having a syncopal episode at work. He reports feeling nauseous and dizzy. The patient is alert and oriented x4. Heart sounds are irregular and rapid with no S1 or S2 sound noted. Lungs are clear, diminished at the bases, and peripheral pulses in the lower extremities are diminished. A 12-lead EKG reveals atrial fibrillation with rapid ventricular rhythm, with a HR of 130. Other vitals are BP 95/60 mmHg, SpO$_2$ 95% on room air, RR 20, and T 98.4 °F (36.9 °C). After notifying the provider of new onset atrial fibrillation and assessment findings, what should the nurse's next action be?

COMPLICATIONS

Complications of HF include dysrhythmia, pleural effusion, hepatomegaly, renal failure, thromboembolism, and sudden death. Medical management is possible with collaborative care of medication compliance and lifestyle modifications; however, HF resistant to medical intervention may require more invasive interventions, including IABP and/or cardiac transplantation.

- Fatigue
- Orthopnea
- Pink frothy sputum
- Pleural effusion
- Pulmonary edema
- Tachycardia
- Tachypnea
- Weakness
- Right-sided HF:
  - Anorexia
  - Edema/anasarca
  - Fatigue
  - Heart murmur
  - Hepatomegaly
  - JVD
  - Nausea
  - Tachycardia
  - Weight gain

 NURSING PEARL

NYHA HF Classes
- Class 1: No limitations on physical activity
- Class 2: Slight limitation on physical activity
- Class 3: Marked limitation on physical activity
- Class 4: Discomfort with any physical activity, symptomatic even at rest

Diagnosis

Labs
- ABG
- BMP with magnesium
- BNP
- CBC
- Cardiac enzymes
- Thyroid function

Diagnostic Testing
- 12-lead EKG
- Cardiac biopsy
- Chest x-ray
- Continuous EKG monitoring
- Coronary angiogram/catheterization (right and/or left sided)
- Stress test
- TTE

 ALERT!

Close monitoring of potassium levels is essential to protect electrical conduction of the heart. This is especially important if patients are taking thiazide or loop diuretics, as they can cause hypokalemia. Replacement electrolytes should be administered as ordered to maintain a potassium level >4 mmol/L.

Treatment

- Cardiac catheterization
- Cardiac transplantation
- Cardiac rehab at time of discharge
- Diet: sodium and fluid restriction
- ICD
- IABP or LVAD
  - Requires transfer to higher level of care for initial implantation/deployment
  - Chronic LVADs managed in PCU
- Medications: ACEIs, ARBs, beta blockers, aldosterone antagonists, diuretics, vasodilators, and digoxin (Table 2.8).
- Pacemaker (Tables 2.4 and 2.5)
- Supplemental oxygen

Nursing Interventions

- Administer prescribed medication as ordered.
- Assess airway, breathing, and circulation.
- Assess the need for noninvasive oxygen or intubation and transfer to higher level of care.
- Assess for elevated or low BP, fluid retention, or electrolyte imbalances.
- Assess for signs of decreased cardiac output as evidence by worsening:
  - Chest pain
  - Dyspnea
  - Edema
  - Fatigue
  - JVD
  - Lung crackles
  - Mental status
  - Orthopnea
  - Palpitations
  - Skin color changes
  - Skin temperature changes (cool/clammy)
- Elevate HOB to alleviate orthopnea and dyspnea and decrease cardiac workload.
- Monitor weight daily and report weight gain >2–3 lbs over 24 hr or over 5 lbs in 1 week. This may indicate high fluid retention.
- Monitor vital signs continuously for changes.
- Maintain oxygen saturation >90%. Titrate oxygen and upgrade oxygen delivery device as needed.
- Monitor strict I/O strictly due to the potential for fluid retention.

Patient Education

- Adhere to a low sodium fluid restricted diet if ordered by the provider.
- Follow physical restrictions and take breaks between activities as needed.
- Take medications as prescribed and follow up with any outpatient appointments after discharge.
- Once discharged, engage in physical activity program as ordered and tolerated. Consider participating in a cardiac rehabilitation program if recommended by your provider.

 NURSING PEARL

Daily weights are essential to monitor fluid retention and volume status. Weight gain of >3 lbs in a 24-hr period indicates fluid retention and volume overload. The provider should be notified if sudden weight gain occurs in a 24-hr period.

 POP QUIZ 2.9

A 59-year-old male with CHF is admitted to the PCU. He complains of worsening fatigue, anorexia, nausea, and new onset of blurred vision. He also notices the presence of halos around objects in his vision. Past medical history is notable for HF, diabetes, and anxiety. Current medications include metformin 1000 mg PO BID, furosemide 80 mg PO daily, captopril 25 mg PO BID, and digoxin 0.125 mg PO daily. Vital signs are as follows: HR 126, BP 96/70, RR 24, SpO$_2$ 94% on 4L of oxygen via nasal cannula and T 98.1 °F (36.7 °C). Given the patient's medications and clinical presentation, what is happening with this patient?

HYPERTENSION AND HYPERTENSIVE CRISIS

Overview

- *Hypertension* is defined as an abnormal elevation in BP. See Table 2.7 for stages of hypertension.
- Hypertension can be managed with lifestyle modifications and medications.
- A *hypertensive crisis* is a marked elevation in BP that is associated with end-organ damage as evidence by pulmonary edema, myocardial ischemia, acute renal failure, aortic dissection, or neurological deficits including mental status changes and/or stroke.

- Hypertensive crisis cannot be managed outside of the hospital and is considered a medical emergency.
- The increased SVR places additional pressure on vasculature and organ structures resulting in end-organ damage.
- While it is imperative to lower BP during a hypertensive crisis, it must be lowered gradually to prevent refractory ischemia. The goal is to lower MAPs by 20% to 25% in the first 1 to 2 hr.

Signs and Symptoms

- Often asymptomatic with symptom manifestation only if severe
- Severe hypertension symptoms:
  - Activity intolerance
  - Agitation
  - Angina
  - Anxiety
  - Altered level of consciousness (if hypertensive encephalopathy)
  - AV nicking (finding on ophthalmic exam)
  - Dizziness
  - Headache
  - Nausea and vomiting
  - Pain (chest, back, or abdomen)
  - Palpitations
  - Restlessness
  - Retinopathy, papilledema
  - Transient focal neurological deficits
  - Vision changes

COMPLICATIONS

Complications of hypertension and a hypertensive crisis include renal failure, hemorrhagic stroke, arterial dissection, MI, visual disturbances, and/or loss of vision, CAD, left ventricular hypertrophy, HF, and death. In patients with hypertensive crisis and no evidence of organ damage, BP must be gradually lowered over 48 hr as tolerated to maintain cerebral perfusion and prevent ischemia stroke. If organ damage or aortic dissection is present, BP should be lowered to <140 mmHg in the first hr of treatment.

Table 2.7 Stages of Hypertension	
Normal	Systolic <120
	Diastolic <80
Elevated	Systolic 120–129
	Diastolic <80
Stage 1: Hypertension	Systolic 130–139
	Diastolic 80–89
Stage 2: Hypertension	Systolic >140
	Diastolic ≥90
Stage 3: Hypertension (Hypertensive Crisis)	Systolic >180
	Diastolic ≥120

Source: Data from American Heart Association

Diagnosis

Labs
- BMP
- Cardiac enzymes
  - CK
  - CK-MB
  - Troponin
- CBC
- Lipid panel
- TSH
- Uric acid
- Urinalysis

Diagnostic Testing
- 12-lead EKG
- Echocardiogram
- Head CT scan
- Brain MRI
- Ophthalmic exam: AV Nicking
- Renal ultrasound

 ALERT!

Hyperthyroidism is a common secondary cause for hypertension. In patients with hyperthyroid induced hypertension, first-line treatment should start with thyroid regulation before progressing to antihypertensive medications.

Treatment

- First 1 to 2 hr for hypertensive emergency: lower MAP by 20% to 25% or BP to 160/100 mmHg
- Lifestyle modifications:
  - Alcohol intake reduction
  - Anxiety and stress reduction
  - Diet
    - DASH diet
    - Sodium reduction
    - Fluid restriction
  - Physical activity
  - Smoking cessation
  - Weight loss
- Medication (Table 2.8)
  - ACEIs
  - Alpha adrenergic inhibitors
  - ARBs
  - Beta adrenergic blockers
  - Beta blockers
  - Calcium channel blockers
  - Diuretics
  - Vasodilators
- Transition from IV to oral medication within 12 to 24 hr (if possible)

 ALERT!

Nitroprusside is the gold standard treatment in the management of hypertensive crisis. Watch for signs of cyanide toxicity: blurred vision, tinnitus, altered mental status, hyperreflexia, or seizure. Risk of toxicity is elevated with prolonged therapy >48 hr and in patients with renal failure.

Nursing Interventions

- Administer antihypertensive medications as ordered.
- Assess airway, breathing, and circulation.
- Assess neurologic status, including level of consciousness and for focal deficits.
- Assess for signs of stroke. See Chapter 10 for more information on stroke.

 NURSING PEARL

If IV beta blockers are administered rapidly, patient can become severely bradycardic. Though this resolves quickly, avoid rapid administration of IV beta blocker.

- Assess for tissue ischemia, coronary ischemia, T-wave inversion, and cerebral ischemia related to overly aggressive lowering of BP.
- Implement anxiety and stress reduction practices as needed.
- Limit caffeine intake for accurate BP readings.
- Monitor BP and vital signs as ordered.
- Monitor I/O to optimize fluid balance.
- Monitor sodium intake and fluid as ordered.
- Monitor weight daily.

Patient Education

- Adhere to dietary recommendations as ordered for lipid and sodium control.
- Continuously update (if alert and oriented) on current status, plan of care, and upcoming tests or procedures.
- Follow the DASH diet.
- Follow exercise and weight management recommendations.
- Follow up as appropriate with outpatient appointments.
- If referred by provider, participate in cardiac rehab program.
- Increase physical activity as recommended.
- Limit alcohol intake.
- Pursue smoking cessation as advised.
- Take medications as prescribed.

 POP QUIZ 2.10

A patient with newly diagnosed hypertension was admitted to the PCU 3 days ago. His BP on admission was 189/102 mmHg. With medication therapy, his BP is now 141/84 mmHg, HR 102, RR 16, SpO$_2$ 96% on 4 L nasal cannula and T 96.8 °F (36 °C). With the healthcare team's permission, the patient's wife brought food and snacks into the hospital from home. As the nurse enters the room around lunchtime, the patient and his wife have finished eating takeout Chinese food with multiple soy sauce packets on the bedside table. The wife asks if she can bring in a breakfast sandwich from the drive-thru the next morning. What should the nurse's first action be?

POST ICU CARE

Overview

- Patients in the ICU have likely undergone procedures or have been diagnosed with critical illnesses which required additional specialized monitoring.
- As such, patients transferred to the PCU from the ICU should be monitored closely for hemodynamic instability, post-procedure complications, or other changes in status.

 COMPLICATIONS

Patients newly admitted to the PCU must be closely watched for decompensation and worsening condition, requiring transfer back to the ICU. To prevent this, close hemodynamic monitoring and assessment of post-procedure complications are essential. Early detection and treatment of deteriorating conditions can prevent an unnecessary rebound to the ICU.

Signs and Symptoms

- Complications associated with cardiac catheterization and angiography:
  - Bruising and/or hematoma noted around access site
  - Loss of peripheral pulse distal to the insertion site
  - Redness/swelling around access site
  - Skin cool to touch and pale distal to insertion site
  - Severe back pain
- Hemodynamic instability:
  - Angina/chest pain
  - Dysrhythmia development
  - Diaphoresis
  - Dyspnea
  - Dizziness
  - Mental status changes
  - Nausea/vomiting
  - Palpitations
  - Tachycardia/bradycardia

Diagnosis

Labs

The following labs typically assessed daily:

- CBC
- Coagulation
  - PT/PTT
  - INR
- CMP/BMP

Diagnostic Testing

- 12-lead EKG
- Chest x-ray
- Doppler ultrasound
- Echocardiogram

 ALERT!

If the patient becomes hemodynamically unstable or may require a higher level of care, notify the provider immediately and consider calling a rapid response to assemble all necessary disciplines to address rapid response situation and facilitate quick transfer to higher level of care.

Treatment

- If patient is experiencing hemodynamic instability, identify cause and treat with appropriate therapy:
  - ACLS protocol and ICU transfer, as indicated
  - Antiarrhythmic drugs
  - Antihypertensives (hypertension)
  - Fluid volume replacement
  - Vasodilators (hypotension)
- Monitor for complications post procedure.
- Other common reasons for readmission to ICU:
  - HF exacerbation
  - Hemorrhage/surgical emergency
  - Hyperkalemia unresponsive to treatment
  - Loss of consciousness/unresponsiveness
  - New infection/sepsis
  - New MI or stroke
  - Poor ventilation/inability to protect airway
  - Reemergence of hemodynamically unstable dysrhythmia (V-tach, A-fib with RVR, etc.) requiring cardioversion

 ALERT!

Stent thrombosis following PCI can occur early (as an acute event in the first 24 hr or as a subacute event between 24 hr and 1 month post procedure), late (between 1 and 12 months post procedure) and very late (after 12 months post procedure). Stent thrombosis at any stage is thought to occur due to ineffective anticoagulation. Be sure the patient receives the ordered anticoagulation before and after procedure and educate the patient on the importance of continuing their anticoagulation for at least a year as directed by their provider.

Nursing Interventions

- Administer medications as ordered.
- Monitor vital signs as ordered.
- Perform a detailed head-to-toe physical assessment every shift.
  - Access site status (increased bruising, swelling, hematoma, etc.)
  - Color, sensation, and movement of extremities distal to invasive access sites
  - Edema and signs of fluid overload monitoring
  - Peripheral pulses
- Closely monitor continuous telemetry.
- Continuous SpO_2 monitoring.

 NURSING PEARL

Sudden decrease or loss of pulse in extremities distal to arterial access sites can indicate serious complications and develop into a surgical emergency. If decrease in perfusion is prolonged, loss of limb is possible. Therefore, it is essential that peripheral pulses and physical assessment be conducted at frequent and regular intervals.

Patient Education

- Notify the nurse for any of the following symptoms:
  - New onset or worsening chest pain, dizziness, confusion, palpitations, nausea/vomiting, diaphoresis or dyspnea, active bleeding from access site, increased swelling, or pain in access site, and cold, numb, or tingly extremities.
- Work with PT to engage in physical activities as ordered and tolerated to maintain or regain lost mobility from ICU admission.
- Perform intermittent suctioning ×10 to encourage airway secretion clearance.

POP QUIZ 2.11

If a patient transferred from the ICU becomes hemodynamically unstable, what should the nurse's next actions be?

VALVULAR HEART DISEASE

Overview

- Valvular disease is an umbrella term which describes mitral stenosis, mitral regurgitation, mitral prolapse, aortic stenosis, aortic regurgitation, and tricuspid or pulmonic valve stenosis.
  - Stenosis describes a narrowing of the heart valve.
  - Regurgitation describes the accumulation of leaflets on the valves which prevent complete closure and backward flow of blood.
  - Prolapse describes a bulging of the valve which also prevents complete closure.
- Treatment of valvular heart disease ranges from medical management to open heart surgery.

COMPLICATIONS

Patients with valvular insufficiencies are at risk for developing HF. Timely identification, condition monitoring, and treatment are essential to improve patient outcomes. As conditions progress, patients may need surgery to replace or repair the valve to prevent further decompensation.

Signs and Symptoms

- Dependent on the valve involved and type of impairment. Symptoms can include the following:
  - Cardiogenic shock
  - Dyspnea with or without exertion
  - Fatigue
  - HF
  - Heart sound changes
    - Absent or accentuated S1
    - Absent S2
    - Holosystolic, pansystolic, mid-systolic or diastolic murmur
    - S3/S4 gallop
  - Palpitations
  - Peripheral edema
  - Pulmonary edema

Labs
- Blood cultures
- CBC
- CMP

Diagnostic Testing
- 12-lead EKG
- Cardiac catheterization
- Continuous bedside monitoring
- Echocardiogram

ALERT!

Acute mitral valve regurgitation can progress quickly to cardiogenic shock. Prompt identification and intervention is needed to prevent escalation of care.

Treatment

- Balloon valvuloplasty
- Fluid and sodium restriction
- Medications
  - Antibiotics: if indicated in infective carditis or for rheumatic fever
  - Antihypertensives: beta blockers
  - Anticoagulation
  - Antidysrhythmic medications
  - Diuretics
  - Vasodilators
- Surgical valve replacement or repair

Nursing Interventions

- Administer medications as ordered.
- Assess surgical or insertion site for bleeding, hematoma, and signs of infection.
- Assess and treat pain with scheduled and PRN medications.
- Improve activity tolerance.
- Maintain appropriate positioning to decrease cardiac workload: semi-Fowler's, HOB >30°.
- Monitor continuous telemetry and pulse oximetry.
- Monitor vital signs as ordered.
- Perform incentive spirometry.
- Perform detailed regular assessments, including:
  - Auscultation of heart and lungs
  - Mental status
  - Pain
  - Systemic perfusion and oxygenation

NURSING PEARL

As valvular disease progresses, care may shift to managing HF, endocarditis, or dysrhythmia. These additional conditions may warrant additional interventions, including PICC line insertion for IV antibiotic administration, ICD, pacemaker, or VAD depending on severity of condition.

Patient Education

- Adhere to heart healthy diet to limit sodium intake and decrease workload of the heart as recommended.
- Decrease alcohol intake to reduce cardiac strain.
- Monitor BP and HR daily.
- Monitor weight daily to assess for fluid retention.
- Pursue smoking cessation.
- Take coagulation and other medications as prescribed.
- Use prophylactic antibiotic treatment for dental or invasive procedures.

POP QUIZ 2.12

A patient with mitral valve stenosis has been newly diagnosed with atrial fibrillation. The nurse knows that atrial fibrillation can cause what complication if left untreated?

VASCULAR DISEASE

Overview

- Vascular disease includes coronary artery stenosis, arterial and venous occlusion, and peripheral vascular insufficiency.
- Symptom presentation and treatment differs for each condition; however, the overall goal is to improve circulation and perfusion.
- *Carotid artery stenosis* is an atherosclerotic disease that leads to partial blockage and causes ischemic stroke or TIA-like symptoms.

COMPLICATIONS

Complications for vascular diseases include the development of nonhealing ulcers and wounds, tissue necrosis, pain, infection, embolism (DVT, PE, or stroke), and amputation. Appropriate medical management and lifestyle modifications must be implemented to prevent disease progression, which can result in vision changes, aphasia, and stroke.

- *Arterial occlusion* is a medical emergency where arterial blood flow is stopped, resulting in ischemia of distal organs and tissues.
- *Venous occlusion* occurs when a vein becomes narrowed, blocked, or pinched, resulting in tissue necrosis and death.
- *Peripheral vascular insufficiency* and disease is an atherosclerotic disease that leads to partial or total occlusion of the abdominal aorta, iliac arteries, lower limbs, and/or upper extremities.
- *Peripheral vascular insufficiency* can progress to both stenosis and/or occlusion of peripheral vessels. thereby resulting in renal vascular disease, ischemic bowel, and cerebral vascular disease, depending on location of occlusion.

 ALERT!

Risk factors for developing peripheral vascular insufficiency include age >50, BMI >30, type 1 and 2 diabetes, family history of cardiovascular disease, HIV, hypertension, hyperlipidemia, and tobacco use. The nurse should take note of risk factors upon obtaining patient history or examination and prepare for appropriate treatment.

Signs and Symptoms

- Carotid artery stenosis (stroke symptoms which resolve rapidly, within 48 hr of onset):
  - Cranial nerve deficits
  - Limb weakness
  - Slurred speech
  - Visual changes/disturbances
- Arterial occlusion
  - Acute onset of skin color change: white spots/nonblanchable areas
  - Immediate or rapid onset
  - Severe and disproportionate pain
- Venous occlusion
  - Blisters
  - Pain (dull, delayed, or less severe as compared to arterial occlusions)
  - Pallor (red/bluish or purple skin coloration)
  - Pustules
  - Tissue necrosis
- Peripheral vascular insufficiency
  - Bruits
  - Coolness of extremity
  - Intermittent claudication (cramping pain with exertion)
  - Nonhealing ulcers
  - Organ ischemia depending on location of occlusion
  - Pain in the calf and/or foot
  - Renal or GI dysfunction
  - Skin changes including hair loss to extremity

 NURSING PEARL

The six Ps of peripheral arterial disease include pain, pallor, pulses that are absent or diminished, paresthesia, paralysis, and poikilothermia. If these signs and symptoms are identified during assessment, notify the provider immediately.

Diagnosis

Labs

- CBC (will usually show a decreased hematocrit)
- Coagulation studies may be elevated or decreased
  - ACT
  - D-dimer
  - PT/INR
  - PTT
- BMP with magnesium
- Urinalysis, for proteinuria and hematuria

Diagnostic Testing

- ABI
  - Normal 0.9 to 1.3
  - ABI <0.9 indicates peripheral artery disease
  - ABI <0.4 indicates severe ischemia
- CT angiography
- Doppler duplex ultrasonography
- MRA
- Peripheral angiography

ALERT!

Medication noncompliance, especially with anticoagulants, can place the patient at risk for thrombus and clot formation. Taking an accurate and thorough history and physical is essential to understanding the full clinical presentation and appropriate treatment plan.

Treatment

- Endovascular interventions:
  - Catheter-directed thrombectomy
  - Balloon angioplasty
  - Peripheral artery stenting
- Surgical interventions:
  - Carotid endarterectomy
    - ○ Performed to decrease the risk of stroke
  - Femoral-popliteal bypass
- Medications:
  - Anticoagulation agents (Table 3.1)
  - Thrombolytics (Table 5.1)
  - Analgesics (Table A.2)
  - Vasodilators (Table 2.8)
  - Reversal agents (Vitamin K, Table 5.6)

Nursing Interventions

- Administer medications as ordered.
- Assess affected extremities for adequate circulation and perfusion.
- Assess and treat pain.
- Draw and monitor serial labs as ordered
- If the patient undergoes a surgical or endovascular procedure to treat their peripheral vascular insufficiency, see Cardiac Catheterization section for assessment and care of surgical sites.
  - Hemodynamic changes
    - ○ Assess EKG monitoring system for development of dysrhythmias and/or rate changes.
    - ○ Monitor BP.
    - ○ Monitor for both hypotension and hypertension.
  - Neurological assessments should be performed frequently—especially for patients with carotid artery disease—to identify any serious changes.
    - ○ Assess orientation status (alert to person, place, time, and situation), cranial nerves, pupillary response, and GCS.
    - ○ If any symptoms consistent with a stroke are identified, notify provider and follow institution procedure (e.g., notify attending, call code stroke or rapid response, etc.)
    - ○ New dysarthria or aphasia, facial droop, hypertension
    - ○ New onset blurred vision or visual field deficits
    - ○ New onset visual loss, nystagmus, rapid neurological decline, or sudden change in mental status
    - ○ Unequal pupils and unresponsiveness to sternal rubs, deep suctioning, painful or verbal stimuli (see Chapter 6 for additional review of stroke)

NURSING PEARL

Sudden decrease or loss of pulse in extremities undetected by palpation and/or Doppler ultrasound is a serious complication and surgical emergency. If a decrease in perfusion is prolonged, tissue necrosis and loss of limb is possible. Therefore, it is essential that neurovascular and neuromotor checks be conducted at frequent and regular intervals in patients with vascular disease.

- Oxygenation
  - ○ Assess airway, breathing, and circulation.
  - ○ Position patient with HOB >30° (if allowed per activity orders).
  - ○ Use appropriate oxygen delivery system to achieve oxygen saturation >90%.
  - ○ Use continuous SpO_2 monitoring.
  - ○ Notify providers of changes in oxygen demand immediately.
- Positioning
  - ○ Keep limb straight post endovascular procedure for duration directed by provider.
  - ○ Maintain extremity level with heart or below heart with reverse Trendelenburg position.

Patient Education

- Follow the DASH diet.
- Followup as appropriate with outpatient appointments.
- Follow exercise and weight management recommendations.
- Follow diabetes management and treatment recommendations closely.
- Increase physical activity as recommended.
- If referred by provider, participate in cardiac rehab program.
- Pursue smoking cessation as advised.
- Take medications as prescribed.

 POP QUIZ 2.13

A 60-year-old female patient is admitted to the PCU. Past medical history includes chronic A-fib, PAD, CAD, anxiety, and depression. She presents with an uncontrolled nosebleed. Laboratory studies are notable for an INR of 14. When interviewing the patient, she admits it is possible that she mixed her medication together and accidentally doubled her dose of Coumadin. The patient has nasal packing in place, and head CT results are pending. Vital signs are as follows: BP 113/75, HR 84, RR 16, T 98.4°F (36.9°C), and SpO_2 94% on room air. What should the nurse's next action be?

Table 2.8 Cardiovascular Medications

Indications	Mechanism of Action	Contraindications, Precautions, and Adverse Effects
ACEIs (e.g., lisinopril, enalapril, and captopril)		
• Left-sided HF • Hypertension	• Inhibit the conversion of angiotensin I to angiotensin II • Reduce vascular resistance to improve function of the left ventricle • Dilate veins, which decreases venous return	• Use with caution in patients experiencing hemodynamic instability and acute kidney injury. • Medication may need to be discontinued if patient develops new onset cough. • Monitor for signs of hyperkalemia and hypotension. • Avoid the use of two renin–aldosterone system inhibitors, especially in patients with renal failure. • Use with insulin or other antidiabetic agents may enhance hypoglycemic effect.
Alpha adrenergic blockers (e.g., prazosin and doxazosin)		
• BP control and management	• Vasodilate by blocking alpha 1 and 2 receptors	• Medication is contraindicated in hypotension. • Use with caution in patients with cataracts and older adults. • Adverse effects include hypotension, tachycardia, weakness, and tremors.

(continued)

Table 2.8 Cardiovascular Medications *(continued)*

Indications	Mechanism of Action	Contraindications, Precautions, and Adverse Effects
Antiarrhythmics, Class 1-A (procainamide, disopyramide, and quinidine)		
• A-fib • V-tach • CPR	• Inhibit sodium transport through myocardial cells, prolonging the recovery period after repolarization thereby slowing the impulse and allowing for conversion	• Use with caution when administering in cardiogenic, hemorrhagic shock, hypotension, renal, or hepatic dysfunction. • Do not administer in patients with second- or third-degree AV block or systemic lupus erythematosus.
Antiarrhythmics, Class 1-B (lidocaine)		
• Treatment of V-tach or V-fib	• Inhibit an influx of sodium in myocardial tissue, increasing recovery period after repolarization and allowing for conversion out of dysrhythmia	• Use with caution in geriatric patients, HF, hepatic disease, and hypotension.
Antiarrhythmics, Class 1-C (flecainide, propafenone)		
• Prevention of ventricular dysrhythmias • Prevention or conversion of A-fib, atrial flutter, or SVT	• Inhibit sodium channels and shortens action potential of purkinje fibers without impacting other myocardial tissues, thus preventing or converting dysrhythmias	• Hepatic and renal disease can alter excretion of flecainide. • Do not administer in patients with cardiogenic shock. • Use with caution with prolonged QRS or PR interval.
Antiarrhythmics, Class II, beta blockers (e.g., atenolol and, metoprolol)		
• Left- and right-sided HF • BP and HR control and management	• Block the effects of epinephrine and norepinephrine in the body to decrease HR, contractility, and vascular resistance • Reduce BP via vasodilation, thereby decreasing afterload	• Use with caution in patients with asthma, as it may cause bronchospasm. • Do not use in patients with heart blocks, sick sinus syndrome, or other bradycardias. • Use with other HR reducers can cause bradycardia.
Antiarrhythmics, Class II and Class III (sotalol)		
• Maintenance of NSR with symptomatic A-fib or atrial flutter	• Beta-blocking effects and Class III antiarrhythmic activity to lengthen refractory period in cardiac tissue, allowing for maintenance of an NSR	• Do not abruptly discontinue. • Use with caution in hypotensive patients or patients with renal impairment.

(continued)

Table 2.8 Cardiovascular Medications *(continued)*

Indications	Mechanism of Action	Contraindications, Precautions, and Adverse Effects
Antiarrhythmics, Class III (e.g., amiodarone and ibutilide)		
• Rate control with multiple tachydysrhythmias	• Delay of repolarization • Depress SA and AV node automaticity • Vasolytic effects resulting in slowed HR	• Amiodarone is not recommended in the context of HF cardiogenic shock due to negative inotropic effects. • Use with caution in patients with underlying heart block or hepatic impairment.
Antiarrhythimcs, Class IV, calcium channel blockers (e.g., diltiazem)		
• Rate control with supraventricular tachydysrhythmias • Antihypertensive	• Inhibit calcium influx across myocardial and smooth muscle • Slow AV conduction	• Use with caution in patients with hypotension or HF.
Antiarrhythmics, miscellaneous (e.g., adenosine)		
• Narrow complex, monomorphic tachycardia • Wide complex tachycardia	• Stimulate adenosine-sensitive potassium channels in the atrial and sinoatrial node, causing outflow of potassium, resulting in sinus bradycardia	• Adenosine is contraindicated in patients with sinus node disease. • Use with caution in patients with Wolff–Parkinson–White syndrome. • This medication is not effective for A-fib, atrial flutter, or ventricular tachycardia.
Antiarrhythmic, unclassified-cardiac glycosides (e.g., digoxin)		
• Left-sided symptomatic HF • Irregular heartbeat (such as atrial fibrillation)	• Slow conduction through the AV node to improve cardiac contractility in left-sided HF by eliciting a positive inotropic effect	• Hold for patients with digoxin toxicity, tachy/brady dysrhythmias, bradycardia, and AV block. • Hypokalemia, hypomagnesemia, and hypercalcemia exacerbate digoxin toxicity. • Do not administer to patients with Wolff–Parkinson–White syndrome or hypertrophic subaortic stenosis. • Use with caution in patients with impaired renal function, thyroid disease, and MI. • Medication may increase risk of digitalis toxicity when used with potassium-depleting diuretics. Use with digoxin and sympathomimetics or succinylcholine increases risk of cardiac dysythmias.
Anticholinergics (e.g., atropine and glycopyrrolate)		
• Bradycardia • Decrease oral secretions preoperatively or at end of life	• Competitively inhibit autonomic cholinergic receptors • Block parasympathetic actions on the heart, resulting in increased SA node rate	• Flushing of the face may occur, which does not indicate anaphylaxis. • Risk of tachycardia if dose above 2–3 mg.

(continued)

Table 2.8 Cardiovascular Medications *(continued)*

Indications	Mechanism of Action	Contraindications, Precautions, and Adverse Effects
Antidiuretic hormones (e.g., vasopressin)		
• Hypotension • Cardiogenic or septic shock • During cardiac arrest and after resuscitation • Central diabetes insipidus • GI bleeding	• Initiates antidiuretic effect by increasing water absorption at the renal collecting ducts • Stimulate contraction of smooth muscle and capillaries, small arterioles, and venules, resulting in increased BP	• Use with caution in patients with heart and renal failure, seizure disorders, migraines, asthma, CHF, CAD, and in older adults. • Adverse reactions include water intoxication, myocardial/mesenteric ischemia, hyponatremia, hypertension, headache, nausea, diarrhea, tremor, and abdominal pain.
Antiplatelets (e.g., aspirin and clopidogrel)		
• A-fib/A-flutter • CAD • PVD • Acute coronary syndrome • Postoperative antithrombotic prophylaxis	• Inhibit platelet aggregation	• Use with caution in patients with underlying conditions which may cause bleeding, including hepatic impairment and trauma. • Monitor for signs of bleeding. • Adverse effects include generalized bleeding, GI bleeding, and Steven Johnson syndrome (aspirin).
ARBs (e.g., valsartan and losartan)		
• Left-sided HF • Hypertension • Patients who cannot tolerate ACEIs due to renal function or other side effects	• Block the binding of angiotensin I to angiotensin II receptors	• Use with caution in patients experiencing hemodynamic instability and acute kidney injury. • Avoid use of two renin–aldosterone system inhibitors, especially in patients with renal failure. • Use with insulin or other antidiabetic agents may enhance hypoglycemic effect.
Beta blocker with alpha blockade (e.g., labetalol)		
• Hypertension, rate control	• Block beta 1 receptors in the heart • Block beta 2 receptors in the bronchial and vascular smooth muscle • Block alpha 1 receptors in vascular smooth muscle • Vasodilation and decreased PVR to decrease BP	• Medication is contraindicated in patients with severe bradycardia, AV block, cardiogenic shock, or prolonged hypotension or asthma. • Use with caution in pheochromocytoma, cerebrovascular disease, diabetes, hepatic disease, or while operating machinery. • Do not abruptly discontinue.
Calcium supplements (calcium chloride)		
• Treatment for hypocalcemia	• Supplement low-circulating calcium • Assist with maintaining homeostasis	• Calcium supplements are contraindicated in hypercalcemia and V-fib. • Do not give intramuscularly or subcutaneously. • Use with caution in hyperparathyroidism, nephrolithiasis, and sarcoidosis.

(continued)

Table 2.8 Cardiovascular Medications *(continued)*

Indications	Mechanism of Action	Contraindications, Precautions, and Adverse Effects
Corticosteroids (e.g., prednisone and dexamethasone)		
• Cardiac inflammation of autoimmune etiology	• Suppress inflammation and normal immune response	• Medication is contraindicated in patients who are pregnant, have active, untreated infections, or together with live virus vaccines. • Use with caution in hypothyroidism and liver disease. • Adverse effects include thromboembolism, peptic ulcers, anorexia, nausea and vomiting, decreased wound healing, bruising, hyperglycemia, osteoporosis, and increased susceptibility to infection.
Diuretics: aldosterone antagonists (e.g., spironolactone)		
• Left- and right-sided HF • For patients with fluid overload	• Block the effects of aldosterone in the body, thereby blocking sodium reabsorption, causing diuresis without loss of potassium	• Use with caution in patients who have renal failure, as medication is potassium sparing; hyperkalemia may occur. • Monitor magnesium levels as long-term use may cause increase in renal tubular reabsorption of magnesium, causing hypermagnesemia, especially in patients taking magnesium supplements. • Use with angiotensin II receptor antagonists, ACEIs, or ARBs may cause increased serum potassium levels and increased creatinine in patients with HF.
Diuretics: loop diuretics (e.g., furosemide)		
• Left-sided HF with fluid overload • Right-sided HF for symptom management but in lower doses • Hypertension • Edema associated with liver cirrhosis and renal disease	• Inhibit sodium and chloride reabsorption at proximal and distal tubules and loop of Henle causing excretion of sodium, potassium, magnesium, calcium, bicarbonate, and water	• Monitor for dehydration, AKI, GFR <30, and hypotension. • Monitor for pancreatitis, ototoxicity, and aplastic anemia. • Monitor for hypokalemia, hyponatremia, hypochloremia alkalosis, hyperglycemia, hyperuricemia, and hypocalcemia. • Monitor for digitalis toxicity when administering digoxin with loop diuretics. • Monitor and correct potassium levels when used with medications that potentiate hypokalemia: corticosteroids, insulin, and beta antagonists.
Diuretics: thiazide (hydrochlorothiazide)		
• Fluid overload • Pulmonary hypertension • HF • Hypertension	• Increase water excretion by inhibiting reabsorption of sodium and chloride at the distal tubules	• Diuretics are contraindicated in anuria and renal failure. • Use with caution in hepatic disease, hypotension, hypovolemia, and diabetes. • Adverse effects include photosensitivity, hypokalemia, and hyperglycemia.

(continued)

Table 2.8 Cardiovascular Medications *(continued)*

Indications	Mechanism of Action	Contraindications, Precautions, and Adverse Effects
Immunosuppressants (azathioprine)		
• Autoimmune induced cardiac inflammation	• Suppress cell mediated immunity and altered antibody function	• Medication is contradicted in concurrent use with mycophenolate. • Use caution in infection, cancer, radiation therapy, and severe renal impairment. • Adverse effects include chills, fever, nausea and vomiting, anorexia, hepatotoxicity, and pulmonary edema.
Inotropic agents (dobutamine, dopamine)		
• Left-sided HF • Patients who require positive inotropic support	• Improve stroke volume and cardiac output by beta adrenergic agonist action • Increases myocardial contractility (positive inotropic effects), chronotropy, and systemic vascular resistance	• Monitor electrolytes and renal function, as it may cause hypokalemia. • Monitor due to increased risk for ventricular dysrhythmias, especially in patients with atrial fibrillation. • Use with alpha blockers, vasodilators, and other adrenergic sympathomimetics may antagonize CV effects. • Do not use with beta blockers, as they will negate each other's effects.
IVIG		
• Autoimmune induced cardiac inflammation	• Inactivate autoreactive T-cells	• There are no contraindications. • Use with caution in critical illness. • Adverse effects include headache, fever, chills, fatigue, nausea, vomiting, tachycardia, pleural effusion, and acute renal failure.
Nitrates (e.g., nitroglycerin and isosorbide nitrates)		
• Stable or unstable angina • Adjunct therapy in MI • Hypertension (IV)	• Increase oxygenation to the coronary arteries, resulting in decreased preload and afterload, thus decreasing workload of the heart • Decrease cardiac workload to alleviate chest pain and lower BP	• Nitrates are contraindicated in patients with cardiac tamponade, constrictive pericarditis, or in patients taking PDE-5 inhibitors. • Use with caution in patients with hypovolemia, head trauma, cardiomyopathy, or cardioversion (transdermal patch). • Adverse effects include hypotension, tachycardia, headache, and dizziness.

(continued)

Table 2.8 Cardiovascular Medications *(continued)*

Indications	Mechanism of Action	Contraindications, Precautions, and Adverse Effects
Sympathomimetic agents (e.g., epinephrine, norepinephrine, phenylephrine)		
• Acute hypotension • Cardiogenic shock • Sepsis or septic shock • During cardiac arrest and after resuscitation	• Epinephrine: nonselective adrenergic agonist and act on both alpha and beta receptors resulting in cardiac stimulation and arteriolar vasoconstriction • Norepinephrine: act on alpha-adrenergic receptors to increase systemic BP and coronary artery blood flow • Phenylephrine: alpha-1 adrenergic agonist result in potent vasoconstriction	• Use with caution in hypovolemic, hypertension, hyperthyroid, and closed angle glaucoma. • Caution should be observed to avoid extravasation. • Adverse effects include peripheral vasoconstriction or ischemia, tissue necrosis, PVCs, ST-T wave changes, and bradycardia.
Vasodilators (e.g., nitroglycerin and nitroprusside)		
• Hypertensive emergency • Stable or unstable angina • Adjunct therapy in MI • Hypertension • Acute HF • Mitral regurgitation	• Acts directly on arterial and venous smooth muscle resulting in peripheral vasodilation and decreased left ventricular afterload, which lowers BP • Decreases myocardial oxygen demand	• Do not administer in aortic coarctation, AV shunt, or high output acute HF. • Nitroprusside can cause cyanide toxicity. Monitor plasma thiocyanate concentrations. • Nitrates are contraindicated in patients with cardiac tamponade, constrictive pericarditis, or in patients taking PDE-5 inhibitors. • Use with caution in patients with hypovolemia, head trauma, cardiomyopathy, or cardioversion (transdermal patch). • Adverse effects include hypotension, tachycardia, headache, and dizziness.

RESOURCES

American Association of Critical Care Nurses. (2018). The cardiovascular system. In T. Hartjes (Ed.), *Core curriculum for high acuity, progressive care, and critical-care nursing* (7th ed., pp. 144–300). Elsevier.

American Heart Association. (2020). *Advanced cardiovascular life support provider manual* (pp 123–142). Author.

American Heart Association. (n.d.). *Understanding blood pressure readings.* https://www.heart.org/en/health-topics/high-blood-pressure/understanding-blood-pressure-readings

Aronow, W. S. (2017, May 5). Treatment of hypertensive emergencies. *Annals of Translational Medicine, 5,* S5. https://www.ncbi.nlm.nih.gov/pmc/articles/PMC5440310/

Fabre, V., & Bartlett, J. G. (2019). *Endocarditis – Injection drug users.* Johns Hopkins ABX Guide. https://www.hopkinsguides.com/hopkins/view/Johns_Hopkins_ABX_Guide/540192/all/Endocarditis___injection_drug_users

Gopal, M., Bhaskaran, A., Khalife, W. I., & Barbagelata, A. (2009). Heart disease in patients with HIV/AIDS—An emerging clinical problem. *Current Cardiology Reviews, 5*(2), 149–154. https://www.ncbi.nlm.nih.gov/pmc/articles/PMC2805817/

Hartung, H. P. (2008). Advances in the understanding of the mechanism of action of IVIg. *Journal of Neurology, 255*(S3), 3–6. https://doi.org/10.1007/s00415-008-3002-0

Medscape. (n.d.). Lanoxin [Drug information]. *Medscape.* https://reference.medscape.com/drug/lanoxin-digoxin-342432.

Moskowitz, A., Chen, K. P., Cooper, A. Z., Chahin, A., Ghassemi, M. M., & Celi, L. A. (2017). Management of atrial fibrillation with rapid ventricular response in the intensive care unit: A secondary analysis of electronic health record data. *Shock, 48*(4), 436–440. https://www.ncbi.nlm.nih.gov/pmc/articles/PMC5603354/

Prescribers' Digital Reference. (n.d.). *Adenosine* [Drug information]. PDR Search. https://www.pdr.net/drug-summary/Adenosine-adenosine-24200

Prescribers' Digital Reference. (n.d.). *Aldactone* [Drug information]. PDR Search. https://www.pdr.net/drug-summary/Aldactone-spironolactone-978.2934

Prescribers' Digital Reference. (n.d.). *Atropine sulfate* [Drug information]. PDR Search. https://www.pdr.net/drug-summary/Atropine-Sulfate-Injection-atropine-sulfate-684

Prescribers' Digital Reference. (n.d.). *Bivigam (immune globulin intravenous (human)* [Drug information]. PDR Search. https://www.pdr.net/drug-summary/Bivigam-immune-globulin-intravenous--human--3477

Prescribers' Digital Reference. (n.d.). *Captopril* [Drug information]. PDR Search. https://www.pdr.net/drug-summary/Captopril-captopril-2348.4130

Prescribers' Digital Reference. (n.d.). *Cardene I.V. Premixed injection 20 mg* [Drug information]. PDR Search. https://www.pdr.net/drug-summary/Cardene-I-V--Premixed-Injection-20-mg-nicardipine-hydrochloride-2169.8386

Prescribers' Digital Reference. (n.d.). *Cardura (doxazosin mesylate)* [Drug information]. PDR Search. https://www.pdr.net/drug-summary/Cardura-doxazosin-mesylate-1849.6175

Prescribers' Digital Reference. (n.d.). *Coumadin (warfarin sodium)* [Drug information]. PDR Search. https://www.pdr.net/drug-summary/Coumadin-warfarin-sodium-106

Prescribers' Digital Reference. (n.d.). *Cozaar (losartan potassium)* [Drug information]. PDR Search. https://www.pdr.net/drug-summary/Cozaar-losartan-potassium-339.4526

Prescribers' Digital Reference. (n.d.). *Digoxin (digoxin)* [Drug information]. PDR Search. https://www.pdr.net/drug-summary/Digoxin-digoxin-724.8383

Prescribers' Digital Reference. (n.d.). *Diltiazem* [Drug information]. PDR Search. https://www.pdr.net/drug-summary/Diltiazem-Hydrochloride-Injection-diltiazem-hydrochloride-725

Prescribers' Digital Reference. (n.d.). *Diltiazem hydrochloride injection* [Drug information]. PDR Search. https://www.pdr.net/drug-summary/Diltiazem-Hydrochloride-Injection-diltiazem-hydrochloride-725

Prescribers' Digital Reference. (n.d.). *Dobutamine (dobutamine hydrochloride)* [Drug information]. PDR Search. https://www.pdr.net/drug-summary/Dobutamine-dobutamine-hydrochloride-3534.3469

Prescribers' Digital Reference. (n.d.). *Dopamine hydrochloride* [Drug information]. PDR Search. https://www.pdr.net/drug-summary/Dopamine-Hydrochloride-dopamine-hydrochloride-3710.3586

Prescribers' Digital Reference. (n.d.). *Effient (prasugrel)* [Drug information]. PDR Search. https://www.pdr.net/drug-summary/Effient-prasugrel-289.6190

Prescribers' Digital Reference. (n.d.). *Hydrochlorothiazide tablets* [Drug information]. PDR Search. https://www.pdr.net/drug-summary/Hydrochlorothiazide-Tablets-hydrochlorothiazide-1973.1942

Prescribers' Digital Reference. (n.d.). *Imuran (azathioprine)* [Drug information]. PDR Search. https://www.pdr.net/drug-summary/Imuran-azathioprine-745

Prescribers' Digital Reference. (n.d.). *Lasix (furosemide)* [Drug information]. PDR Search. https://www.pdr.net/drug-summary/Lasix-furosemide-2594.8405

Prescribers' Digital Reference. (n.d.). *Levophed (norepinephrine bitartrate)* [Drug information]. PDR Search. https://www.pdr.net/drug-summary/Levophed-norepinephrine-bitartrate-868

Prescribers' Digital Reference. (n.d.). *Lisinopril* [Drug information]. PDR Search. https://www.pdr.net/drug-summary/Prinivil-lisinopril-376.4115

Prescribers' Digital Reference. (n.d.). *Lovenox (enoxaparin sodium)* [Drug information]. PDR Search. https://www.pdr.net/drug-summary/Lovenox-enoxaparin-sodium-521.2354

Prescribers' Digital Reference. (n.d.). *Metoprolol tartrate (metoprolol tartrate)* [Drug information]. PDR Search. https://www.pdr.net/drug-summary/Metoprolol-Tartrate-metoprolol-tartrate-3114.5976

Prescribers' Digital Reference. (n.d.). *Micro-K 10 (potassium chloride)* [Drug information]. PDR Search. https://www.pdr.net/drug-summary/Micro-K-10-potassium-chloride-770

Prescribers' Digital Reference. (n.d.). *Minipress (prazosin hydrochloride)* [Drug information]. PDR Search. https://www.pdr.net/drug-summary/Minipress-prazosin-hydrochloride-999

Prescribers' Digital Reference. (n.d.). *Multaq (dronedarone)* [Drug information]. PDR Search. https://www.pdr.net/drug-summary/Multaq-dronedarone-522.1412

Prescribers' Digital Reference. (n.d.). *Nitroglycerin* [Drug information]. PDR Search. https://www.pdr.net/drug-summary/Nitroglycerin-in-5--Dextrose-nitroglycerin-1148

Prescribers' Digital Reference. (n.d.). *Norpace/norpace CR (disopyramide phosphate)* [Drug information]. PDR Search. https://www.pdr.net/drug-summary/Norpace-Norpace-CR-disopyramide-phosphate-1182

Prescribers' Digital Reference. (n.d.). *Norvasc (amlodipine besylate)* [Drug information]. PDR Search. https://www.pdr.net/drug-summary/Norvasc-amlodipine-besylate-1853.3578

Prescribers' Digital Reference. (n.d.). *Plavix (clopidogrel bisulfate)* [Drug information]. PDR Search. https://www.pdr.net/drug-summary/Plavix-clopidogrel-bisulfate-525.3952

Prescribers' Digital Reference. (n.d.). *Propranolol hydrochloride tablets (propranolol hydrochloride)* [Drug information]. PDR Search. https://www.pdr.net/drug-summary/Propranolol-Hydrochloride-Tablets-propranolol-hydrochloride-1400.8469

Prescribers' Digital Reference. (n.d.). *Sodium nitroprusside* [Drug information]. PDR Search. https://www.pdr.net/drug-summary/Nitropress-sodium-nitroprusside-3404#12

Prescribers' Digital Reference. (n.d.). *Valsartan (valsartan)* [Drug information]. PDR Search. https://www.pdr.net/drug-summary/Valsartan-valsartan-24321

Prescribers' Digital Reference. (n.d.). *Vasotec (enalapril maleate)* [Drug information]. PDR Search. https://www.pdr.net/drug-summary/Vasotec-enalapril-maleate-2344.4124

Prescribers' Digital Reference. (n.d.). *Verapamil hydrochloride injection (verapamil hydrochloride)* [Drug information]. PDR Search. https://www.pdr.net/drug-summary/Verapamil-Hydrochloride-Injection-verapamil-hydrochloride-2813.1935

National Heart Lunch and Blood Institute. (n.d.). *Arrhythmia.* U.S. Department of Health and Human Services, National Heart Lung and Blood Institute. https://www.nhlbi.nih.gov/health-topics/arrhythmia#:~:text=If%20left%20untreated%2C%20arrhythmia%20can,failure%2C%20or%20sudden%20cardiac%20arrest

National Heart Lung and Blood Institute. (n.d.). *Cardiogenic shock.* U.S. Department of Health and Human Services, National Heart Lung and Blood Institute. https://www.nhlbi.nih.gov/health-topics/cardiogenic-shock

National Heart Lung and Blood Institute. (n.d.). *Heart inflammation.* U.S. Department of Health and Human Services, National Heart Lung and Blood Institute. https://www.nhlbi.nih.gov/health-topics/heart-inflammation

PULMONARY SYSTEM

ACUTE RESPIRATORY DISTRESS SYNDROME

Overview

- ARDS is a form of acute respiratory failure that develops when there is damage to the alveolar-capillary membrane causing fluid buildup, hypoxemia, reduced lung compliance, and pulmonary infiltrates.
- ARDS is defined as a PaO_2/FiO_2 ratio of <300.
- It comprises three phases:
  - *Exudative phase*: 7 to 10 days after exposure to lung injury, causing an inflammatory cascade. This cascade causes fluid and hemorrhage in the lung.
  - *Proliferative phase*: Restoration of the epithelial and endothelial barriers is reestablished.
  - *Fibrotic phase*: May not always occur but is associated with fibrous tissue formation, which can lead to prolonged mechanical ventilation and mortality.
- The most common cause of ARDS is systemic inflammatory response syndrome and/or sepsis.
- ARDS can lead to atelectasis, pulmonary edema, decreased pulmonary compliance, and difficulty breathing.
- Patients who develop ARDS cannot be effectively treated without intubation, and mechanical ventilation may need transfer to a higher level of care.

COMPLICATIONS

Complications of ARDS include ventilator-associated pneumonia, barotrauma, atelectasis, pulmonary HTN, lung scarring, multi-organ failure, and death. ARDS often presents with multiple other comorbidities and diagnoses (e.g., sepsis, multisystem trauma, acute pancreatitis, etc.), so collaborative care and management is essential to prevent permanent lung damage and death.

Signs and Symptoms

- Accessory muscle use
- Altered mental status
- Chest pain
- Crackles
- Cyanosis
- Diaphoresis
- Dyspnea
- Fatigue
- Fever
- Hypotension
- Hypoxia
- Increasing oxygen demand
- Respiratory alkalosis
- Retractions
- Tachycardia
- Tachypnea
- Wheezes

ALERT!

In patients transferred from ICU who were mechanically ventilated with high PEEP or increased tidal volumes, ARDS causes overdistention of the alveoli and increases the risk of developing barotrauma. In these transferred patients, watch for symptoms of pneumothorax, tension pneumothorax, and subcutaneous emphysema.

Diagnosis

Labs

- ABG:
  - Expected hypoxemia initially accompanied with acute respiratory alkalosis
  - Severe ARDS indication: ABG progressing to hypercapnic respiratory acidosis
- CMP: May reflect evidence of end-organ injury resulting from severe hypoxia, shock, or systemic inflammation
- CBC: May show elevated WBC if infection is present

Diagnostic Testing

- Bronchoscopy
- Chest CT
- Chest x-ray
- Echocardiogram

Treatment

- Blood transfusion
- Medications (Table 3.1*)
  - Antibiotics (Table A.1)
  - Anticoagulants
  - Corticosteroids
  - Diuretics (Table 2.8)
- Nutrition and fluid support (Table A.3)
- Oxygen and ventilatory support
  - CPAP
  - BiPAP
  - Intubation and mechanical ventilation requiring transfer to higher level of care
- Physical therapy
- Positioning:
  - HOB >30° to improve oxygenation and prevent risk of aspiration
  - Patient likely prone when transferred to ICU

 ALERT!

ARDS can be a complication of COVID-19, which is caused by the SARS-CoV-2 virus. Care parameters are continually evolving. For current information on caring for patients with COVID-19, consult the National Institute of Health (www.covid19treatmentguidelines.nih.gov) and the CDC (www.cdc.gov/coronavirus/2019-ncov/hcp/).

Nursing Interventions

- Administer medication to achieve BP goals.
- Assess and pad bony prominences and areas of skin.
- Consider the use of a diuretic to optimize fluid status.
- Consult physical and occupational therapy to assist the patient with ambulation.
- Consult with respiratory therapy to maintain adequate respiratory status.
- Draw labs as ordered.
- Encourage the patient to cough and deep breathe.
- Increase supplemental oxygen as needed to maintain O_2 SAT >90%.
- Maintain patient comfort.
- Monitor vital signs.
- Obtain accurate I/O.
- Obtain an ABG with any changes in pulmonary changes.
- Perform daily oral care with chlorhexidine.
- Perform pulmonary hygiene and encourage the use of the incentive spirometer hourly.
- Position patient appropriately for maximum ventilation and pressure ulcer prevention.

 NURSING PEARL

Monitor laboratory values carefully and notify providers of any worsening trends. ARDS patients can decompensate quickly and require diligent monitoring and intervention if status worsens.

Patient Education

- Follow up with outpatient follow-up appointments, diagnostic tests, and laboratory draws.
- Participate in pulmonary rehab.

---

* Table 3.1 is located at the end of this chapter.

- Continue using incentive spirometry.
- To use incentive spirometer, place the mouthpiece facing mouth. Exhale deeply, make a tight seal around the mouthpiece with mouth and lips, and inhale as deeply as possible. Repeat 10 times every 1 to 2 hr.
- Engage in physical activity. Start small and work up to regain baseline functioning.
- Supplemental home oxygen may be required at time of discharge. Engage in safe oxygen therapy practices by avoiding smoking and avoiding open flames, flammable products, and heat sources. Avoid products with oil or petroleum, and keep a fire extinguisher close by.

POP QUIZ 3.1

Patients with ARDS who require mechanical ventilation in the ICU are at risk for developing barotrauma. How does barotrauma occur, and what are the clinical manifestations?

ASTHMA (SEVERE)

Overview

- Asthma is a chronic inflammatory disorder of the airway that affects both children and adults.
- Allergens, pollutants, food additives, occupational exposures, stress, exercise, cold air, viral URIs, sinusitis, and menses can trigger severe asthma attacks.
- Airway inflammation in severe asthma attacks results in bronchoconstriction, hyperreactivity, and edema.
- Patients presenting with severe asthma attack usually present in the tripod position with accessory muscle use, anxiety or agitation, and/or wheezing with a respiration rate >30 and HR >120.

COMPLICATIONS

Patients who present with a severe asthma attack are at an increased risk of developing status asthmaticus. These patients should be urgently assessed and prepared for intubation. Without prompt identification and intervention, patients may experience respiratory failure or death.

Signs and Symptoms

- Anxiety
- Accessory muscle use
- Chest tightness
- Cough
- Cyanosis
- Diminished breath sounds
- Dyspnea
- Hypoxemia
- Tachycardia
- Tachypnea
- Wheezing

Diagnosis

Labs

- ABG: In asthma, reflect hypoxemia or hypercarbia
- CBC: In asthma, eosinophils elevated
- IgE levels (antibody that protects from bacteria, viruses, and allergens): In asthma attack, IgE elevated

Diagnostic Testing

- Chest x-ray
- SpO$_2$ monitoring
- Peak expiratory flow rate

ALERT!

ABG values should be used in conjunction with physical assessment and vital sign trends to determine whether transfer to higher level of care for mechanical ventilation is indicated.

Treatment

- Medications (Table 3.1)
  - Inhaled anticholinergic agents
  - Inhaled beta-2 adrenergic agonists
  - Corticosteroids
- Maintain patient airway
- Oxygen and ventilatory support:
  - Intubation and mechanical ventilation
  - Nasal cannula
  - Nonrebreather
  - Simple mask
- Trigger removal (if allergic cause)
- Monoclonal antibody therapy in patients with positive skin tests

Nursing Interventions

- Administer medication as ordered.
- Administer supplemental oxygen; titrate up as appropriate on L/min and device.
- Prepare to call for a rapid response if the patient's condition rapidly deteriorates or a higher level of care is indicated.
- Closely trend ABG results.
- Closely monitor vital signs.
- Closely monitor for worsening signs of respiratory distress, including the following:
  - Increasing oxygen requirement with minimal response to medication or supplemental oxygen
  - Hypoxemia
  - New inability to complete sentences or communicate verbally due to reduced oxygenation
  - Retractions
  - Seated in the tripod position
- Draw labs as ordered.
- Maintain patient comfort.
- Provide pain medication as needed.
- Perform daily oral care.
- Position patient appropriately for maximum ventilation and pressure ulcer prevention.
- Remove anxiety triggers if possible.

 NURSING PEARL

Patients experiencing severe asthma attack may experience anxiety. Provide therapeutic communication and support to acknowledge any feelings of anxiety. Worsening anxiety may worsen the severity of asthma attack.

Patient Education

- After an acute asthma exacerbation, review medication regimen with provider.
- Review asthma control plan:
  - Keep rescue inhalers on hand in case of acute attack.
  - Change occupation if allergen or trigger exposure is work related.
  - Control asthma triggers by self-monitoring symptoms and removing from the source of allergen if possible. This may include avoiding tobacco, dust mites, animals, specific foods, or pollen.
  - Ensure proper inhaler use. To use most inhalers, use thumb and fingers to hold the inhaler upright with the mouthpiece down, pointing toward mouth. Remove the mouthpiece cover and gently shake. Hold the mouthpiece away from mouth and exhale deeply. Use the inhalation method recommended by provider (open mouth vs. closed mouth) and breathe in slowly (3–5 seconds) while pressing down at the top of the cannister to dispense medication. Hold breath for 10 seconds before removing the mouthpiece and exhaling slowly. Repeat this process for the recommended number of puffs. Once finished, wipe mouthpiece and reapply cap.

 POP QUIZ 3.2

A patient experiencing a severe asthma exacerbation saw minimal improvement after Atrovent (ipratropium) administration. Throughout the shift, the patient's respiratory status progressively declined. What is the next intervention in severe asthma exacerbation?

- Identify and control asthma triggers:
  - Avoid allergen (e.g., tobacco, dust mites, animals, pollen) if possible.
  - Get allergy testing if etiology is unknown.
  - Self-monitor symptoms.
- Continuously review/educate on current situation and plan of care.
- Take medications as prescribed.
- Engage in weight reduction practices.
- Engage in smoking cessation protocols.

CHRONIC OBSTRUCTIVE PULMONARY DISEASE EXACERBATION

Overview

- *COPD* is a chronic restrictive airway disease classified by airflow limitation.
- COPD consists of both bronchitis (inflammation of the bronchioles) and emphysema (destruction of the alveoli secondary to irritant exposure such as smoke or particulates).
- COPD exacerbation can rapidly progress to acute respiratory failure requiring mechanical ventilation.
- Patients intubated due to a severe COPD exacerbation are likely to fail extubation.

Signs and Symptoms

- Accessory muscle use
- Chest tightness
- Chronic productive cough
- Central cyanosis
- Clubbing of the nails
- Dyspnea and tachypnea
- Hypercapnia
- Hypoxia
- Increased anteroposterior diameter
- Peripheral edema
- Low SpO_2
- Muscle atrophy
- Weight loss
- Wheezing

Diagnosis

Labs

- ABGs: May show hypercarbia or hypoxia
- Blood and sputum cultures: May show organism growth
- CBC: Elevated WBC possible if infection present

Diagnostic Testing

- Chest CT
- Chest x-ray
- Pulmonary function tests

 COMPLICATIONS

Complications of COPD include acute exacerbations, acute and/or chronic respiratory failure, pulmonary HTN, right-sided HF, weight loss, and bacterial infections. Close monitoring and management of symptoms can help decrease the risk of developing these complications and improve quality of life.

 ALERT!

Patients with no history of smoking or secondhand smoke inhalation who are diagnosed with COPD should be worked up for alpha-1 antitrypsin deficiency. This is a genetic disorder that can cause COPD and is the most common cause of COPD in nonsmokers.

 NURSING PEARL

Typically, there are two findings seen in COPD:

- *Blue Bloaters*: A patient whose skin appears ashen/blue and has a $PaCO_2 > 45$ mmHg with $PaO_2 < 60$ mmHg
- *Pink Puffers*: A patient whose skin remains pink but seems to gasp (or puff) for air and whose $PaCO_2$ is normal and $PaO_2 > 60$ mmHg

 ALERT!

Patients with COPD may have a baseline SpO_2 value <90%. This makes SpO_2 an unreliable diagnostic tool for assessing respiratory status. ABGs are a much more accurate indicator of respiratory status in this population; they accurately provide values for PaO_2, CO_2, and HCO_3, indicating acid–base imbalances and hypercapnia.

Treatment

- Airway suctioning as needed for secretions
- Chest physiotherapy
- Lung transplantation (end-stage treatment)
- Medications (Table 3.1)
  - Antibiotics, if indicated (Table A.1)
  - Anticholinergics
  - Bronchodilators
  - Corticosteroids
- Nutritional supplementation
- Pulmonary rehab
- Self-care
  - Physical exercise
  - Diaphragmatic breathing
  - Smoking cessation
- Supplemental oxygen and ventilatory support
  - Nasal cannula
  - Simple mask
  - Nonrebreather
  - Intubation and mechanical ventilation

Nursing Interventions

- Administer medication as ordered.
- Administer noninvasive ventilation and mechanical ventilation, if necessary.
- Closely monitor ABGs and serial laboratory studies.
- Closely monitor vital signs.
- Maintain patient comfort by achieving patient pain goals.
- Perform chest physiotherapy.
- Prepare patient for intubation, if indicated.
- Position patient appropriately for maximum ventilation and pressure ulcer prevention.
- Remove anxiety triggers if necessary to improve ventilation.

 NURSING PEARL

Chest physiotherapy can be delivered manually, with a vest, or a programmable bed. Chest physiotherapy can help loosen airway secretions, which can be suctioned to maintain a patent airway.

Patient Education

- Attend pulmonary rehabilitation as ordered by provider.
- Avoid exposure to airway irritants.
- Use home oxygen therapy as indicated.
- Follow up with all scheduled appointments.
- Start smoking cessation program and avoid secondhand smoke.
- Take medications as ordered.
- Use supplemental oxygen as needed.
- Get vaccinated for seasonal flu and pneumonia.

 POP QUIZ 3.3

What is the most common cause of COPD in patients with no past history of smoking or history of exposure to secondhand smoke?

OBSTRUCTIVE SLEEP APNEA

Overview

- OSA occurs when the airway becomes fully or partially occluded while the patient is sleeping, resulting in an obstruction of airflow.
- This occurs when there is not sufficient space to accommodate airflow in a portion of the upper airway.

- Complications of sleep apnea can range from poor, nonrestorative sleep to significant long-term effects on CV health, mental illness, and quality of life.
- Risk factors for sleep apnea include obesity, alcohol use, smoking, anatomic structure, male gender, use of sedatives, habitual snoring, use of sedatives, and family history.
- There are many treatment options for OSA, ranging from lifestyle modifications to surgical procedures.

Signs and Symptoms

- Apnea during sleep
- Daytime fatigue
- Decreased attention and concentration
- Dry mouth and headache
- Frequent loud snoring
- Gasping for air while sleeping
- Nocturia
- Sexual dysfunction

Diagnosis

Diagnostic Testing
- Sleep studies

Treatment

- Lifestyle modifications
  - Diet modification to achieve healthy BMI
  - Healthy sleeping habits
  - Physical activity
  - Smoking cessation program, if indicated
- Airway devices
  - CPAP
  - Mouth pieces
- Surgical procedures
  - Nerve stimulator implant
  - Orofacial therapy
  - Tonsillectomy
  - Tracheostomy

Nursing Interventions

- Apply supplemental oxygen for an SpO_2 goal >90%.
- Consult with respiratory therapist.
- Develop sleep plan and schedule with patient.
- Encourage consistent use of oral or nasal airway device.
- Encourage lifestyle modifications to improve OSA.
- Perform sleep hygiene.
- Monitor and treat complications.
- Monitor continuous SpO_2 values while patient is sleeping.

 COMPLICATIONS

Complications of untreated OSA include atrial fibrillation, cancer, cardiac and vascular disease (MI, HF, stroke), metabolic disorders (type 2 diabetes and glucose intolerance), and glaucoma. OSA has a high mortality rate and should be treated seriously when diagnosed to prevent further complications and systemic damage.

 ALERT!

Sleep studies are the gold standard to diagnose OSA. Additionally, lab values can be helpful to rule out other contributing medical or metabolic conditions.

 NURSING PEARL

CPAP compliance is low; over 50% of patients do not continue usage after the first month. However, patients who are compliant with CPAP have better outcomes compared to those who do not use CPAP.

Patient Education

- Encourage compliance with airway devices.
  - Follow the user instructions to assemble a CPAP home device. Insert appropriately sized filters and attach the CPAP hose to the mask. Program CPAP pressure settings as determined by the results of a sleep study test and provider. Set up the humidifier and be sure to use distilled water.
  - Fit the CPAP to face and secure snuggly with the straps.
  - Turn on the device and enjoy a restful sleep.
  - Be sure to clean CPAP regularly.
- Modify diet as ordered by provider.
- Maintain healthy sleep patterns.
- Maintain physical activity as ordered by provider.
- Begin smoking cessation plan if needed.

POP QUIZ 3.4

What medications should be avoided overnight in patients with OSA?

PLEURAL SPACE COMPLICATIONS

Overview

- Pleural space complications include chylothorax, empyema, hemothorax, pneumothorax, and pleural effusion.
- *Chylothorax* is an accumulation of chyle in the pleural area of the lung.
  - Chyle is a milky white substance that is produced in the small intestine. This can be absorbed by the lymphatic system and deposited in the lung.
  - Often, this is the result of thoracic trauma, neoplasm, or infection.
- *Empyema* is the collection of pus in the pleural area of the lung.
- *Hemothorax* is the presence of blood in the pleural space, usually caused by trauma.
- *Pneumothorax* is the presence of air in the pleural space. Pneumothorax can be further classified as spontaneous or traumatic/tension.
- *Pleural effusion* is defined as the excessive buildup of fluid in the pleural area. Often, this can result from pneumonia, HF, malignancy, cirrhosis, and/or ascites.

COMPLICATIONS

If significant, hemothorax can result in hemodynamic instability, shock, hypoxia, and death. Complications of pneumothorax include pneumoperitoneum, pneumopericardium, pulmonary edema, empyema, respiratory failure or arrest, cardiac arrest, and pleural effusion complications include empyema, sepsis, and pneumothorax.

Signs and Symptoms

- Small or large chylothorax
  - Small chylothorax asymptomatic and detected through nonrelated imaging
  - Large chylothorax usually unilateral and most common in right lung; possible symptoms include:
    - Chest pressure
    - Decreased breath sounds
    - Dullness to percussion
    - Decreased exercise capacity
    - Progressive dyspnea
- Empyema symptoms are consistent with pneumonia but linger for extended period of time:
  - Cough
  - Crackles
  - Dullness to percussion
  - Egophony
  - Increased palpable fremitus
  - Fever
  - Pleuritic, sharp chest pain on inspiration
  - Sputum production

- Hemothorax:
  - Absent or decreased breath sounds
  - Chest wall asymmetry
  - Cardiac arrest
  - Hypoxia
  - Hypotension
  - Respiratory distress and arrest
  - Tachypnea
  - Tracheal deviation
- Pleural effusion can be asymptomatic or present with the following:
  - Cough
  - Decreased tactile fremitus
  - Dullness noted on percussion
  - Dyspnea on exertion
  - Egophony
  - Fever
  - Pleural rub
  - Sharp pain with breathing or cough
- Spontaneous pneumothorax: Symptoms may include the following:
  - Absent chest wall movement
  - Asymmetric lung expansion
  - Acute dyspnea with increased work of breathing
  - Cyanosis
  - Decreased tactile fremitus or breath sounds
  - Hyperresonance on percussion
  - JVD
  - Pulsus paradoxus
  - Sharp pleuritic ipsilateral chest pain
  - Respiratory failure
  - Tachycardia
  - Tachypnea
  - Acute respiratory failure and hemodynamic instability (tension/traumatic pneumothorax)

ALERT!

Any accumulation of fluid or air in the pleural space can compromise lung function, placing the patient at risk for adverse events. Treatment requires early identification and evacuation of invading fluid or air from the pleural space.

ALERT!

Alert the provider if absence of breath sounds is noted on assessment, especially in the context of vital sign changes or increasing oxygen demand. These findings require immediate intervention.

Diagnosis

Labs
- ABG to show respiratory compromise, acidosis, or hypercarbia
- CBC to show elevated WBC

Diagnostic Testing
- Chest CT
- Chest x-ray
- Ultrasound

Treatment

- Supplemental oxygen with titration as needed to maintain oxygen saturation >90%
- Medications as ordered:
  - Analgesics (Table A.2)
  - Antibiotics, if indicated (Table A.1)
  - Diuretics, if indicated (Table 2.8)
- Chest tube inserted into chest wall to drain air or fluid

(continued)

Treatment *(continued)*

- Thoracentesis: Procedure in which large-bore needle inserted into pleural wall space and drains accumulating fluid
- Needle decompression: Emergency procedure used to stabilize patients with tension pneumothorax
- Thoracotomy: Open surgical procedure to gain access to the pleural space so surgeons can remove fluid from around the lungs and insert drains as needed to stabilize patient

Nursing Interventions

- Assess and maintain chest tube integrity.
  - Assess for air leak.
  - Attach to low wall suction or water seal as ordered.
  - Maintain clean, dry, and occlusive chest tube dressings.
  - Change chest tube dressing per facility protocol (usually every 72 hr or when soiled).
  - Monitor chest tube output volume, color, and consistency.
  - Notify the provider for any rapid increase in drainage amount.
- Promote pulmonary hygiene.
  - Titrate oxygen and delivery device as needed.
  - Turn, cough, and take a deep breathe.
  - Use incentive spirometer.
  - Move patient out of bed to chair.
- Promote hemodynamic stability.
  - Administer blood transfusion.
  - Administer medications (Table 3.1).
  - Administer IV fluids.
- Notify the provider if the patient's oxygen saturation does not improve, despite increasing supplemental oxygen. Prepare for transfer to higher level of care.
- Update patient and/or family on current clinical status, plan of care, and upcoming procedures.

 NURSING PEARL

Indications for an urgent thoracotomy for a hemothorax include 300 to 500 mL/hr of output for 2 to 4 consecutive hr after chest tube insertion, or >1,500 mL over 24 hr. This is a complication of hemothorax and may indicate active bleeding of a great vessel injury, chest wall injury, or cardiac tamponade. These conditions indicate active bleeding. Notify the provider immediately and prepare for transfer to higher level of care.

Patient Education

- Ask questions about the purpose of external medical devices including the following:
  - Bedside telemetry
  - Chest tube systems
  - Incentive spirometer
- Ask questions about medication for hemothorax, chylothorax, pleural effusion, or empyema.
- Notify the nurse immediately if any of the following occurs:
  - Bleeding, drainage, or pain around chest tube insertion sites
  - Chest pain
  - Dyspnea
  - Feelings of anxiety or impending doom

 POP QUIZ 3.5

When discussing treatment options for a hemothorax, the nursing student states a needle decompression can be used to treat a hemothorax. How should the nurse respond?

PNEUMONIA

Overview

- Pneumonia is defined as an acute inflammation of the lungs caused by a variety of agents that may lead to alveolar consolidation.
- Pneumonia may be categorized by the following:

- Aspiration of foreign substance, food, or liquid into lung causing injury
- Bacterial infection
- Viral infection
- Fungal infection

Signs and Symptoms

- Accessory muscle use
- Bronchial or diminished breath sounds
- Chest pain
- Fever and chills
- Productive cough
- Tachycardia
- Weakness, malaise

Diagnosis

Labs

- ABG to indicate hypoxia or acidosis
- Blood and sputum cultures to identify organism present and guide treatment through antibiotic susceptibility
- CBC: Elevated WBC counts indicate infectious process presence

Diagnostic Testing

- Bronchoscopy with bronchoalveolar lavage
- Chest x-ray
- Chest CT scan
- Thoracentesis

Treatment

- IV fluids as needed (Table A.3)
- Supplemental oxygen and ventilatory support
- Identify/treat cause:
  - Aspiration: Antibiotics (Table A.1)
  - Bacterial: Antibiotics
  - Fungal: Antifungals
  - Viral: Antivirals, lung support
- Adjunct medications as indicated (Table 3.1)
  - Anticholinergics
  - Bronchodilators
  - Corticosteroids
  - Expectorants
  - Antipyretics (Table A.2)
- Adequate nutrition through PO intake or tube feeding alternatives as necessary

Nursing Interventions

- Administer antibiotics as ordered.
- Apply supplemental oxygenation if needed. Titrate oxygen and delivery device as needed.
- Collect blood, sputum, and urine cultures.
- Encourage activity, mobility, and incentive spirometer use to help improve recovery.
- Frequently monitor airway patency.
- Monitor and follow up on labs as ordered.
- Monitor fever curve and provide cooling interventions as needed.

COMPLICATIONS

Untreated pneumonia can progress to sepsis, empyema, lung abscess, multiple organ dysfunction syndrome, and respiratory failure. Timely diagnosis and treatment can prevent progression to any of these complications.

ALERT!

Do not start broad-spectrum antibiotics until cultures have been collected. Beginning antibiotics before drawing or collecting cultures can yield inconclusive or inaccurate results, making identification of the causative agent difficult.

(continued)

Nursing Interventions *(continued)*

- Perform chest physiotherapy.
- Position patient in an upright position to promote adequate ventilation.
- Promote hemodynamic stability.
  - Administer IV fluids, if indicated.
  - Support BP as needed.
- Promote pulmonary hygiene.
  - Encourage cough and deep breathing.
  - Encourage incentive spirometer.
- Pulmonary toileting, secretion mobilization, and clearance are essential to help improve oxygenation and perfusion.

Patient Education

- Vaccinate against flu and pneumonia at discharge if available or in outpatient setting before the start of flu season.
- Work with primary care provider to identify resources or medications to support smoking cessation.
- In cases of aspiration pneumonia, restrict diet as ordered. This may include preparing thicker consistency meals.
- If diagnosed with aspiration pneumonia, follow up with the following:
  - Swallow study
  - Speech therapy consults and swallowing rehab

POP QUIZ 3.6

What is one essential daily intervention that should be performed to prevent the development of ventilatory-associated pneumonia?

PULMONARY EMBOLISM

Overview

- A *PE* is a partial or complete blockage of the pulmonary arteries due to a blood clot, fat, air, or foreign material.
- If the PE is caused by a blood clot, the origin of the clot most often comes from a DVT in the leg or a venous clot.
- Fat emboli are usually a complication secondary to a long bone or pelvic fracture.
- Air emboli may occur after surgery or through an IV or central line.
- Septic emboli may occur if the patient experiences a bacterial or viral infection.

COMPLICATIONS

Complications of a PE are severe and include the following:

- Cardiac arrest
- Dysrhythmia
- Pulmonary infarction
- Pulmonary HTN
- Respiratory arrest
- Death

Signs and Symptoms

- Chest pain
- Cough
- Crackles
- Dyspnea
- Feelings of impending doom
- Fever
- Hemoptysis
- Hypoxemia
- Mental status changes
- Petechiae on truck and head of body (fat emboli)

ALERT!

Risks for PE include DVT/VTE, atrial fibrillation, MI, CVA, surgery, trauma, prolonged immobilization, pregnancy, hormonal birth control, smoking, and obesity.

- Pleural friction rub
- Pulmonary HTN
- Right ventricular hypertrophy
- Syncope
- Tachycardia

Diagnosis

Labs

- ABG: Expect hypoxemia or hypercarbia
- CBC: May show elevated platelet counts
- Coagulation studies:
  - D-dimer
  - INR
  - PT
  - PTT
- Troponins

Diagnostic Testing

- Chest x-ray
- Chest CT scan with and without contrast
- Pulmonary angiography
- Venous ultrasound
- Ventilation and perfusion lung scan
- CT angiography
- Echocardiogram

Treatment

 NURSING PEARL

First-choice anticoagulants include unfractionated or low-molecular-weight heparin for inpatient treatment. Patients are usually bridged to warfarin when ready for discharge.

- Medication (Table 3.1):
  - Fibrinolytic agents (Table 5.1)
  - Heparin (Table 3.1)
  - Low-molecular-weight heparin
  - Warfarin (Table 3.1)
  - Opioids (Table A.2)
- Oxygen and ventilatory support
- Surgery:
  - Inferior vena cava filter
  - Pulmonary embolectomy

Nursing Interventions

 ALERT!

Monitor patients with long bone fractures closely. Severe long bone fractures can leak fat emboli into the vascular space, which can travel to the lungs and result in a PE and respiratory compromise in an otherwise stable patient.

- Administer medications as ordered.
- Discuss potential procedures.
  - Chest tube insertion
  - Surgery
- Educate on follow-up care after discharge.
- Monitor and follow up on labs as ordered.
- Patients on a heparin drip will have serial PTTs drawn until a therapeutic level is obtained.
- Monitor for dysrhythmia on continuous cardiac monitoring.
- Monitor for hematoma or signs of bleeding due to anticoagulation therapy.
- Notify healthcare team of worsening status or condition.
  - Anxiety
  - Chest pain
  - Dyspnea

(continued)

Nursing Interventions *(continued)*

- Position patient in semi-Fowler's position.
- Promote adequate oxygenation.
  - Titrate supplemental oxygen as needed.
  - Continuous SpO_2 monitoring.
- Promote hemodynamic stability.
  - Administer blood transfusion, if indicated.
  - Support BP as needed.
- Support patient's emotional well-being.

Patient Education

- Ambulate and exercise as tolerated and ordered.
- Anticoagulation medication increases risk for bleeding. Take precautions to fall-proof the home environment by wearing appropriate footwear or nonskid socks, removing rugs and other tripping hazards, installing handrails, and using nonslip mats in bathrooms or other areas of concern.
- Continue outpatient lab draws to monitor long-term anticoagulation therapy as needed.
- Take precautions to prevent DVT, specifically postsurgery:
  - Ambulation as allowed; elevate lower extremities when not ambulatory.
  - Wear graduated compression stockings or SCDs.

PULMONARY HYPERTENSION

Overview

- *Pulmonary HTN* occurs when the pressure in the blood vessels that carry blood from the Ht to the lungs is higher than normal.
- Pulmonary HTN often presents with right-sided HF.
- Though drug therapy has advanced to improve quality of life, there is no cure.

COMPLICATIONS

Complications of pulmonary HTN include PE, HF, pericardial effusion, hepatic damage, dysrhythmia, bleeding, and anemia. With no curative treatment, careful medical management is required to keep the patient's condition from progressing.

Signs and Symptoms

- Ascites
- Cardiac murmurs and gallops
- Chest pain and dyspnea on exertion
- Fatigue and lethargy
- Ortner's syndrome: hoarseness, cough, and hemoptysis
- Peripheral edema
- JVD
- Pleural effusion
- Right ventricular dysfunction
- Syncopal episodes

Diagnosis

Labs
- ABG to show hypoxemia
- BNP to show elevation, indicating right ventricular overload (end-organ damage)
- CMP to show elevated liver and kidney function tests (end-organ damage)
- CBC to show low Hg or HCT due to medication therapy

Diagnostic Testing
- Chest x-ray
- Chest CT scan
- Cardiac catheterization
  - Pulmonary artery pressure >25 mmHg
  - Cardiac output
  - Left ventricular filling pressure
- Echocardiogram
- Pulmonary function tests
- Pulmonary angiography
- Ventilation and perfusion lung scan

Treatment
- Oxygen and ventilatory support
- Medications
  - Diuretics (Table 2.8)
  - Anticoagulation (Table 2.8)
  - Calcium channel blockers (Table 2.8)
  - Prostacyclin analogs (Table 3.1)
    - Epoprostenol
    - Iloprost
    - Treprostinil
- Surgery
  - Atrial septostomy
  - Pulmonary thromboendarterectomy
  - Lung transplant

Nursing Interventions
- Administer medications as ordered.
- Maintain patient comfort.
- Monitor and follow up on labs as ordered.
- Monitor for dysrhythmia on continuous monitoring.
- Position patient in semi-Fowler's position.
- Promote hemodynamic stability and oxygenation via medication management.
- Titrate oxygen and delivery device as needed to maintain oxygen saturation >90% or to ordered goal.

Patient Education
- Adhere to medication schedule and watch for signs and symptoms of complications.
- Attend all follow-up care after discharge.
- Be able to identify signs and symptoms of complications and know when to seek medical expertise.
- Maintain care of PICC or port if discharged with an invasive line.
- Notify healthcare team of worsening condition.
  - Chest pain
  - Dyspnea
- Supplemental home oxygen may be required at time of discharge. Engage in safe oxygen therapy practices by avoiding smoking, open flames, flammable products, and heat sources. Avoid products with oil or petroleum and keep a fire extinguisher close by.
- Take medications as prescribed and do not discontinue without speaking with provider.

ALERT!

Pulmonary HTN has either an unknown etiology or a genetic component. Currently, other causes of pulmonary HTN are unknown at this time. This, in combination with vague nonspecific symptoms, makes diagnosis difficult.

NURSING PEARL

When patients with pulmonary hypertension exert themselves, higher levels of oxygen may be required for support. Consider preemptively increasing oxygen supplementation before physical exertion such as ambulating to the bedside commode or working with PT.

POP QUIZ 3.7

What treatment options exist for patients whose pulmonary HTN is unresponsive to conventional medical management?

RESPIRATORY DEPRESSION

Overview

- Respiratory depression can result from certain medical conditions (chronic lung disease or OSA), trauma to the head or chest, medications, severe obesity, alcohol abuse, or drug abuse.
- Reversal of respiratory depression depends on the cause of the respiratory depression.

Signs and Symptoms

- Altered mental status
- Cyanosis
- Dyspnea
- Fatigue
- Headache
- Slow, shallow breathing

Diagnosis

Labs
- ABG to indicate hypoxia or hypercarbia

Diagnostic Testing
- Chest x-ray
- Pulse oximetry
- Sleep study
- PFTs

Treatment

- Oxygen and ventilatory support
- Medication
  - Flumazenil
  - Naloxone

Nursing Interventions

- Administer reversal medications as ordered.
- Continuously monitor pulse oximetry.
- Frequently assess the rate and rhythm of the patient's respirations.
- Frequently monitor airway patency.
- Insert an oral airway if needed to maintain an open, patent airway.
- Monitor and follow up on labs as ordered.
- Monitor vital signs, especially RR and BP.
- Position patient in an upright position to promote adequate ventilation.
- Promote hemodynamic stability and support BP as needed.
- Promote oxygenation.
- Titrate oxygen and delivery device as needed.

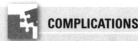 **COMPLICATIONS**

Respiratory depression can lead to respiratory failure and death. Early identification and treatment of causative factors is essential to prevent complications and death.

 ALERT!

Medication-induced respiratory depression can rapidly progress to respiratory failure and arrest. Naloxone and flumazenil are common reversal agents for narcotics and benzodiazepines, which can cause respiratory depression.

 NURSING PEARL

Naloxone has a short half-life. Patients experiencing medication-induced respiratory depression may need multiple doses to overcome the sedating effect.

Patient Education

- Avoid drinking and taking narcotics or other respiratory depressants together.
- Discuss lifestyle modifications if alcohol/drug induced.
- Engage in diet modification and physical activity if overweight.
- If diagnosed with OSA, wear CPAP device nightly.

POP QUIZ 3.8

A patient presents to the PCU from the PACU. The patient is complaining of 10/10 pain at the incision site and requests additional pain medication, but quickly falls asleep and frequently needs sternal rubs to provide responses to the nurse's questions. The patient's vital signs are as follows: HR 92, BP 115/82 mmHg, RR: 8, SpO_2 92% on 4LNC, T 96.8 °F (36.0 °C). What should the nurse's next action be?

RESPIRATORY FAILURE

Overview

- *Acute respiratory failure* occurs when the lungs are unable to exchange oxygen and CO_2 to oxygenate the body, resulting in hypoxia and/or hypercapnia.
- This usually occurs rapidly due to the buildup of fluid in the lung.
- Respiratory failure can be broken down into two categories:
  - *Hypoxic respiratory failure* occurs when there is not enough oxygen circulating in the blood. Hypoxic respiratory failure can be caused by pneumonia, ARDS, asthma, PE, or edema.
  - *Hypercapnic respiratory failure* occurs when too much CO_2 builds up in the blood. This can be caused by central nervous system depression due to drug or alcohol use, COPD, Guillain-Barre syndrome, MS, myasthenia gravis, or an increase in ICP.

COMPLICATIONS

Respiratory failure causes impaired gas exchange and systemic oxygen deprivation. Complications include cerebral ischemia, renal failure, MI, cardiac arrest, and death. Recognizing respiratory decompensation and initiating emergency therapy is essential to improving patient outcome.

Signs and Symptoms

- Accessory muscle use
- Altered mental status
- Anxiety/agitation
- Cyanosis
- Diaphoresis
- Dyspnea
- Retractions
- Slow, shallow breathing

Diagnosis

Labs

- ABG: Typically reveal hypoxia and/or hypercapnia
- Blood and sputum cultures
- BMP
- CBC

Diagnostic Testing

- Bronchoscopy
- Chest CT
- Chest x-ray

(continued)

Diagnostic Testing (continued)

- Echocardiogram
- Pulmonary function tests
- Possible other tests to determine underlying conditions that may have caused the acute respiratory failure

Treatment

- Correct hypoxemia, respiratory acidosis, and hypercapnia using supplemental oxygen and ventilation therapy:
  - Noninvasive positive pressure ventilation:
    - CPAP: Administers FiO_2 at a continuous pressure to assist with increased work of breathing and hypoxic respiratory failure
    - BiPAP: Administers FiO_2, as well as two settings for inspiratory and expiratory pressure
      - Oxygenates and ventilates patients with hypoxic or hypercarbic respiratory failure
      - Last resort treatment prior to mechanical ventilation
      - No BiPAP therapy to unconscious or unresponsive patients
  - Mechanical ventilation and ECMO: Immediate transfer to higher level of care
- Medications (Table 3.1):
  - Antibiotics (Table A.1)
  - Anticholinergics
  - Bronchodilators
  - Corticosteroids

 ALERT!

Be alert to changes in the patient's work of breathing such as tachypnea, tripod positioning, worsening dyspnea, difficulty responding to questions in full sentences, retractions, accessory muscle use, and/or anxiety. Be proactive and initiate appropriate noninvasive positive pressure ventilation before complete decompensation and respiratory failure.

Nursing Interventions

- Administer medications as ordered.
- Assess vital signs frequently, specifically the patient's respiration rate and SpO_2.
- Consult with respiratory therapist to provide adequate ventilation.
- Frequently monitor airway patency.
- Maintain continuous pulse oximetry.
- Monitor and follow up on labs as ordered.
- Pad bony prominences on the patient's face prior to placing a CPAP or BiPAP mask to prevent pressure ulcers.
- Perform chest physiotherapy to loosen and remove secretions.
- Perform frequent pulmonary assessments.
- Position patient in an upright position to promote adequate ventilation.
- Promote oxygenation. Titrate oxygen and delivery device as needed.
- Position patient appropriately to maximize ventilation with HOB >30° or prone, depending on clinical condition.
- Turn every 2 hr.

 ALERT!

BiPAP is contraindicated in patients who are unable to maintain their airway or remain conscious. If BiPAP is initiated, careful assessment and monitoring of the patient's mental status and alertness is necessary to ensure ventilation is effective.

Patient Education

- Acute respiratory failure can occur quickly, often due to other comorbid conditions. Do not delay contacting medical professional if concerns regarding care or status arise.
- Discuss pulmonary rehabilitation.

 POP QUIZ 3.9

How can patients in severe respiratory failure benefit from being positioned?

- Maintain pulmonary toileting and airway secretion clearance during recovery.
- Seek emergency medical care if experiencing worsening or difficult breathing that is unrelieved by any intervention. Educate on follow-up care with primary care or pulmonology.
- Take medications as prescribed.

THORACIC SURGERY

Overview

- Thoracic surgery includes any surgical procedure that occurs on the organs of the chest, including the lungs, Ht, esophagus, and trachea.
- Any thoracic surgery has the potential to require intensive monitoring due to the nature of the surgery or complications that occur during the surgery.
- Patients who have had thoracic surgeries such as VATS, lobectomy, and pneumonectomy are commonly admitted into the PCU.
  - VATS procedures can be used for diagnostic and therapeutic purposes, including biopsy collection, cancer staging, fluid drainage, and tissue resection.
  - Lobectomy is the removal of a lobe of the lung.
  - Pneumonectomy is the removal of the entire lung.
- Other thoracic surgery patients transferred to progressive care units include those who have had esophagectomy, pneumonectomy, decortication, pleurectomy, and lung transplants.

 COMPLICATIONS

Thoracic surgery has many complications, including agitation after anesthesia, anxiety, cyanosis, decreased ventilation, diaphoresis, dyspnea, increased oxygen requirements or work of breathing, tachycardia tachypnea, cardiac dysrhythmias, atelectasis, pneumonia, respiratory failure, and death. Close monitoring of ventilatory and hemodynamic status postprocedure can help identify complications and initiate treatment.

Diagnosis

Labs

- Labs to identify patient's status prior to procedure and postoperatively:
  - ABG
  - CBC
  - Clotting factors: PT, PTT, INR
  - CMP
  - Type and screen

Diagnostic Testing

- Bronchoscopy with lavage
- Chest x-ray
- Chest CT scan
- Ultrasound

Treatment

- Postoperative analgesia (Table A.2)
- Postoperative supplemental oxygen as needed

ALERT!

Atelectasis following thoracic surgery can be an emergency requiring intubation or emergent chest tube placement.

Nursing Interventions

- Ambulate once cleared from bed rest.
- Assess and manage postoperative pain with medication and nonpharmacologic interventions.
  - Medication intervention may include continuous IV infusion of fentanyl, hydromorphone, or morphine.
  - Patients may also receive epidurals or thoracic blocks with combinations of bupivacaine/hydromorphone or bupivacaine/fentanyl.
  - Ketorolac or acetaminophen may be adjunctive medications to assist with pain management.

(continued)

Nursing Interventions *(continued)*

- Incisional pain may be managed with ice packs or lidocaine patches.
- Nonpharmacologic interventions for pain management include massage, acupressure, music therapy, pet therapy (if allowed by institution and patient condition), or methods of distraction using conversation, relaxation techniques, meditation, television, or any other calming activity.
- Assess, clean, and maintain chest tubes and drains.
- Assess drain output for increasing and/or change in output (e.g., increasing volumes, drainage that changes from dark to bright/frank blood).
- Assess surgical site for symptoms of infection including redness, swelling, purulent and/or foul-smelling drainage, and systemic changes (hypotension, tachycardia, and fever).
- Assist patient with cough and deep breathing exercises. Splint and support surgical sites as needed.
- Collect blood and sputum cultures when an infection is suspected.
- Encourage the use of incentive spirometry, if possible, postoperatively.
- Engage in DVT/VTE prophylaxis per institutional protocol. This usually includes anticoagulation, SCDs, ambulation, and bed mobility (q2h turns, calf pumps, leg lifts, etc.).
- Maintain oral hygiene care per institutional protocol.
- Maintain pulmonary hygiene with oral suctioning.
- Trend lactate, ABG, CBC, and BMP.

NURSING PEARL

Always assess chest tubes from insertion site at the patient to the atrium to ensure there are no kinks in the line. Also check that suction is on (if ordered). Note and report any air leaks to the provider.

Patient Education

- Ambulate and engage in physical activity as early as possible.
- Discuss need for follow-up care after discharge. Keep scheduled appointments and lab draws to monitor health status.
- Maintain care of surgical incision. Monitor for new pain, redness, swelling, or warmth to touch around surgical site. Also monitor for new or purulent drainage.
- Maintain proper pulmonary toileting and airway clearance.

POP QUIZ 3.10

When discussing care of a patient following thoracic surgery with a nursing student, the student describes atelectasis as an emergency, requiring chest tube placement and possible intubation and transfer. How should the nurse respond?

Table 3.1 Pulmonary Medications

Indication	Mechanism of Action	Contraindications, Precautions, and Adverse Effects
Anticholinergics (e.g., ipratropium)		
<ul><li>Asthma, COPD, acute respiratory failure</li><li>Bronchospasm</li><li>Bronchoconstriction</li></ul>	<ul><li>Block the effects of acetylcholine to help relax the muscles causing bronchoconstriction</li><li>Reduce the production of mucus</li><li>Inhibit cholinergic receptors in bronchial smooth muscle</li></ul>	<ul><li>Medication is contraindicated in cross sensitivity to atropine or bromide.</li><li>Inhaled anticholinergics can produce a paradoxical bronchospasm, which can be life-threatening in some patients; however, it is rare and usually occurs with the first use of new cannister.</li><li>Use caution in soy or peanut allergy, in patients with known dysrhythmia, or in BPH, or urinary obstructions.</li><li>Adverse effects include hypotension, GI irritation, allergic reaction, headache, nervousness, dysrhythmia, and urinary retention.</li></ul>

(continued)

Table 3.1 Pulmonary Medications *(continued)*

Indication	Mechanism of Action	Contraindications, Precautions, and Adverse Effects
Anticoagulants (e.g., warfarin)		
• Blood clots such as DVTs and PEs	• Inhibit vitamin K availability to reduce the effects of clotting factors	• Patients taking warfarin are at increased risk of bleeding; ensure bleeding and fall precautions are maintained. • Clotting factors must be checked regularly.
Anticoagulants: Heparin, fractionated (enoxaparin)		
• Treatment and prophylaxis of thromboembolic disorders	• Prevent growth of existing thrombus • Prevent formation of new thrombus	• Medication is contraindicated in uncontrolled bleeding and severe thrombocytopenia. • Use caution in renal or hepatic disease, GI bleed/ulcerative disease, head injury, or bleeding disorders. • Adverse effects include bleeding.
Anticoagulants: Heparin, unfractionated (heparin)		
• PE, DVT • Postoperative antithrombotic prophylaxis	• Are used to treat and prevent the formation of blood clots by accelerating the activity of antithrombin III to inactivate thrombin	• Use cautiously in patients who have an increased risk for bleeding. • Medication is contraindicated for patients with severe thrombocytopenia. • Monitor CBC and clotting factors with special attention to PTT when administering as a continuous infusion. • Use cautiously in patients with hepatic disease, as they are often at higher risk of bleeding.
Beta-2 agonists/bronchodilators (albuterol)		
• Reverse and prevent airway obstruction related to COPD and asthma	• Relax airway smooth muscle and decrease obstruction and inflammation, resulting in improved airway clearance	• Use caution in patients with cardiac disease, diabetes, glaucoma, hyperthyroidism, and HTN. • Adverse effects include paradoxical bronchospasm, anxiety, nervousness, chest pain, dysrhythmia, and palpitations.
Corticosteroids (e.g., prednisone, dexamethasone, methylprednisolone)		
• Asthma, COPD, anaphylaxis, inflammatory states: ARDS, pneumonia, respiratory failure	• Inhibit steps in the inflammatory pathway to prevent inflammation of the lungs and reduce mucus production	• Patients receiving corticosteroids for an extended time or in high doses are at increased risk of immunosuppression, making them more prone to infection. • Avoid using in patients with Cushing's syndrome. • Use caution in untreated infection, diabetes, glaucoma, immunodepression, and liver disease. • Adverse effects include headache, hoarseness, diaphoresis, and bronchospasm. • Medication may reduce glucose tolerance, causing hyperglycemia in diabetic patients.

(continued)

Table 3.1 Pulmonary Medications *(continued)*

Indication	Mechanism of Action	Contraindications, Precautions, and Adverse Effects
Expectorants (e.g., dextromethorphan, guaifenesin)		
• Pneumonia, respiratory failure, ARDS	• Help alleviate congestion, reduce viscosity, and clear mucus from airways	• Do not give for persistent or chronic cough due to smoking, asthma, or COPD. • Medication is contraindicated in alcohol intolerance. • Use caution in prolonged cough accompanied by fever, rash, or headache and in diabetic patients. • Adverse effects include dizziness, headache, nausea, vomiting, diarrhea, and rash.
Prostacyclin analogs (e.g., epoprostenol, treprostinil, and iloprost)		
• Treatment of pulmonary atrial HTN	• Promote vasodilation and reduce pulmonary vascular resistance	• Medication is contraindicated in pulmonary edema. • Use caution in hypotension or patients at risk for bleeding. • Adverse effects include headache, flushing, tachycardia, nausea, vomiting, dizziness, and myalgia.

RESOURCES

Centers for Disease Control and Prevention. (n.d.). *Healthcare workers: Information on COVID-19.* https://www.cdc.gov/coronavirus/2019-ncov/hcp/

Lewis, S. M. (2011). *Medical-surgical nursing: Assessment and management of clinical problems.* Mosby.

National Heart Lung and Blood Institute. (2019). *Acute respiratory distress syndrome.* U.S. Department of Health and Human Services, National Heart Lung and Blood Institute. https://www.nhlbi.nih.gov/health-topics/acute-respiratory-distress-syndrome

National Heart Lung and Blood Institute. (2020). *Asthma.* U.S. Department of Health and Human Services, National Heart Lung and Blood Institute. https://www.nhlbi.nih.gov/health-topics/asthma

National Heart Lung and Blood Institute. (n.d.). *Pleural disorders.* U.S. Department of Health and Human Services, National Heart, Lung, and Blood Institute. https://www.nhlbi.nih.gov/health-topics/pleural-disorders

National Heart Lung and Blood Institute. (n.d.). *Pulmonary hypertension.* U.S. Department of Health and Human Services, National Heart Lung and Blood Institute. https://www.nhlbi.nih.gov/health-topics/pulmonary-hypertension

National Heart Lung and Blood Institute. (n.d.). *Sleep apnea.* U.S. Department of Health and Human Services, National Heart Lung and Blood Institute. https://www.nhlbi.nih.gov/health-topics/sleep-apnea

National Institutes of Health. (n.d.). *COVID-19 treatment guidelines.* https://www.covid19treatmentguidelines.nih.gov/

OpenAnesthesia. (n.d). *ABG: COPD.* https://www.openanesthesia.org/abg_copd/

Prescribers' Digital Reference. (n.d.). *Albuterol sulfate* [Drug information]. PDR Search. https://www.pdr.net/drug-summary/Albuterol-Sulfate-Inhalation-Solution-0-5--albuterol-sulfate-1426.4211

Prescribers' Digital Reference. (n.d.). *Alteplase* [Drug information]. PDR Search. https://www.pdr.net/drug-summary/Activase-alteplase-1332.3358

Prescribers' Digital Reference. (n.d.). *Amphotericin B* [Drug information]. PDR Search. https://www.pdr.net/drug-summary/Amphotericin-B-amphotericin-B-3117.3010

Prescribers' Digital Reference. (n.d.). *Clopidogrel bisulfate* [Drug information]. PDR Search. https://www.pdr.net/drug-summary/Plavix-clopidogrel-bisulfate-525.3952

Prescribers' Digital Reference. (n.d.). *Dextromethorphan hydrobromide/guaifenesin* [Drug Information]. PDR Search. https://www.pdr.net/drug-summary/Robitussin-Maximum-Strength-Cough-Chest-Congestion-DM-dextromethorphan-hydrobromide-guaifenesin-3199.2055

Prescribers' Digital Reference. (n.d.). *Enoxaparin sodium* [Drug information]. PDR Search. https://www.pdr.net/drug-summary/Lovenox-enoxaparin-sodium-521.2354

Prescribers' Digital Reference. (n.d.). *Epoprostenol sodium* [Drug information]. PDR Search. https://www.pdr.net/drug-summary/Flolan-epoprostenol-sodium-188.3624

Prescribers' Digital Reference. (n.d.). *Fluconazole* [Drug information]. PDR Search. https://www.pdr.net/drug-summary/Diflucan-fluconazole-1847.3044

Prescribers' Digital Reference. (n.d.). *Flumazenil* [Drug information]. PDR Search. https://www.pdr.net/drug-summary/Flumazenil-flumazenil-1729

Prescribers' Digital Reference. (n.d.). *Guaifenesin* [Drug information]. PDR Search. https://www.pdr.net/drug-summary/Maximum-Strength-Mucinex-guaifenesin-1642.1918

Prescribers' Digital Reference. (n.d.). *Heparin sodium* [Drug information]. PDR Search. https://www.pdr.net/drug-summary/Heparin-Sodium-Injection-heparin-sodium-1263.107

Prescribers' Digital Reference. (n.d.). *Iloprost* [Drug information]. PDR Search. https://www.pdr.net/drug-summary/Ventavis-iloprost-1709

Prescribers' Digital Reference. (n.d.). *Ipratropium bromide* [Drug Information]. PDR Search . https://www.pdr.net/drug-summary/Atrovent-HFA-ipratropium-bromide-1743

Prescribers' Digital Reference. (n.d.). *Methylprednisolone sodium succinate* [Drug information]. PDR Search. https://www.pdr.net/drug-summary/Methylprednisolone-Sodium-Succinate-methylprednisolone-sodium-succinate-24315

Prescribers' Digital Reference. (n.d.). *Morphine sulfate* [Drug information]. PDR Search. https://www.pdr.net/drug-summary/Morphine-Sulfate-Oral-Solution-morphine-sulfate-1228

Prescribers' Digital Reference. (n.d.). *Naloxone hydrochloride* [Drug information]. PDR Search. https://www.pdr.net/drug-summary/Narcan-naloxone-hydrochloride-3837

Prescribers' Digital Reference. (n.d.). *Prednisone* [Drug information]. PDR Search. https://www.pdr.net/drug-summary/Prednisone-Tablets-prednisone-3516.6194

Prescribers' Digital Reference. (n.d.). *Treprostinil* [Drug information]. PDR Search. https://www.pdr.net/drug-summary/Remodulin-treprostinil-1004.3120

Prescribers' Digital Reference. (n.d.). *Warfarin sodium* [Drug information]. PDR Search. https://www.pdr.net/drug-summary/Coumadin-warfarin-sodium-106

Robriquet, L., Georges, H., Leroy, O., Devos, P., D'escrivan, T., & Guery, B. (2006). Predictors of extubation failure in patients with chronic obstructive pulmonary disease. *Journal of Critical Care, 21*(2), 185–190. https://doi.org/10.1016/j.jcrc.2005.08.007

Siegel, M. D. (2020). Acute respiratory distress syndrome: Clinical features, diagnosis, and complications in adults. *UpToDate.* https://www.uptodate.com/contents/acute-respiratory-distress-syndrome-clinical-features-diagnosis-and-complications-in-adults/print?search=noncardiogenic-pulmonary&source=search_result&selectedTitle=4~99&usage_type=default&display_rank=4

Tarbox, A. K., & Swaroop, M. (2013). Pulmonary embolism. *International Journal of Critical Illness and Injury Science, 3*(1), 69–72. https://doi.org/10.4103%2F2229-5151.109427

Yale School of Medicine. (n.d). *Common tests for patients with pulmonary hypertension.* https://medicine.yale.edu/intmed/pulmonary/clinical/pvdp/tests/

4

ENDOCRINE SYSTEM

DIABETES MELLITUS TYPE 1

Overview

- Diabetes mellitus type 1 is caused by an autoimmune response in which the body attacks and destroys pancreatic cells that produce insulin.
- This results in a failure to produce insulin, which leads to uncontrolled hyperglycemia.
- Typically, diabetes mellitus type 1 develops in childhood or adolescence.
- Risk factors for developing diabetes mellitus type 1 are not well understood, but are thought to have a genetic component.

Signs and Symptoms

- Symptoms of patients with diabetes mellitus type 1 may include:
  - Blurred vision
  - Fatigue
  - Impaired wound healing
  - Mood changes (more common with uncontrolled, undiagnosed, or fluctuating blood glucoses)
  - Polydipsia
  - Polyuria
  - Polyphagia
  - Recurrent infections
  - Unexplained weight loss prior to diagnosis
  - Weakness
- Refer to the sections on hypo- and hyperglycemia for signs and symptoms of those specific disorders.

Diagnosis

Labs

- Fasting blood glucose: NPO for at least 8 hr before the test
  - Normal: <100 mg/dL
  - Prediabetes: 100 to 125 mg/dL
  - Diabetes: 126 mg/dL or higher
- HbA1C: Average blood sugar for the past 2 to 3 months
  - Normal: <5.7%
  - Prediabetes: 5.7% to 6.5%
  - Diabetes: 6.5% or higher
- Two-hr oral glucose tolerance test: Checks blood sugar levels before and 2 hr after a sweet drink

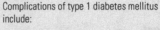

COMPLICATIONS

Complications of type 1 diabetes mellitus include:

- Hypoglycemic episodes, which can lead to loss of consciousness and/or seizures.
- Ketoacidosis.
- Nephropathy.
- Neuropathy.
- Retinopathy.
- Systemic vascular damage, which causes decreased blood circulation due to narrowed blood vessels. This can lead to impaired wound healing.

(continued)

Labs (continued)

- Normal: <140 mg/dL
- Prediabetes: 140 mg/dL to 199 mg/dL
- Diabetes: 200 mg/dL or higher
- Random plasma glucose in a patient with classic symptoms of hyperglycemia or hyperglycemic crisis: ≥200 mg/dL
- Urinalysis
  - Positive glucose
  - Positive ketones
- BMP to assess electrolyte abnormalities and kidney function

 ALERT!

HbA1c provides evidence about a patient's average blood glucose levels during the previous 2–3 months, which is the predicted half-life of red blood cells. This value is checked in both type 1 and type 2 diabetes and should be <6.5%. Follow-up with regularly scheduled appointments and lab draws to appropriately monitor this value.

Treatment

- Lifestyle modifications:
  - 30 minutes or more of daily physical activity
  - Frequent daily blood glucose monitoring
  - Follow low-carbohydrate diet
  - Long-term plans to achieve and maintain a healthy weight and BMI
- Medications: Insulin replacement (Table 4.1* and Figure 4.1)

Nursing Interventions

- Administer appropriate insulin or oral medication dosages as directed by the provider based on the patient's blood glucose.
- Assess the skin for nonhealing or open wounds, especially on the patient's feet.
- Check the patient's blood glucose ACHS.
- Monitor and follow-up on labs as ordered.
- Monitor daily carbohydrate intake.
- Monitor vital signs.
- Refer to social worker to ensure patient has accessibility to medications and blood glucose monitoring supplies.

 NURSING PEARL

Diabetes can cause problems during pregnancy for women and their developing babies. Women who want to become pregnant should consult a diabetes nurse educator and/or endocrinologist to formulate a care plan that promotes a healthy pregnancy and newborn.

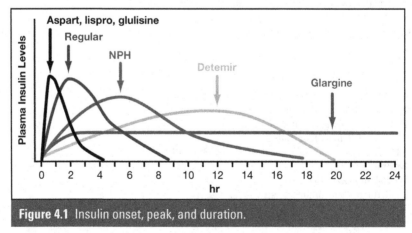

Figure 4.1 Insulin onset, peak, and duration.

Source: Reproduced with permission of Leslie DeGroot, MD, Editor-in-chief, Endotext.org from Hirsch, IB, Skyler, JS. The management of type 1 diabetes. www.endotext.org. Version of December 18, 2015, published by MDTEXT.COM INC. South Dartmouth, MA 02748.

---

* Table 4.1 is located at the end of this chapter.

Patient Education

- After discharge, monitor blood glucose before meals, at bedtime, and when feeling symptomatic.
- Conduct daily skin assessments at home. If unable to visualize areas of skin, use mirrors or seek assistance from another person in the house.
- Eat a low-carbohydrate diet and keep track of daily carbohydrate intake.
- Engage in exercise or physical activity for at least 30 minutes a day.
- Rotate insulin injection site, which may include the abdomen, upper arm, thigh, lower back, hips, or buttocks.
- Understand the signs of hyper- and hypoglycemic episodes and how to care for each.
  - Early hypoglycemic symptoms include behavioral changes (anxiety and irritability), diaphoresis, fatigue, hunger, palpitations, and tachycardia. Late hypoglycemic symptoms include confusion, lethargy, slurred speech, seizures, and coma.
    - Treat with 15 to 20 g of fast-acting carbohydrates (such as regular sodas, fruit juice, sugar candy, glucose gel, or tablet) and recheck blood glucose 15 minutes later.
    - If blood glucose values after rechecking remain below 70 mg/dL, repeat the above steps until blood glucose is higher than 70 mg/dL.
    - If unable to take food or drink by mouth, use of the emergency glucagon kit is indicated. Be sure family and friends know how to use the kit or know to call 911 for assistance.
  - Hyperglycemic symptoms may manifest as altered mental status, abdominal pain, fatigue and lethargy, frequent urination, and thirst, and vomiting.
  - Monitor blood glucose daily before meals, at bedtime, and when feeling symptomatic using a home blood glucose monitoring device.
  - Treat elevated blood glucose values with a prescribed diabetes management plan. This may include increasing short-acting insulin dose or diet to manage hyperglycemia.
    - If hyperglycemia persists despite following the diabetes management plan outlined by provider, ask for a referral to an endocrinologist for recommendations or changes to the treatment plan.
    - If severe hyperglycemia or symptoms of DKA persist, proceed to the nearest ED.

POP QUIZ 4.1

What should family be instructed to do if they find their diabetic family member symptomatic for hypoglycemia or in an altered or unresponsive state, unable to take anything by mouth?

DIABETES MELLITUS TYPE 2

Overview

- Diabetes mellitus type 2 occurs when the cells in the body become resistant to insulin and the pancreas cannot make enough insulin to meet the body's demands, leading to an accumulation of glucose.
- It was once thought that diabetes mellitus type 2 was a disorder that affected adults only. However, with an increasing prevalence of childhood obesity, diabetes mellitus type 2 is now seen in pediatric populations as well.
- Diabetes mellitus type 2 is the most prevalent form of diabetes and can be directly related to BMI, diet, and exercise.

COMPLICATIONS

Complications of diabetes mellitus type 2 include hypo- and hyperglycemic episodes, ketoacidosis, loss of consciousness, seizure, renal damage, systemic vascular damage, and neuropathy.

Signs and Symptoms

Refer to the Diabetes Mellitus Type 1, Hyperglycemia, and Hypoglycemia sections.

Diagnosis

Labs

- Fasting blood glucose: NPO for at least 8 hr before the test
  - Normal: <100 mg/dL
  - Prediabetes: 100 to 125 mg/dL
  - Diabetes: 126 mg/dL or higher
- HbA1C: Measures average blood sugar for the past 2 to 3 months
  - Normal: <5.7%
  - Prediabetes: 5.7% to 6.5%
  - Diabetes: 6.5% or higher
- Two-hr oral glucose tolerance test: Checks blood sugar levels before and 2 hr after a sweet drink
  - Normal: <140 mg/dL
  - Prediabetes: 140 mg/dL to 199 mg/dL
  - Diabetes: 200 mg/dL or higher
- Random plasma glucose test in a patient with classic symptoms of hyperglycemia or hyperglycemic crisis: ≥200 mg/dL
- Urinalysis
  - Positive glucose
  - Positive ketones
- BMP to assess electrolyte abnormalities and kidney function

 ALERT!

Patients diagnosed with prediabetes may be able to reverse blood glucose to normal ranges with lifestyle modifications. The ADA recommends weight loss and 30 minutes of moderate exercise 5 days a week as methods to reduce the risk of type 2 diabetes in patients diagnosed with prediabetes. Prior to discharge, refer patients to diabetes educator or other appropriate resources for assistance in making these lifestyle modifications.

Treatment

- Lifestyle modifications:
  - 30 minutes or more of daily physical activity
  - Blood glucose monitoring with meals and at bedtime
  - Long-term plans to achieve and maintain a healthy weight and BMI
  - Low-carbohydrate dietary choices
- Medications (see Table 4.1):
  - Alpha-glucosidase inhibitors
  - Biguanides
  - DPP-4 inhibitors
  - Incretin mimetics
  - Insulin replacement
  - Sulfonylureas
  - Meglitinides
  - Thiazolidinediones

 NURSING PEARL

When patients order their first meal following type 2 diabetes diagnosis, they may need assistance in interpreting what they can and cannot eat. Be prepared to offer guidance and consult a diabetes nurse educator to assist with education.

Nursing Interventions

- Administer appropriate insulin or oral medication dosages as directed by the provider based on the patient's blood glucose.
- Assess the skin for nonhealing or open wounds, especially on the patient's feet.

- Conduct frequent blood glucose checks and monitor for both hypoglycemia and hyperglycemia.
- Monitor and follow-up on labs as ordered.
- Monitor daily carbohydrate intake.
- Monitor vital signs.

Patient Education

- Conduct daily skin assessments at home. If unable to visualize areas of skin, use mirrors or seek assistance from another person.
- Count grams of carbohydrate intake and follow the recommended low-carbohydrate diet.
- Engage in daily physical activity of at least 30 minutes.
- Monitor blood glucose before meals, at bedtime, and when feeling symptomatic.
- Rotate site of insulin injections as applicable. Various injection sites may include the abdomen, upper arm, thigh, lower back, hips, or buttocks.
- Understand the signs of hyper- and hypoglycemic episodes and how to care for each.

POP QUIZ 4.2

A patient admitted to the PCU has a fasting glucose of 157. What should be considered with this finding?

DIABETIC KETOACIDOSIS

Overview

- DKA is a life-threatening condition characterized by extreme hyperglycemia, ketosis, and acidosis.
- DKA develops when insulin levels are low, causing the body to respond by converting stores of fat and protein into glucose. This releases ketones into the bloodstream, resulting in severely elevated blood glucose levels.
- DKA is most common in patients with type 1 diabetes, but it has the potential to develop in any poorly controlled diabetic patient.

COMPLICATIONS

DKA is a life-threatening condition. Complications of DKA include diabetic coma, dysrhythmia development, and cardiac arrest. Careful management and replacement of volume and insulin is needed to reverse DKA progression.

Signs and Symptoms

- Abdominal pain
- Anorexia
- Confusion
- Dehydration
- Dry mucous membranes
- Fruity breath
- Hypotension
- Increased thirst
- Kussmaul respirations
- Lethargy
- Normal or elevated serum osmolality
- Polyuria and nocturia
- Poor skin turgor
- Severe hyperglycemia
- Tachycardia
- Weakness
- Vomiting

Diagnosis

Labs

- ABG: Acidosis with pH <7.3
- Blood glucose: Profound hyperglycemia with Blood glucose >250
- CMP:
  - Anion gap >10
  - Bicarbonate >18 mEq
  - Hypernatremia
  - Hyperkalemia
  - Hypermagnesemia
  - Hyperphosphatemia
- Urinalysis: Positive for glucose and ketones

 ALERT!

Frequent monitoring of laboratory values is essential to appropriately manage and reverse metabolic imbalances. Consider drawing from central or arterial line to decrease the number of peripheral sticks the patient will receive.

Treatment

- Continuous insulin infusion titrated based on blood glucose levels and facility protocol
- DKA patients profoundly dehydrated and require careful fluid resuscitation
- Electrolyte replacement: Potassium, magnesium, bicarbonate, and phosphate lab values drawn frequently and treated per provider order
- IV fluids:
  - First hr: 0.9% NaCl at 15 to 20 mL/kg as ordered by provider
  - Fluid replacement after first hr depends on hemodynamic and hydration status and electrolyte values
  - Patients with hypernatremia receive 0.45% NaCl at 4 to 14 mL/kg/hr (250–500 mL/hr)
  - Patients with hyponatremia continue receiving 0.9% NaCl at 4 to 14 mL/kg/hr (250–500 mL/hr) per physician order
- Possible transfer to ICU for close monitoring (depends on facility)
- Switch to subcutaneous insulin injection when: Blood glucose level is <200 and two of the following laboratory values are met:
  - Serum bicarbonate ≥ to15 mEq/L
  - Venous pH >7.3
  - Calculated anion gap ≤12 mEq/L

Nursing Interventions

- Administer medications, IV insulin, IV fluid, and electrolyte replacement as ordered based on laboratory values.
- Monitor blood glucose hourly (or per institution policy).
- Monitor vital signs.
- Monitor and follow-up on labs as ordered.
- Monitor intake and output.
- Promote adequate nutrition.
  - If patients are receiving IV insulin, keep NPO for glucose control.
  - If insulin drip is discontinued and the patient is transitioning to PO intake, monitor carbohydrate counts for all orally ingested foods.

 NURSING PEARL

Blood glucose should be monitored hourly while a patient is on an insulin drip. However, blood glucose checks can be extended to q2h per facility protocol if the patient's blood glucoses are stable and the drip has consistently remained at the same rate. Hypoglycemia can occur rapidly if not closely monitored.

Patient Education

- Assess blood glucose before meals and at bedtime (or more frequently as needed).
- If administering subcutaneous insulin, rotate injection site.
- If DKA is suspected at home, consider using a urine dipstick to detect ketones and check blood glucose; seek care as appropriate.

- Monitor for warning signs and symptoms of possible DKA, including signs of hyperglycemia accompanied by fruity breath, deep respirations, and confusion.
- Postdischarge care:
  - Anticipate fluctuations in blood glucose if sick or undergoing stress.
  - Be sure to monitor for symptoms of hypoglycemia, which include confusion, diaphoresis, hunger, irritability, tachycardia, and lightheadedness.
  - Monitor for symptoms of hyperglycemia, which include dyspnea, headache, dehydration, excessive thirst, frequent urination, weakness, and nausea.

POP QUIZ 4.3

A patient was admitted for DKA last night. This morning, they are found to have a Na+ value of 152. They are receiving a continuous insulin infusion at 7 units/hr and 0.9% NS at 125 mL/hr. What should the nurse's next action be?

HYPERGLYCEMIA

Overview

- Hyperglycemia can be a manifestation of insulin resistance or pancreatic insufficiency to produce insulin as seen in both type 1 and type 2 diabetes. Medications are often necessary to lower blood glucose.
- A high blood glucose may also be seen in critically ill patients, even in the absence of preexisting diabetes, due to infection, certain medications (steroids), chronic disease, or nutrition given through an IV or feeding tube.

COMPLICATIONS

Prolonged hyperglycemia can be a symptom of uncontrolled diabetes. Prolonged uncontrolled blood glucose values can result in both microvascular and systemic damage including neuropathy, ophthalmic damage (retinopathy), renal damage (nephropathy), CAD, PVD, and cerebrovascular disease. This systemic damage can ultimately result in renal failure, cardiac dysfunction, blindness, limb ischemia, and death.

Signs and Symptoms

- Altered mental status
- Abdominal pain
- Fatigue
- Lethargy
- Polydipsia
- Polyuria
- Vomiting
- Weight loss

Labs
- BMP
- Fasting blood glucose: >126 mg/dL
- Point of care blood glucose check: >140 mg/dL
- Random plasma glucose: >200 mg/dL
- Urinalysis: Positive glucose

Treatment

- Medications (Table 4.1):
  - If hyperglycemia due to critical illness, infections, glucose-increasing medications (steroids): Chronic disease or tube feeding/TPN treat with insulin
  - If hyperglycemia due to type 1 diabetes: Insulin replacement
  - If hyperglycemia due to type 2 diabetes:
    - Alpha-glucosidase inhibitors
    - Biguanides

(continued)

Treatment *(continued)*

- ○ DPP-4 inhibitors
- ○ Incretin mimetics
- ○ Insulin replacement
- ○ Meglitinides
- ○ Sulfonylureas
- ○ Thiazolidinediones
- Lifestyle modifications:
  - 30 minutes or more of daily physical activity
  - Achieve and maintain healthy weight and BMI
  - Daily blood glucose monitoring (or more frequently, as needed)
  - Low-carbohydrate diet with supportive services as needed

Nursing Interventions

- Administer medications as ordered based on etiology and laboratory values.
- Assess skin for open or nonhealing wounds, paying special attention to the patient's feet.
- Check the patient's blood glucose after administration of insulin or another antihyperglycemic agent. Monitor for symptoms of both hypoglycemia and hyperglycemia.
- Monitor and follow-up on labs as ordered.
- Monitor vital signs.
- Notify the provider if the patient's blood glucose remains elevated despite intervention.
- Perform an ophthalmic examination if the patient complains of vision changes.
- Promote adequate nutrition by monitoring carbohydrate intake.

NURSING PEARL

Consultation with a diabetes nurse educator and dietician may be helpful for newly diagnosed patients with diabetes. This can also be helpful for the family who will support their care.

Patient Education

- Conduct daily skin assessments at home. If unable to visualize areas of skin, use mirrors or seek assistance from another person.
- Count grams of carbohydrate intake and follow the recommended low-carbohydrate diet.
- Engage in daily physical activity of at least 30 minutes.
- Follow-up with appropriate providers, which may include a primary care doctor, endocrinologist, eye doctor, and podiatrist.
- Monitor blood glucose before meals, at bedtime, and when feeling symptomatic.
- Recognize the symptoms of hyperglycemic episodes.
- Rotate site of insulin injections as applicable.

POP QUIZ 4.4

Describe the vascular complications associated with prolonged, untreated, or uncontrolled hyperglycemia.

HYPOGLYCEMIA

Overview

- Hypoglycemia is defined as a blood glucose lower than 70 mg/dL; however, symptoms may not manifest until blood glucose drops below 55 mg/dL.
- While uncommon in patients who do not have diabetes, hypoglycemia can occur transiently after long periods without eating, during severe illness, or following insulin overcorrection or overdose.

COMPLICATIONS

Untreated hypoglycemia can result in seizure, coma, or death. It is essential to identify and treat hypoglycemia before patients progress to these severe complications.

Signs and Symptoms

- Early:
  - Behavioral changes: Anxiety, irritability
  - Diaphoresis
  - Fatigue
  - Hunger
  - Palpitations
  - Tachycardia
- Late:
  - Coma
  - Confusion
  - Lethargy
  - Seizure
  - Slurred speech

Labs

- Blood glucose check: <70 mg/dL
- BMP
- HbA1C
- Liver function test

ALERT!

Patients with persistent hypoglycemia may learn to live and function with a lower blood glucose. This means that a patient may be asymptomatic with a blood glucose <70 mg/dL. This can be very dangerous and can cause a delay in recognition of the condition until late signs/symptoms develop. Notify the provider of any low glucose level even if the patient is asymptomatic.

Treatment

- Medications (Table 4.1):
  - D50 or D5W IV if patient is NPO or unable to tolerate oral intake
  - Glucagon IM
- PO intake of a readily absorbable carbohydrate if the patient is able to tolerate oral intake

Nursing Interventions

- Administer a dextrose medication or a 15-g carbohydrate snack.
- If the patient is NPO, consider adding maintenance IV fluids with dextrose until the patient is able to tolerate PO intake.
- Monitor and follow-up on labs as ordered.
- Monitor vital signs.
- Promote adequate nutrition. Check to make sure the patient is adequately eating meals.
- Perform frequent blood glucose checks 15 minutes after an intervention. If blood glucose remains below 70 mg/dL, repeat with another intervention.
- Be sure to follow institutional protocol, as hypoglycemia treatments may vary.
- Continue to check blood glucose hourly thereafter until the blood glucose has stabilized.
- Notify the provider, who may alter the patient's treatment plan.

NURSING PEARL

Patients with hypoglycemia may need a consult with a dietitian to evaluate diet choices or eating patterns. If a new diagnosis of type 1 or type 2 diabetes is made, a consult to a diabetes nurse educator should be made.

Patient Education

- Always carry a carbohydrate snack or glucose tablet.
- Be sure to monitor blood glucose levels closely at home.
- Consider wearing a diabetic alert bracelet.
- Discuss frequent follow-up care with endocrinology postdischarge.
- Monitor disease progress through regularly scheduled checkups and careful glucose monitoring.
- Understand the signs and symptoms of hypoglycemic episodes and how to intervene.

POP QUIZ 4.5

A patient is admitted with a blood glucose of 58 mg/dL. After being treated with 4 oz of orange juice, the patient's repeat blood glucose is 65. What should the nurse's next action be?

Table 4.1 Endocrine Medications

Indications	Mechanism of Action	Contraindications, Precautions, and Adverse Effects
Alpha-glucosidase inhibitors (acarbose and miglitol)		
• Hyperglycemia • Type 2 diabetes	• Taken with meals to prevent hyperglycemia by slowing down carbohydrate digestion and absorption	• Medication is contraindicated in hypoglycemia, type 1 diabetes, and dual therapy with other oral antidiabetic medications and in patients with chronic intestinal disease or creatinine >2 mg/dL. • Adverse effects include GI disturbances.
Biguanides (e.g., metformin)		
• Hyperglycemia • First-line treatment for type 2 diabetes	• Decrease hepatic gluconeogenesis production • Decrease intestinal absorption of glucose • Increase peripheral uptake and utilization	• Medication is contraindicated in patients with renal or liver failure, unstable heart failure, acidosis, severe alcohol abuse, and DKA. • Adverse effects include decreased B12 levels, GI disturbances, metallic taste, and weight loss. • Use caution in concurrent use with IV contrast, as medication has a nephrotoxic effect; hold metformin 48 hr prior to and after any procedure using IV contrast.
Dextrose injection, 50% (D50) (also available as 5% dextrose in water, 240 mL [D5W])		
• Parenteral (IV) treatment of hypoglycemia	• Glucose replacement and supplementation	• Medication is contraindicated in hyperglycemia. • Adverse effects include hyperglycemia.
DPP-4 inhibitors (e.g., alogliptin and sitagliptin)		
• Taken daily to prevent hyperglycemia by increasing insulin production • Type 2 diabetes	• Stimulate insulin secretion and suppress glucagon secretion • Inhibit gastric emptying	• Medication is contraindicated in type 1 diabetes, DKA, and patients with pancreatitis. • Use caution in older adult patients and those with renal impairment. • Adverse effects include hypoglycemia.
Glycogenolytic agents (glucagon)		
• Parenteral (IM) treatment of hypoglycemia	• Stimulate hepatic production of glucose from glycogen stores	• Medication is contraindicated in hypersensitivity and pheochromocytoma. • Use caution in insulinoma or pheochromocytoma history, starvation, and adrenal insufficiency. • Adverse effects include anaphylaxis, hypotension, nausea, and vomiting.

(continued)

Table 4.1 Endocrine Medications *(continued)*

Indications	Mechanism of Action	Contraindications, Precautions, and Adverse Effects
Incretin mimetics (exenatide)		
• Blood glucose control in type 2 diabetes	• Mimic the action of incretin and promote endogenous insulin secretion	• Medication is contraindicated in hypersensitivity, type 1 diabetes, DKA, ESRD, and severe GI disease. • Use caution in pediatric populations. • Adverse effects include pancreatitis, nausea, vomiting, and diarrhea.
Insulin: Intermediate-acting (NPH)		
• Hyperglycemia control • Can be used in both type 1 and type 2 diabetes	• Bind to a glycoprotein receptor specific to insulin on surface of target cells • Onset 1–2 hr • Duration 12 hr	• Adverse effects include hypoglycemia and lipohypertrophy (with long-term use).
Insulin: Long-acting (e.g., glargine)		
• Hyperglycemia control • Once-daily dosing • Can be used in both type 1 and type 2 diabetes	• Bind to a glycoprotein receptor specific to insulin on the surface of a target cell • Onset 1.5–2 hr • Duration 12–24 hr	• Use caution in infection, stress, and changes in diet. • The most common adverse effect is hypoglycemia. • Long-term use may cause lipohypertrophy.
Insulin: Rapid-acting (e.g., lispro and aspart)		
• Treatment of hyperglycemia • Given to correct elevated blood glucose prior to meals or preemptively before carbohydrate intake • Can be used in both type 1 and type 2 diabetes	• Bind to a glycoprotein receptor specific to insulin on the surface of a target cell • Onset 5–15 min • Duration 4–6 hr	• Contraindications include hypoglycemia. • Use caution in infection, stress, and changes in diet. • The most common adverse effect is hypoglycemia. • Medication is given subcutaneously. • Long-term use may cause lipohypertrophy.
Insulin: Short-acting (e.g., regular insulin)		
• Treatment of hyperglycemia • Can be used in both type 1 and type 2 diabetes • Can be used as an IV infusion to treat DKA and HHS	• Bind to a glycoprotein receptor specific to insulin on the surface of target cell • Onset 30–60 min • Duration 6–8 hr	• Contraindications include hypoglycemia. • Use caution in infection, stress, and changes in diet. • The most common adverse effect is hypoglycemia.

(continued)

Table 4.1 Endocrine Medications *(continued)*

Indications	Mechanism of Action	Contraindications, Precautions, and Adverse Effects
Meglitinides (e.g., repaglinide and nateglinide)		
• Taken with meals to prevent hyperglycemia by stimulating the body to produce more insulin • Type 2 diabetes	• Stimulate insulin secretion by the pancreatic beta cells	• Contraindications include hypoglycemia, type 1 diabetes, and dual therapy with other oral antidiabetics. • Use caution in patients with infections, liver and cardiovascular disease, lactic acidosis, and in the geriatric population. • Adverse effects include hypoglycemia.
Sodium-glucose cotransporter-2 inhibitors (SGLT2) (e.g., canagliflozin, dapagliflozin, and empagliflozin)		
• Blood glucose control in type 2 diabetes	• Prevent reabsorption of glucose filtered in the tubular lumen of the kidney through inhibiting SGLT2	• Medication is contraindicated in patients with severe rental impairments or who are on dialysis. • Use caution in DKA, type 1 diabetes mellitus, dehydration, hypotension, infection, or in geriatric populations. • Adverse effects include hypoglycemia, yeast infection, frequent urination, electrolyte imbalances, dehydration, nausea, and weakness.
Sulfonylureas (e.g., glyburide and glipizide)		
• Hyperglycemia • Second-line treatment for type 2 diabetes	• Stimulate endogenous insulin secretion by native pancreatic cells, increasing the body's sensitivity to its own insulin	• Medication can be used in combination with other oral hypoglycemic agents in patients who fail initial therapy with lifestyle interventions and metformin. • There is risk for potential allergic reactions in patients with a history of sulfa allergies. • Use caution in patients with chronic kidney disease as it is renally excreted. • Adverse effects include hypoglycemia.
Thiazolidinediones (e.g., rosiglitazone and pioglitazone)		
• Hyperglycemia • Third-line treatment for type 2 diabetes	• Improve sensitivity to insulin and decrease insulin resistance	• Medication is contraindicated in patients with heart failure or any evidence of fluid overload, history of fracture, or at high risk for fracture, acute liver disease, type 1 diabetes, and pregnancy. • Adverse effects include heart failure, elevated liver enzymes, anemia, and fractures. • Pioglitazone is contraindicated in patients with a history of or active bladder cancer.

RESOURCES

American Diabetes Association. (n.d.). *Hypoglycemia (low blood glucose).* https://www.diabetes.org/healthy-living/
medication-treatments/blood-glucose-testing-and-control/hypoglycemia
Deglin, J. H., Vallerand, A. H., & Sanoski, C. A. (2011). *Davis's drug guide for nurses.* F.A. Davis.
DiMeglio, L. A., Evans-Molina, C., & Oram, R. A. (2018). Type 1 diabetes. *Lancet, 391*(10138), 2449–2462. https://
doi.org/10.1016/S0140-6736(18)31320-5
American Diabetes Association. (n.d.). *Diagnosis.* https://www.diabetes.org/a1c/diagnosis
Gosmanov, A. R., Gosmanova, E. O., & Dillard-Cannon, E. (2014). Management of adult diabetic ketoacidosis.
Diabetes, Metabolic Syndrome and Obesity: Targets and Therapy, 7, 255–264. https://doi.org/10.2147/DMSO.
S50516
Huether, S. E., & McCance, K. L. (2012). *Understanding pathophysiology.* Elsevier/Mosby.
Lewis, S. M. (2011). *Medical-surgical nursing: Assessment and management of clinical problems.* Mosby.
Prescribers' Digital Reference. (n.d.). *Acarbose* [Drug Information]. PDR Search. https://www.pdr.net/
drug-summary/Precose-acarbose-1315
Prescribers' Digital Reference. (n.d.). *Canagliflozin* [Drug Information]. PDR Search. https://www.pdr.net/
drug-summary/Invokana-canagliflozin-3094
Prescribers' Digital Reference. (n.d.). *Exenatide* [Drug Information]. PDR Search. https://www.pdr.net/
drug-summary/Byetta-exenatide-61
Prescribers' Digital Reference. (n.d.). *Glucagon rDNA origin* [Drug Information]. PDR Search. https://www.pdr.net/
drug-summary/Glucagon-glucagon--rDNA-origin--290.2553
Prescribers' Digital Reference. (n.d.). *Insulin aspart rDNA origin* [Drug Information]. PDR Search. https://www.pdr.
net/drug-summary/NovoLog-insulin-aspart--rDNA-origin--456.3612
Prescribers' Digital Reference. (n.d.). *Insulin glargine* [Drug Information]. PDR Search. https://www.pdr.net/
drug-summary/Basaglar-insulin-glargine-3870.8201
Prescribers' Digital Reference. (n.d.). *Insulin lispro* [Drug Information]. PDR Search. https://www.pdr.net/
drug-summary/Humalog-insulin-lispro-291.3757
Prescribers' Digital Reference. (n.d.). *Miglitol* [Drug Information]. PDR Search. https://www.pdr.net/
drug-summary/Glyset-miglitol-1872
Prescribers' Digital Reference. (n.d.). *NPH, human insulin isophane rDNA origin* [Drug Information]. PDR Search.
https://www.pdr.net/drug-summary/Humulin-N-NPH--human-insulin-isophane--rDNA-origin--2911.4411
Prescribers' Digital Reference. (n.d.). *Pioglitazone* [Drug Information]. PDR Search. https://www.pdr.net/
drug-summary/Actos-pioglitazone-556.397
Prescribers' Digital Reference. (n.d.). *Regular, human insulin rDNA origin* [Drug Information]. PDR Search. https://
www.pdr.net/drug-summary/Humulin-R-regular--human-insulin--rDNA-origin--2912.3423
Prescribers' Digital Reference. (n.d.). *Rosiglitazone maleate* [Drug Information]. PDR Search. https://www.pdr.net/
drug-summary/Avandia-rosiglitazone-maleate-175.404
Prescribers' Digital Reference. (n.d.). *Saxagliptin* [Drug Information]. PDR Search. https://www.pdr.net/
drug-summary/Onglyza-saxagliptin-111.5959
Sommerfield, A. J., Deary, I. J., & Frier, B. M. (2004). Acute hyperglycemia alters mood state and impairs cognitive
performance in people with type 2 diabetes. *Diabetes Care, 27*(10), 2335–2340. https://doi.org/10.2337/
diacare.27.10.2335

ANEMIA

Overview

- Anemia indicates a reduction in the number or volume of RBCs, or a reduction in hemoglobin and hematocrit circulating throughout the body.
- Anemia primarily causes a reduction in blood oxygen carrying capacity, resulting in hypoxia.
- Sickle cell anemia is a common inherited form of anemia. Hallmark findings include a crescent or "sickle" shaped RBC which has decreased oxygen carrying capacity and can obstruct blood flow to other areas of the body.
- Timely recognition and intervention are key to prevent severe complications.
- Three etiologies of anemia include (Table 5.1):
  - Blood loss
  - Reduced RBC production
  - Increased RBC destruction

 COMPLICATIONS

Severe untreated anemia can affect age groups differently. In younger populations, impaired neurologic development may occur. In pregnancy, severe anemia can lead to early labor and premature birth. Complications for severe anemia, such as multiorgan failure or death, are more common in the geriatric population due to preexisting comorbidities in this population.

 NURSING PEARL

Preparation for a stem cell transplant causes anemia, but low RBCs persist following the transplant until the new bone marrow is able to produce the appropriate number of RBCs.

Table 5.1 Conditions That Cause Anemia

Blood Loss	Increased RBC Destruction	Reduced RBC Production

• Acute
 • Chronic
 • May be related to:
   • Coagulopathies
   • Frequent phlebotomy
   • Surgery
   • Trauma
	• Damage by artificial valves
	 • Immune destruction (e.g., hemolytic transfusion reaction)
	 • Inherited disorders (e.g., sickle cell)
	 • RBC membrane defects
	 • Splenic destruction
		• Aplastic anemia
		 • Bone marrow malignancies
		 • Chemotherapy or radiation
		 • Chronic inflammatory conditions
		 • Chronic kidney disease
		 • Nutritional deficiencies:
		   • B12
		   • Folate
		   • Iron
		 • Stem cell transplant

Signs and Symptoms

- Mild anemia: May be asymptomatic
- Severe anemia symptoms may include any of the following:
  - Altered mental status
  - Brittle nails
  - Chest pain
  - Decreased exertional tolerance
  - Delayed growth
  - Dizziness
  - Dyspnea especially on exertion
  - Fatigue, weakness, and lethargy
  - Hair loss
  - Headache
  - Hypotension
  - Jaundice
  - Koilonychia (spooning nails)
  - Pallor
  - Petechiae
  - Pica
  - Splenomegaly or hepatomegaly
  - Tachycardia
- Symptoms specific to sickle cell may include any of the following:
  - Acute and/or chronic pain
  - Dactylitis (swelling of hands and feet)
  - Infections and fevers
  - Priapism
  - Vision problems

ALERT!

Sickle cell anemia may present in the inpatient setting as a sickle cell crisis, which may be triggered by infection, hypoxia, acidosis, dehydration, and other stressors. Sickle cell crises may present in a combination of three categories (Table 5.2). Identification of appropriate phase of crisis can help guide treatment.

Diagnosis

Labs
- Vitamin B12: <180 ng/L
- Blood films/smears: May show abnormally sized RBCs
- Bilirubin: May be >1.2 mg/dL in hemolytic anemia
- CBC
  - Hemoglobin: May be <13 g/dL in men and <12 g/dL in women
  - Hematocrit: <38% in men and <35% in women
- Coombs's test: May be positive
- Iron/ferritin: <30 ng/mL
- Folate: <2.7 ng/mL

Table 5.2 Manifestations of Sickle Cell Crisis

Hematologic aplastic crisis	• Exacerbation of anemia with significant drop in hemoglobin • Sickle cells have a 10- to 20-day half-life • Sickle cells frequently sequestered by spleen • Symptomatic anemia
Infectious crisis	• Elevated risk of secondary infections (e.g., pneumonia, blood stream infections, meningitis, and osteomyelitis) • Sickle cell occlusions in the spleen reduce immunologic function
Vaso-occlusive crisis	• Microvascular occlusions caused by sickled RBCs • Severe pain possible in abdomen, chest, bones, and joints • Tissue and organ ischemia

- High-performance liquid chromatography (sickle cell)
- Reticulocyte count: <0.5%
- Serum iron: May be <60 mcg/dL
- Stool, guaiac test: May be positive
- Total iron binding capacity

 ALERT!

If severe anemia results in angina, myocardial infarction, heart failure, or dysrhythmias, cardiology should be consulted immediately for evaluation.

Diagnostic Testing
- Chest x-ray
- CT
- Upper endoscopy (if suspected GI hemorrhage)
- Pelvic ultrasound

Treatment

- Treatment is dependent on etiology (Table 5.3)
- Deficiency: Vitamin B12, iron or folate: PO or IV replacement of B12, folate or iron (Table 5.6*) and blood transfusion (Table 5.3)
- Aplastic anemia: Bone marrow transplant
- Chronic disease:
  - Renal failure: Erythropoietin (Table 5.6)
  - Autoimmune or rheumatologic conditions: Manage the causative disease
- Red blood destruction (hemolytic anemia):
  - Sickle cell: Blood transfusions, exchange transfusions, antibiotics, opioids, hydroxyurea, IV hydration, oxygen therapy, stem cell/bone marrow transplant
  - Medication mediated: Discontinue medication immediately (if possible)
  - DIC: Antifibrinolytic agents (Table 5.6)
  - Faulty mechanical valves: Valve replacement surgery
  - Persistent despite treatment: Splenectomy may be indicated

Table 5.3 Vitamin and Mineral Related Anemias

Anemia	Vitamin/Mineral Deficiency
Iron deficient anemia	Iron deficiency
Megaloblastic anemia	Folate deficiency
Pernicious anemia	B12 deficiency

Table 5.4 General Indications for Blood Product Transfusion

Condition	Treatment
• Patients with Hgb <7 g/dL	• Packed RBCs
• Patients with platelets <20,000/μL • Platelets <50,000/μL and actively bleeding	• Platelets
• Plasma coagulation factors deficient • Reversal of anticoagulation	• Fresh frozen plasma
• Diagnosis of DIC • Factor VIII replacement • Fibrinogen levels <100 mg/dL	• Cryoprecipitate

Note: Transfusion criteria and target lab levels may vary in different types of patient populations.

---

* Table 5.6 is located at the end of this chapter.

Nursing Interventions

- Administer oxygen, medications (Table 5.6), IV hydration (Table A.3), and blood products as ordered.
- Assess airway, breathing, and circulation.
- Assess for signs of hemorrhage or occult bleeding.
- Assess for signs of infection.
- Assess for signs of respiratory distress or hypoperfusion.
- Assess for worsening signs of fatigue, weakness, and lethargy.
- Draw and monitor serial CBCs to assess RBC, hemoglobin, and hematocrit.
- Elevate extremities to prevent swelling.
- Monitor electrolyte and blood levels following transfusion of blood products.
- Monitor perfusion and oxygenation.
- Monitor vital signs for signs of worsening condition.
- Position patient with HOB at 30° or higher to improve oxygenation and perfusion.
- Prepare patient for administration of blood transfusion for severe anemia
- Promote appropriate diet choices for deficiency anemias.
- Provide therapeutic communication and support; discuss condition specific to anemia diagnosis and assess for willingness to accept blood transfusions.

NURSING PEARL

If patient is experiencing iron deficiency anemia, there is an increased risk of constipation and black tarry stools with iron replacement therapy.

Patient Education

- After discharge, avoid extreme temperatures and changes in altitudes that could cause a vaso-occlusive crisis.
- Avoid smoking due to nicotine's ability to attach to hemoglobin and cause decreased oxygen delivery.
- Avoid offending drug or drug class if hemolytic anemia is a result of medication therapy.
- Follow up regularly with hematologist for routine monitoring.
- Identify iron rich foods:
  - Dark green leafy vegetables
  - Dried fruit
  - Iron-fortified cereals, breads, and pastas
  - Legumes
  - Red meat, pork, or poultry
  - Seafood
- Incorporate vitamin C-containing foods to enhance iron absorption (iron deficiency anemia):
  - Broccoli
  - Grapefruit
  - Kiwi
  - Leafy green vegetables
  - Melons and oranges
- If compromised spleen, follow infection prevention techniques:
  - Handwashing
  - Staying up to date on vaccinations
  - Taking prophylactic antibiotics as prescribed
- Recognize an increased risk of black tarry stools and constipation with iron replacement therapy.
- Recognize fortified foods are necessary to treat vitamin B12 deficiency.
- Self-monitor for symptoms of worsening anemia.
- Take medications and iron or vitamin supplements as indicated by provider.

POP QUIZ 5.1

A patient with iron deficiency anemia receiving IV iron infusions is admitted to the PCU from the ED with abdominal pain, fatigue, and weakness. The patient's baseline vital signs included heart rate (HR) 80 and blood pressure (BP) 120/70 mmHg; however, the BP is now 90/62 mmHg and HR is 130. The patient urgently requests a bedpan and has a bowel movement: 300 mL of black tarry loose watery stool that has a strong odor. Patient states this is not consistent with usual bowel movements. What could be the cause of this large volume black tarry stool?

Overview

- Transfusion of blood products include whole blood, RBCs, platelets, and plasma.
- Any consenting adult over the age of 18 is able to refuse blood transfusions.
- In nonemergent situations, patients should have an active type and screen prior to receiving blood.
- Once administered, monitor vital signs frequently to assess for a possible blood transfusion reaction.

 COMPLICATIONS

Complications of blood product transfusion include allergic reaction, circulatory overload, transfusion related lung injury, infections (HIV, hepatitis B, and C), electrolyte abnormalities, DIC, renal failure, hemolysis, and death. Frequent monitoring and assessment are needed to identify and treat any transfusion reaction.

Signs and Symptoms

Signs and symptoms of a blood product transfusion reaction:
- Chills
- Dyspnea
- Fever
- Hypotension
- Hypothermia
- Itching
- Respiratory distress
- Urticaria

Diagnosis

Labs
- Labs diagnostic for transfusion reaction or need for transfusion (Table 5.4)
  - Bilirubin
  - BMP
  - CBC
  - Haptoglobin
  - Negative ABO: Test for other antibodies
  - Type and screen
    - Antiglobulin testing
    - Direct antiglobulin (Coombs) test
  - LDH
  - Urinalysis

ALERT!

If a transfusion reaction is suspected, stop the transfusion, notify the provider, administer IV fluids, obtain patient labs, and send the blood product back to the blood bank for additional testing.

Treatment

- Blood product administration for the following:
  - Any disease process or condition resulting in blood volume loss or depletion
  - Anemia
  - Cancer
  - Surgery
  - Trauma
- Administration of blood products requires:
  - Large bore IV (20 gauge or larger)
  - Active type and screen
  - Consent
- If a transfusion reaction is suspected:
  - Immediately stop blood transfusion.
  - Disconnect blood tubing from patient IV.
  - Draw back to remove blood from IV or central line tubing.

(continued)

Treatment *(continued)*

- Flush IV line with 0.9% saline flush.
- Administer maintenance fluid (usually 0.9% normal saline) at ordered rate (Table A.3).
- Support ventilation with oxygen supplementation as needed.
- Notify the provider.
- Obtain vital signs and labs.
- Send the blood product back to the blood bank for additional testing.
- If itching/urticaria, administer antihistamine as ordered.

Nursing Interventions

- Apply supplemental oxygen as needed.
- Assess for worsening signs of transfusion reaction.
- Monitor vitals for signs of worsening condition related to transfusion reaction.
- Monitor perfusion and oxygenation.
- Position patient with HOB at 30° or higher to improve oxygenation.
- Provide therapeutic communication and support by addressing and managing anxiety experienced by patients after experiencing a reaction.

 NURSING PEARL

If a patient experiences a blood transfusion reaction, notify the patient and/or family members and advise them to notify any medical providers in the future that they have experienced a transfusion reaction.

Patient Education

- Self-monitor for symptoms of worsening or delayed transfusion reaction.
- Follow diet and lifestyle recommendations under the Anemia: Patient Education section to prevent worsening anemia.
- Follow up with all outpatient lab draws and appointments as scheduled.
- Take prescribed medications after discharge to help restore and maintain RBCs or deficient vitamins/minerals to baseline values.

 POP QUIZ 5.2

A 45-year-old patient with a history of ESRD is admitted to the PCU with worsening abdominal pain, nausea, and vomiting. He has a left arm fistula and a 22 gauge IV in the right hand. On admission, the patient started vomiting black coffee ground emesis. The patient was later found to have a GI bleed. The provider orders two units of packed RBCs. What is the first action to administer these blood products?

Overview

- A coagulopathy is any alteration in baseline hematologic function, which results in impaired clot formation.
- Anticoagulation medications including warfarin, platelet inhibitors, and heparin can result in coagulopathies, which can range from abnormal lab results to a medical emergency.
- Close monitoring of coagulation lab results is necessary to effectively titrate continuous anticoagulation medication infusions to prevent over-anticoagulation.

COMPLICATIONS

Complications of medication-induced coagulopathies include hemorrhage and bleeding anywhere in the body. Symptoms range from mild (petechiae and ecchymosis) to severe and life-threatening (intracranial hemorrhage, GI bleed, retroperitoneal bleed, etc.). Appropriate diagnosis and treatment are necessary to prevent further deterioration of condition.

- Heparin coagulopathy can progress to a state known as HIT. Patients with HIT are in an extremely hypercoagulable state and have a 30% mortality rate.

Signs and Symptoms

- Shared symptoms of coagulopathies induced by warfarin, platelet inhibitors, and heparin include:
  - Bleeding
    - GI
    - Hematemesis
    - Intracranial
    - Ocular
    - Retroperitoneal
  - Exfoliative dermatitis or skin necrosis
- Symptoms specific to platelet inhibitors and HIT (Table 5.5)

COMPLICATIONS

Onset of thrombocytopenia HIT is typically 5 to 10 days following initiation of therapy; however, symptoms can begin in <24 hr if the patient has antibodies due to prior heparin exposure.

Diagnosis

Labs
- BMP
- CBC: Platelets <150,000/mcL
- Coagulation: May be elevated due to decreased platelet counts
  - PT/INR
  - PTT
- D-dimer
- Fibrinogen
- PF4 ELISA (HIT)
- Serotonin release assay (HIT)
- TEG

Diagnostic Testing
- 4Ts Score for HIT:
  - 4Ts scoring system includes screening for the four hallmark signs of HIT, including magnitude of thrombocytopenia, timing of thrombocytopenia with respect to heparin exposure, thrombosis or other sequelae of HIT, and likelihood of other causes of thrombocytopenia.
  - The patient will receive a score between 0 and 2 for each category. A score of 0 to 3 indicates low probability, 4 to 5 indicates intermediate probability, and 6 to 8 indicates a high probability of HIT.
- Spleen ultrasound
- Other imaging helpful to identify potential hemorrhage, bleeding, or thrombosis:
  - CT scan
  - MRI
  - Ultrasound

Table 5.5 Platelet Inhibitors and HIT Symptoms

Platelet Inhibitors	HIT
• Agranulocytosis	• Chest pain
• Angioedema	• Chills
• Aplastic anemia	• Development of new blood clot
• Bronchospasm	• Dyspnea
• Erythema multiforme	• Ecchymosis
• Hepatic failure	• Enlargement or extension of blood clot
• Pancreatitis	• Fever
• Pancytopenia	• Hypertension
• Peptic ulcer	• Sudden onset of pain, redness, and swelling of an arm or leg
• Thrombotic thrombocytopenic purpura	• Rash or sore around injection site
• Stevens–Johnson syndrome	• Tachycardia
	• Weakness, numbness, painful extremity movement

Treatment

- Warfarin-induced coagulopathy: Vitamin K administration
- Platelet inhibitor-induced coagulopathy: No specific antidote
  - Time for drug to wear off
  - Symptom treatment as needed
    - Monitor for symptoms of bleeding.
    - Administer blood products as needed.
- HIT: Discontinuation/removal of heparin administration and heparin dosed agents from patient (heparin-flushed lines, etc.)
  - Alternate anticoagulation medications: Enoxaparin, argatroban, and bivalirudin

Nursing Interventions

- Apply supplemental oxygen if indicated.
- Assess abdomen for potential signs of retroperitoneal bleeding.
  - Abdominal or back pain
  - Bruising on flanks
- Assess airway, breathing, and circulation.
- Assess for coffee ground emesis or black stool.
- Assess neurologic status for potential change, possibly indicative of intracranial bleed.
- Draw and monitor CBC and clotting factor laboratory trends.
- Maintain activity precautions until coagulopathy is reversed.
- Monitor perfusion and oxygenation.
- Monitor vital signs for changes related to hypovolemia or excessive bleeding: Tachycardia and hypotension.
- Position patient with HOB at 30° or higher to assist with improved oxygenation and perfusion.
- Provide therapeutic communication and support to allow the patient to express possible feelings of anger, fear, or anxiety from medication-induced coagulopathy.

Patient Education

- Follow activity orders based on coagulopathy levels.
- If due to an accidental medication overdose at home, use an organizational system to prevent medication errors in the future.
- If HIT develops, notify all future providers of a previous history of a reaction to heparin.
- Self-monitor for symptoms of bleeding; notify provider immediately for any new signs of bleeding.

 POP QUIZ 5.3

A patient diagnosed with a PE is receiving a continuous heparin infusion and develops HIT. What would the nurse anticipate would be the next order from the provider?

Table 5.6 Hematology, Immunology, and Oncology Medications

Indications	Mechanism of Action	Contraindications, Precautions, and Adverse Effects
Antifibrinolytic therapy (tranexamic acid)		
• DIC, bleeding after trauma, hemorrhage	• Hemostatic agent to bind to the lysine binding site for fibrin on the plasmin molecule	• Antifibrinolytic therapy is contraindicated in intracranial bleed and thrombolytic disease. • Use caution in renal impairment, seizure disorders, and surgery. • Adverse effects include thrombosis, thromboembolism, pulmonary embolism, renal thrombosis, visual impairments, and seizures.

(continued)

Table 5.6 Hematology, Immunology, and Oncology Medications *(continued)*

Indications	Mechanism of Action	Contraindications, Precautions, and Adverse Effects
Antihistamine (diphenhydramine hydrochloride)		
• Treatment of allergic reactions, including transfusion reactions • Anaphylaxis	• Competitively inhibit the effects of histamine on H1-receptor sites in the GI tract, large blood vessels, and bronchial muscle suppressing the formation of edema and itching resulting from histaminic activity	• Antihistamine is contraindicated in asthma and COPD. • Use caution in closed angle glaucoma, increased intraocular pressure, bladder obstruction, GI obstruction, ileus, urinary retention, hepatic, or cardiac disease. • Adverse effects include oversedation, seizure, hemolytic anemia, agranulocytosis, dermatitis, confusion, dysarthria, euphoria, neuritis, constipation, blurred vision, urinary retention, and wheezing.
Antimetabolites/antineoplastic agents (hydroxyurea)		
• Treatment of abnormally shaped hemoglobin	• Increase hemoglobin F or fetal hemoglobin which is larger and more flexible than other forms of hemoglobin • Decrease propensity of sickle cells to form clots	• Women who are pregnant or might become pregnant should not handle the medication. • Individuals touching the medication should wear disposable gloves. • It is recommended to use effective contraception while taking hydroxyurea and for females to discontinue if planning to become pregnant in the next 3 months. • Live vaccines should not be administered while taking hydroxyurea, as they can cause life-threatening infection.
Corticosteroids (e.g., hydrocortisone)		
• Allergic reactions including anaphylaxis • Drug hypersensitivities	• Decrease formation and release of endogenous inflammatory mediators including prostaglandins, kinins, and histamine	• Avoid abrupt discontinuation, which may result in Cushing's syndrome. • Monitor for secondary fungal infections. • Monitor for secondary infections related to immunosuppression.
Direct thrombin inhibitor (argatroban, bivalirudin)		
• Anticoagulant option for HIT and DIC	• Inhibit and neutralize the actions of thrombin, including thrombin trapped within established clots	• Direct thrombin inhibitors are contraindicated in active bleeding, spinal anesthesia, diverticulitis, endocarditis, aneurysm, hypertension, inflammatory bowel disease, lumbar puncture, and hepatic disease. • Do not abruptly discontinue. • Use caution in patients with angina and/or prolonged PTT. • Adverse effects include bleeding, dysrhythmias including atrial fibrillation, bradycardia, ventricular tachycardia and cardiac arrest, pulmonary edema, chest pain, MI, and thrombosis.

(continued)

Table 5.6 Hematology, Immunology, and Oncology Medications *(continued)*

Indications	Mechanism of Action	Contraindications, Precautions, and Adverse Effects
Erythropoietin agents (epoetin alfa)		
• Anemia associated with CKD, malignancy, renal failure, or medication therapy in HIV-infected patients	• Stimulate bone marrow to make more RBCs	• Erythropoietin agents are contraindicated in albumin or mammalian cell-derived product hypersensitivity, and uncontrolled hypertension. • Use caution in history of seizures. • Adverse effects include seizures, CHF, MI, stroke, and hypertension.
Folic acid supplements		
• Prevention and treatment of megaloblastic and macrocytic anemia	• Supplementation to assist with protein synthesis and RBC function • Stimulate production of RBCs, WBCs, and platelets to restore normal hematopoiesis	• Antianemics are contraindicated in pernicious, aplastic, or normocytic anemias. • Use caution in undiagnosed anemias. • Adverse effects include rash, irritability, difficulty sleeping, malaise, confusion, and fever.
Iron supplements (e.g., ferrous sulfate, ferumoxytol, iron sucrose injection, etc.)		
• Low hemoglobin • Inadequate iron reserves	• Increase hemoglobin production • Allow for transportation of oxygen via hemoglobin	• Administer on empty stomach with orange juice to increase absorption. • Iron supplements are contraindicated in dialysis, hypotension, anaphylaxis, hemochromatosis, hemoglobinopathy, hemosiderosis, 24 hr prior to an MRI, hepatic or gastric disease, and during pregnancy/lactation. • Adverse effects include angioedema, cyanosis, wheezing, hypotension, constipation, black tarry stools, peripheral edema, chest pain, dyspnea, tachycardia, and hypertension. • To prevent teeth color staining, rinse mouth with water or brush teeth after taking liquid form. • Administer iron 2 hr prior or 4 hr after calcium or antacids for optimal iron absorption. • Iron may decrease concentration of levothyroxine. Administer iron 4 hr after levothyroxine.
Vitamin B12 supplements (cyanocobalamin)		
• Vitamin B12 deficiency, pernicious anemia	• Vitamin supplementation to assist in metabolic processes including fat and carbohydrate metabolism and protein synthesis, cell production, and hematopoiesis	• Medication is contraindicated in cobalt hypersensitivity. • Use caution in renal dysfunction, folic or iron deficiency, polycythemia vera, hypokalemia, bone marrow suppression, and uremia. • Adverse effects include pulmonary edema, heart failure, aluminum toxicity, thrombosis, thrombocytosis, hypokalemia, and polycythemia.

(continued)

Table 5.6 Hematology, Immunology, and Oncology Medications *(continued)*		
Indications	**Mechanism of Action**	**Contraindications, Precautions, and Adverse Effects**
Vitamin K (phytonadione)		
• Hyperprothrombinemia	• Has identical action to vitamin K: facilitates binding of proteins to help blood coagulate	• Medication is less effective in patients with hepatic disease. • Frequently monitor coagulation lab values to prevent overcorrection.

RESOURCES

Harewood, J. (2021, July 18). *Hemolytic transfusion reaction.* https://www.ncbi.nlm.nih.gov/books/NBK448158/
Laposata, M. (2019, January 17). Coagulopathies and bleeding disorders; hemorrhage, clotting abnormalities, microvascular bleeding. *Cancer Therapy Advisor.* https://www.cancertherapyadvisor.com/home/decision-support-in-medicine/critical-care-medicine/coagulopathies-and-bleeding-disorders-hemorrhage-clotting-abnormalities-microvascular-bleeding/
National Heart Lung and Blood Institute. (n.d.). *Blood transfusion.* U.S. Department of Health and Human Services, National Heart Lung and Blood Institute. https://www.nhlbi.nih.gov/health-topics/blood-transfusion#:~:text=Four%20types%20of%20blood%20products,given%20by%20volunteer%20blood%20donors
Prescribers' Digital Reference. (n.d.). *Argatroban* [Drug information]. PDR Search. https://www.pdr.net/drug-summary/Argatroban-Injection-in-0-9--Sodium-Chloride-argatroban-1458
Prescribers' Digital Reference. (n.d.). *Coumadin* [Drug information]. PDR Search. https://www.pdr.net/drug-summary/Coumadin-warfarin-sodium-106#11
Prescribers' Digital Reference. (n.d.). *Droxia (hydroxyurea)* [Drug information]. PDR Search. https://www.pdr.net/drug-summary/Droxia-hydroxyurea-898
Prescribers' Digital Reference. (n.d.). *Epogen (epoetin alfa)* [Drug information]. PDR Search. https://www.pdr.net/drug-summary/Epogen-epoetin-alfa-2887
Prescribers' Digital Reference. (n.d.). *Feraheme* [Drug information]. PDR Search. https://www.pdr.net/drug-summary/Feraheme-ferumoxytol-1201.3477#14
Prescribers' Digital Reference. (n.d.). *Folic acid tablets (folic acid)* [Drug information]. PDR Search. https://www.pdr.net/drug-summary/Folic-Acid-Tablets-folic-acid-1634
Prescribers' Digital Reference. (n.d.). *Heparin sodium injection* [Drug information]. PDR Search. https://www.pdr.net/drug-summary/Heparin-Sodium-Injection-heparin-sodium-1263.107
Prescribers' Digital Reference. (n.d.). *Lysteda* [Drug information]. PDR Search. https://www.pdr.net/drug-summary/Lysteda-tranexamic-acid-1247.8307
Prescribers' Digital Reference. (n.d.). *Nascobal* [Drug information]. PDR Search. https://www.pdr.net/drug-summary/Nascobal-cyanocobalamin-2286
Prescribers' Digital Reference. (n.d.). *Plavix* [Drug information]. PDR Search. https://www.pdr.net/drug-summary/Plavix-clopidogrel-bisulfate-525.3952
Prescribers' Digital Reference. (n.d.). *Venofer* [Drug information]. PDR Search. https://www.pdr.net/drug-summary/Venofer-iron-sucrose-805#14
Suddock, J. T. (2021, August 11). *Transfusion reactions.* https://www.ncbi.nlm.nih.gov/books/NBK482202/
UW Medicine Pharmacy Services. (n.d.). *Pre-test probability scoring for hit.* https://depts.washington.edu/anticoag/home/content/pre-test-probability-scoring-hit-0

NEUROLOGIC SYSTEM

ENCEPHALOPATHY

Overview

- *Encephalopathy* is an umbrella term that describes any diffuse disease that alters brain function or structure.
- There are many underlying causes of encephalopathy:
  - *Hypoxic-ischemic brain injury* most often results from injuries such as cardiac arrest, stroke, or head trauma.
  - *Toxic-metabolic brain injury* most often results from poisoning, illicit drug use, excessive alcohol intake, exposure to heavy metals or solvents, or severe metabolic abnormalities caused by organ failure.
  - *Infectious brain injury* can occur from bacteria, viruses, or fungi, which may cause meningitis or encephalitis.
  - *Hepatic brain injury* most often results from elevated ammonia levels seen in severe liver failure.
- While some causes of encephalopathy can be treated, others are progressive and can result in severe complications.

 COMPLICATIONS

Encephalopathy can result in permanent brain damage, coma, seizures, altered mental status, dementia, or death. Early intervention and treatment are essential.

Signs and Symptoms

- Hypoxic/ischemic encephalopathy:
  - Myoclonic activity or status epilepticus
  - Poor neurologic exam: Patient typically unresponsive or brain-dead
- Toxic-metabolic encephalopathy (hypoglycemic, hypercapnic, uremic, vitamin deficiency, and dialysis related):
  - Asterixis
  - Cheyne–stokes respiration
  - Generalized CNS depression
  - Muscle tone loss
  - Pupillary changes (constricted but reactive)
  - Seizures
- Infectious encephalopathy:
  - Behavioral changes
  - Cognitive decline
  - Hallucinations
  - Lymphadenopathy (EBV encephalitis)
  - Microcephaly (prenatal exposure to the Zika virus)
  - Rash (HSV encephalitis)
  - Splenomegaly (EBV encephalitis)

(continued)

Signs and Symptoms *(continued)*

- Hepatic encephalopathy:
  - Behavioral changes
    - Euphoria or anxiety
    - Inappropriate behavior
    - Lethargy or apathy
  - Decreased awareness or level of consciousness or coma
  - Difficulty concentrating
  - Mental status changes

Diagnosis

Labs
- ABG: May indicate acidosis, hypercarbia, or hypoxia
- Ammonia: May be typically elevated >45 units/dL
- Blood cultures: May be positive with infection
- CBC: May be elevated WBC count if an infection is present
- CMP: May show electrolyte abnormalities or decreased renal or liver function

Diagnostic Testing
- EEG
- Brain MRI
- Head CT scan
- Spinal fluid culture

 ALERT!

CSF findings indicative of viral encephalopathy include normal glucose levels, moderately elevated proteins, and lymphocytosis.

Treatment

- All encephalopathy forms primary therapy: general supportive and preventative care:
  - Antipsychotics, such as haloperidol, for agitation or severe behavior changes (Table 11.1)
  - Medications to prevent progression depending on etiology (specific treatments in the following section for each etiology)
  - Physical, occupational, and speech therapy in addition to cognitive retraining to assist patient in regaining baseline functioning
  - Seizure management medications
- Specific treatment dependent on etiology
- Hypoxic/ischemic encephalopathy: correct cause if possible:
  - Correct metabolic abnormalities
  - If septic, administration of antibiotics
  - If toxic ingestion or overdose, delivery of antidote if available
  - Stabilize hemodynamics
  - Therapeutic-induced hypothermia: target temperature 89.6 °F to 93.2 °F (32 °C–34 °C) in the initial hr after cardiac arrest to improve neurologic outcome of resuscitated patients
- Toxic-metabolic encephalopathy:
  - Treatment varies due to the underlying etiology:
    - Metabolic abnormality correction to maintain balance of electrolytes, water, amino acids, excitatory and inhibitory neurotransmitters, and metabolic substrates
    - Normal blood flow, temperature, osmolality, and pH required for optimal CNS function
  - Review/discontinue medications with potential toxicity to the CNS
  - Thiamine (Table 11.1) for patients with a history of alcoholism, malnutrition, cancer, hyperemesis gravidarum, or renal failure on hemodialysis
- Infectious encephalopathy
  - Predisposing condition correction
  - Appropriate medication regimen for etiology of infectious encephalopathy
  - Antimicrobial or antifungal therapy with no delay, if possible
  - Amoebic encephalitis
    - No definitive treatment

- ○ Used to treat over 90% of cases: miltefosine (Table 6.1*), azole antifungals, and pentamidine (Table A.1)
- Bacterial encephalitis or meningitis:
  - ○ Ampicillin, cephalosporins (cefotaxime, ceftriaxone, cefepime), vancomycin, meropenem (Table A.1)
  - ○ Dexamethasone (Table A.4), if applicable
- Fungal encephalitis or meningitis:
  - ○ high dose, intravenous antifungal medications;
  - ○ duration of treatment dependent on patient's immune system and type of fungus causing the infection
- Viral encephalitis (Table 6.1)
  - ○ HSV encephalopathy: Acyclovir
  - ○ CMV encephalopathy: Gancyclovir
  - ○ CMV ganciclovir-resistant encephalopathy: Foscarnet
- Hepatic encephalopathy:
  - Predisposing condition correction
  - Medications such as lactulose or rifaximin (Table 7.1) to lower blood ammonia levels

Nursing Interventions

- Administer medications as prescribed.
- Assess for changes in behavior or mood.
- Assess for worsening signs of CNS depression.
- Assess vital signs for signs of worsening condition or respiratory compromise.
- Maintain sleep hygiene.
- Monitor for changes in perfusion and oxygenation.
- Monitor for changes in neurologic status. Frequently reorient to environment, time, date, and situation as needed.
- Monitor for diarrhea (expected side effect from lactulose) and resultant electrolyte imbalances and dehydration.
- Position patient with HOB at 30° or higher.
- Provide a safe, calm environment.
  - Consider using 1:1 sitter for patient safety.
  - Observe patient frequently.
  - Physically restrain patient as the last resort.
  - Place patient in a low bed.
  - Provide a fall mat.
  - Use a bed/chair alarm.
- Provide family counseling.

Patient Education

- Follow up outpatient with neurology or primary team responsible for care during hospitalization.
- If applicable, pursue alcohol and drug cessation. Seek additional support through AA, therapist, or other supportive programs.
- Self-monitor for symptoms or worsening condition if possible.

SEIZURES

Overview

- A *seizure* is a sudden change in behavior, awareness, and/or abnormal movements caused by the uncontrolled and excessive electrical discharge of neurons in the brain.

POP QUIZ 6.1

A patient with hepatic encephalopathy is refusing lactulose this morning. Their ammonia level is 62 μ/dL. Their neurologic status has improved; however, they are still only oriented to person and place. What should the nurse's next step be?

COMPLICATIONS

Seizures can progress to status epilepticus, which is a constant state of seizure activity without return to consciousness. This may result in permanent brain damage and death.

(continued)

---

* Table 6.1 is located at the end of this chapter.

Overview *(continued)*

- Largely a clinical diagnosis, seizures can occur due to an underlying medical condition or independently. A thorough history, physical and neurologic examinations, and additional tests are needed to identity an underlying cause.

Signs and Symptoms

- Presentation dependent on the type of electrolyte disturbance
- Generalized seizures:
  - Absence seizure:
    - Brief staring spell
    - Preceded by hyperventilation and flashing lights
  - Atonic seizures:
    - Tonic episode and/or paroxysmal loss of muscle tone that begins suddenly
  - Clonic seizures:
    - Limb jerking (may be asymmetric)
    - Loss of consciousness
    - Sudden loss of muscle tone
  - Myoclonic:
    - Sudden jerking
  - Tonic-clonic seizures:
    - Amnesia of the seizure event
    - Cyanosis
    - Excessive salivation
    - Incontinence
    - Jerking and stiffening
    - Loss of consciousness
    - Tongue or cheek biting
  - Tonic:
    - Sudden onset with an increased tone of extensor muscles
- Partial seizures:
  - Complex partial seizures:
    - Involve behavioral, emotional, affective, and cognitive functions
  - Simple partial seizures:
    - May involve motor, sensory, or autonomic phenomenon
    - No loss of consciousness

Diagnosis

Labs

There are no labs specific to diagnose seizures; however, the following may be helpful to rule out metabolic or infectious causes:

- BMP
- Calcium
- CBC
- Magnesium
- Liver function tests
- Rapid point-of-care glucose (checked at first seizure)
- Toxicology screens

Diagnostic Testing

- Brain MRI
- ECG
- EEG
- Head CT scan
- Lumbar puncture if suggestive of an acute infectious process

Treatment

- Consult to neurology
- Medications (Table 6.1): anti-seizure medication therapy dependent on factors including probability that event represented seizure, suspected or confirmed cause of seizure based on initial evaluation, stability of patient, and estimated risk of recurrent seizure
  - Most seizures remit spontaneously within 2 minutes. Rapid administration of a benzodiazepine or antiseizure medication is usually not required.
  - In critically ill patients with an acute symptomatic seizure, administer antiseizure medications intravenously.
  - Administer antiseizure medications prophylactically to high-risk patients.
- Surgery
- Underlying condition treatment if possible
- Vagal nerve stimulation

ALERT!

Vagal nerve stimulation is an alternative to medication therapy. Vagal nerve stimulation can prevent seizures by preventing excessive neuron discharge.

Nursing Interventions

- Administer medications as ordered.
- Assess airway, breathing, and circulation.
- Assess the need for noninvasive oxygen or intubation in severe situations.
- Continuously assess vital signs.
- During a witnessed seizure:
  - Do not insert anything in mouth.
  - Remove harmful objects near the patient.
  - Turn the patient on their side if able.
  - Protect the patient's head from injury.
- If the seizure was unwitnessed by the PCU staff, ask the patient or family member for a detailed description of the event, postictal period, any triggers, family history of seizures, and any prior seizures.
- Maintain patent IV access.
- Provide a safe environment and initiate seizure precautions:
  - Bed in lowest position with bed rail padding
  - Floor mats
  - Suction and oxygen setup/available

Patient Education

- Avoid swimming alone or working at high elevations.
- Avoid operating heavy machinery or automobiles until seizures are considered controlled as determined by a physician per state guidelines. This may result in feelings of loss of independence and decreased self-esteem. Seek support as needed.
- Decrease stressors if possible.
- Follow up with scheduled appointments and lab draws.
- Keep a seizure calendar to keep a record of seizure events.
- Educate friends, families, and/or coworkers on condition. If a seizure lasting longer than 5 minutes or consciousness is not regained, call 911.
- Modify lifestyle to ensure safety in the event of a seizure. Keep bathroom doors unlocked, take showers instead of baths, and consider replacing glass with safety glass.

POP QUIZ 6.2

The nurse is performing a morning assessment when the patient stops responding to questions and has a blank stare, then makes myoclonic jerking movements. The next step during a seizure is to do what?

(continued)

Patient Education *(continued)*

- Take prescribed seizure medication as instructed.
  - Do not skip a dose.
  - Take a forgotten dose as soon as possible.
  - If more than one dose is forgotten, follow up with provider for guidance.
- Understand the triggers for seizure including sleep deprivation, alcohol intake, medications, infections, or systemic illness.

STROKE

Overview

- A *stroke* occurs when there is a sudden loss or blockage of blood circulation to an area of the brain, causing neurologic dysfunction.
- Three classifications of stroke include ischemic, hemorrhagic, and a TIA.
  - An *ischemic stroke* is caused by an occlusion of a cerebral artery that interferes with the overall blood flow to the brain. This can result from myocardial infarction, atrial fibrillation, deep vein thrombosis, surgical procedures, and certain genetic blood clotting disorders (Factor V Leiden).
  - A *hemorrhagic stroke* occurs when there is bleeding into the brain due to the rupture of a blood vessel. It can be classified as an intracerebral or subarachnoid hemorrhage. Hemorrhagic stroke is caused by an arteriovenous malformation, hypertension, trauma, anticoagulation, and illicit drug use.
  - *Transient ischemic attack* is defined as a brief disruption of blood flow to the brain and is not associated with permanent neurologic disability. TIAs are similar to ischemic strokes, but the symptoms of TIAs are temporary.

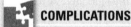 **COMPLICATIONS**

Severe ischemia or hemorrhage can cause diffuse and devastating irreversible brain damage and cell death. This can result in brain death, herniation, and death.

Signs and Symptoms

- Possible symptoms of acute ischemic or hemorrhagic stroke:
  - Aphagia
  - Ataxia
  - Dysarthria
  - Facial droop
  - Hypertension (systolic blood pressure >220 mmHg)
  - Ocular abnormalities
    - Blurred vision or visual field deficits
    - Monocular or binocular blindness
    - Nystagmus
  - Rapid change in level of consciousness
  - Rapid neurologic decline
  - Sudden, altered alertness or obtundation
  - Weakness or paresis that may affect a single extremity, half of the body, or all four extremities
  - Unequal pupils
- TIA: Temporary period of symptoms similar to those of an ischemic stroke

Diagnosis

Labs

- ABG if hypoxia is suspected
- Blood glucose to rule out mental status changes related to hypoglycemia

- CMP to rule out mental status changes related to electrolyte, renal, or liver function abnormalities
- Cardiac biomarkers if a cardiac event is suspected
- CBC:
  - WBC may be elevated if infection is present.
  - Elevated platelet count may indicate high potential for clot formation and possible cause of ischemic stroke.
- PT/INR and PTT: likely elevated if taking anticoagulants
- Pregnancy test for women of child bearing age
- Toxicology screen

Diagnostic Testing
- Brain MRI
- Carotid duplex scanning
- EEG
- Non-contrast head CT scan
- Lumbar puncture

Treatment

- Ischemic stroke:
  - Alteplase (Table 6.1): First-line therapy if initiated within 4.5 hr of symptom onset or time of last known well
  - Antithrombotic therapy with aspirin (Table 2.8) initiated within 48 hr of stroke onset; continued at discharge
  - Blood pressure reduction after the acute phase of ischemic stroke has passed
  - Mechanical thrombectomy
  - Lipid-lowering therapy with high-intensity statin (Table 6.1)
  - Prophylaxis for DVT and PE (Table 3.1)
- Hemorrhagic stroke:
  - Blood pressure management:
    - Patients with acute ICH with SBP between 150 and 220 mmHg: rapid lowering of SBP to a target of 140 mmHg, provided the patient remains clinically stable
    - Patients with acute ICH with SBP >220 mmHg: rapid lowering of SBP to <220 mmHg; then gradual reduction of blood pressure (over a period of hr) to 140 from 160 mmHg, provided the patient remains clinically stable
  - Discontinue all anticoagulant and antiplatelet drugs
  - Hemorrhage extension prevention with appropriate medications or reversal agents (such as vitamin K, FFP, PCC for warfarin, and protamine sulfate for heparin)
  - Management of elevated ICP, which will require higher level of care
  - Seizure management/prophylaxis
  - Surgical intervention
    - Clipping or coiling of aneurysm in hemorrhagic stroke
    - Surgical decompression if previous treatment ineffective
- General care:
  - Continuous monitoring of blood coagulation studies (PT, PTT, INR)
  - IV fluids: agent of choice for intravascular fluid repletion and maintenance fluid therapy: isotonic saline without dextrose (Table A.3)
  - Speech, physical, and occupational therapy
  - Supplemental oxygen or rapid sequence intubation and transfer to higher level of care if indicated (stroke or neuro ICU)

 ALERT!

Contraindications for TPA administration include acute intracranial hemorrhage, history of intracranial hemorrhage, severe uncontrolled hypertension (systolic >185 mmHg and diastolic >110 mmHg), severe head trauma within the last 3 months, thrombocytopenia (platelet count >100,000/mm³), hypercoagulability (INR >1.7 or PT >15 seconds), heparin administration within the last 24 hr, severe hypo- or hyperglycemia, advanced age, recent major surgery to any area of the body, recent GI hemorrhage, and seizures.

Nursing Interventions

- Assess airway, breathing, and circulation.
- Assess blood glucose levels and treat as ordered.
- Assess for elevated or low BP, fluid retention, and electrolyte imbalances.
- Assess for fever and manage as ordered.
- Assess the need for noninvasive oxygen.
- Aspiration precautions:
  - Complete bedside swallow study if patient meets criteria to assess for safe swallowing.
  - Consult speech language pathology if there is a concern for dysphagia.
- Discuss current status and plan of care.
- Draw serial labs as ordered (blood glucose, CBC, PT, PTT, and INR).
- Implement fall prevention interventions including nonslip socks, bed/chair alarms, call bell within reach, bed in the lowest position, frequent assistance with voiding/BM, and peri care.
- Perform serial neurologic exams and GCS as indicated per provider and unit guidelines.
- Perform NIHSS stroke scale upon admission, every 12 hr, if there are any neurologic changes, and/ or per institutional guidelines.
- Prevent pressure injuries.

Patient Education

- Adhere to diet and food regimens as ordered by the provider (Mediterranean diet).
- Attend any follow-up tests or procedures.
- Engage in physical exercise and weight reduction to maintain a healthy lifestyle.
- Follow activity orders.
- Pursue smoking cessation if indicated.
- Take medications as prescribed.
- Work with PT and OT, especially if there is residual weakness or paralysis to learn how to complete ADLs and work toward getting back to baseline.

POP QUIZ 6.2

A 63-year-old male is transferred to the PCU following ICU admission for ischemic stroke. Residual symptoms have started to resolve; however, the patient still experiences left-sided weakness, left-sided facial droop, and ataxia. The patient's daughter has visited for the first time today, bringing the patient's favorite dessert, a chocolate milkshake. Before giving the patient their chocolate milkshake, what should the nurse confirm has taken place?

Table 6.1 Neurologic Medications		
Indications	Mechanism of Action	Contraindications, Precautions, and Adverse Effects
Alkylphosphocholines(miltefosine)		
• Amoebic encephalitis	• Interact with membrane lipids at the site of the organism, inhibiting mitochondrial process to result in cell death	• Medication is contraindicated in pregnancy and Sjogren-Larsson syndrome. • Medication may impact male fertility. • Use caution in renal or hepatic disorders. • Contraception is required during treatment and for 5 months following the last dose to protect from possible risk to fetal development. • Adverse effects include nausea, vomiting, dizziness, headache, testicular pain, abdominal pain, and itching.

(continued)

Table 6.1 Neurologic Medications *(continued)*

Indications	Mechanism of Action	Contraindications, Precautions, and Adverse Effects
Anticonvulsants: benzodiazepines(e.g., alprazolam, clonazepam, diazepam, lorazepam, midazolam)		
• Seizure treatment and management	• Potentiate the effect of GABA to increase inhibition of the reticular activating system	• Do not abruptly discontinue. • Adverse effects include fatigue, nausea, vomiting, weight changes (loss or gain), sexual dysfunction, agitation, unsteady gait, slurred speech, or sedation. • Use caution in use with active suicidal ideation, psychosis or bipolar disorder, CNS depression, pulmonary disease, alcoholism or substance abuse, liver or renal disease, and geriatric populations.
Anticonvulsants (e.g., valproate, levetiracetam, phenytoin)		
• Seizure management	• Decrease excitation • Enhance inhibition of neurons and/or alter electrical activity by affecting ion channels in the cell membrane	• Adverse effects include CNS depression, drowsiness, diplopia, ataxia, nystagmus, cognitive function changes, and rash.
Antivirals (acyclovir)		
• HSV encephalitis	• Prevent replication of HSV DNA through competitive inhibition, inactivating viral DNA, and terminating growing HSV DNA	• Medication is contraindicated in milk protein hypersensitivity. • Use caution in dehydration, renal impairment, seizures, electrolyte imbalance, hepatic disease, hypoxemia, and neurologic diseases. • Adverse effects include seizures, renal failure, tissue necrosis, angioedema, visual impairment, DIC, vasculitis, psychosis, hepatitis, jaundice, hypotension, and coma.
Antivirals (foscarnet)		
• Ganciclovir-resistant CMV encephalitis infections in transplant recipients or patients with AIDS	• Prevent viral DNA replication at binding sites	• Use caution in anemia, neutropenia, cardiomyopathy, nephrotoxicity, renal failure, sodium restriction, dehydration, cardiac disease, electrolyte imbalance, and seizure.
Antivirals (ganciclovir)		
• CMV encephalitis	• Inhibit viral DNA synthesis by competitive inhibition	• Use caution in anemia, bone marrow suppression, chemotherapy, leukopenia, neutropenia, thrombocytopenia, dehydration, and renal failure/impairment.

(continued)

Table 6.1 Neurologic Medications *(continued)*

Indications	Mechanism of Action	Contraindications, Precautions, and Adverse Effects
Fibrinolytic therapy (e.g., alteplase, streptokinase, tenecteplase, reteplase)		
• Known clot in ischemic stroke • ACS	• Breaks up and dissolves clot	• Contraindications include active internal bleeding (hemorrhagic stroke), history of CVA, recent surgery, bleeding disorders, and uncontrolled hypertension. • Use caution in patients with recent surgery or trauma, severe hepatic or renal disease, and concurrent anticoagulation therapy. • Adverse effects include generalized risk for bleeding (most notably in intracranial hemorrhage), GI bleeding, and retroperitoneal bleeding.
HMG-CoA reductase inhibitors/statins (e.g., atorvastatin, simvastatin)		
• Treatment of hypercholesterolemia, including hyperlipidemia, hyperlipoproteinemia, or hypertriglyceridemia • Myocardial infarction prophylaxis • Stroke prophylaxis	• Inhibit HMG-CoA reductase to lower amount of mevalonate (precursor of sterols including cholesterol), which reduces cholesterol in hepatic cells, increases hepatic uptake of LDL cholesterol from circulation, and reduces total cholesterol, LDL cholesterol, and serum triglycerides	• Medication is contraindicated in active hepatic disease, including cholestasis, hepatic encephalopathy, hepatitis, jaundice, or unexplained persistent elevations in serum aminotransferase concentrations. • Myopathy is a potential serious side effect; discontinue if patient develops elevated CPK or rhabdomyolysis. • Adverse reactions include hepatic failure, myoglobinuria, myalgia, diarrhea, nausea, and dyspepsia.
Mineral and electrolyte replacement (zinc)		
• Supplementation in zinc deficiency related to hepatic encephalopathy	• Replace in deficient states • Assist with enzymatic reactions required for normal growth and tissue repair	• Use caution in renal failure. • Adverse effects include gastric irritation, nausea, and vomiting.

RESOURCES

Centers for Disease Control and Prevention. (2020, September 29). *Parasites*. U.S. Department of Health and Human Services, Centers for Disease Control and Prevention. https://www.cdc.gov/parasites/naegleria/treatment.html

Centers for Disease Control and Prevention. (2021, August 2). *Stroke*. U.S. Department of Health and Human Services, Centers for Disease Control and Prevention. https://www.cdc.gov/stroke/types_of_stroke.htm#hemorrhagic

Ferenci, P. (2017, April 18). Hepatic encephalopathy. *Gastroenterology Report, 5*(2), 138–147. doi:10.1093/gastro/gox013

Fugate, J. E., & Rabinstein, A. A. (2015, July). Absolute and relative contraindications to IV RT-PA for acute ischemic stroke. *The Neurohospitalist, 5*(3), 110-121. https://www.ncbi.nlm.nih.gov/pmc/articles/PMC4530420/

Hashburn, R., Tunkel, A., & Mitty, J. (n.d.). Initial therapy and prognosis of bacterial meningitis in adults. *UptoDate*. https://www.uptodate.com/contents/initial-therapy-and-prognosis-of-bacterial-meningitis-in-adults#H13

National Institute of Neurological Disorders and Stroke. (n.d.). Encephalopathy information page. U.S. Department of Health and Human Services, National Institute of Neurological Disorders and Stroke. https://www.ninds.nih.gov/Disorders/All-Disorders/Encephalopathy-Information-Page

Parija, S. C., Dinoop, K., & Venugopal, H. (2015). *Management of granulomatous amebic encephalitis: Laboratory diagnosis and treatment. Tropical parasitology, 5,* 23–28. https://www.ncbi.nlm.nih.gov/pmc/articles/ PMC4326989/.

Prescribers' Digital Reference. (n.d.). *Depakene* [Drug information]. PDR Search. https://www.pdr.net/drug-summa ry/Depakene-valproic-acid-979

Prescribers' Digital Reference. (n.d.). *Depakote tablets* [Drug information]. PDR Search. https://www.pdr.net/drug-s ummary/Depakote-Tablets-divalproex-sodium-1075.5693

Prescribers' Digital Reference. (n.d.). *Enulose* [Drug information]. PDR Search. https://www.pdr.net/drug-summar y/Enulose-lactulose-635#14

Prescribers' Digital Reference. (n.d.). *Foscavir* [Drug information]. PDR Search. https://www.pdr.net/drug-summar y/Foscavir-foscarnet-sodium-3639#11

Prescribers' Digital Reference. (n.d.). *Impavido (miltefosine)* [Drug information]. PDR Search. https://www.pdr.net/ drug-summary/Impavido-miltefosine-3607

Prescribers' Digital Reference. (n.d.). *Keppra injection* [Drug information]. PDR Search. https://www.pdr.net/drug-s ummary/Keppra-Injection-levetiracetam-1055.6058

Prescribers' Digital Reference. (n.d.). *Klonopin* [Drug information]. PDR Search. https://www.pdr.net/drug-summa ry/Klonopin-clonazepam-3064.5869

Prescribers' Digital Reference. (n.d.). *Lyrica* [Drug information]. PDR Search. https://www.pdr.net/drug-summary/ Lyrica-pregabalin-467.8329

Prescribers' Digital Reference. (n.d.-l). *Phenytoin sodium injection* [Drug information]. PDR Search. https://www.pd r.net/drug-summary/Phenytoin-Sodium-Injection-phenytoin-sodium-1151.8322

Prescribers' Digital Reference. (n.d.). *Plavix* [Drug information]. PDR Search. https://www.pdr.net/drug-summary/ Plavix-clopidogrel-bisulfate-525.3952

Prescribers' Digital Reference. (n.d.). *Simvastatin* [Drug information]. PDR Search. https://www.pdr.net/drug-sum mary/Zocor-simvastatin-402.3285

Prescribers' Digital Reference. (n.d.). *Acyclovir* [Drug information]. PDR Search. https://www.pdr.net/drug-summa ry/Acyclovir-acyclovir-sodium-670#10

Prescribers' Digital Reference. (n.d.). *Alteplase* [Drug information]. PDR Search. https://www.pdr.net/drug-summa ry/Activase-alteplase-1332.3358

Prescribers' Digital Reference. (n.d.). *Cytovene* [Drug information]. PDR Search. https://www.pdr.net/drug-summa ry/Cytovene-ganciclovir-sodium-1025#11

7

GASTROINTESTINAL SYSTEM

BOWEL OBSTRUCTION

Overview

- A bowel obstruction involves a partial or complete blockage of forward motility of bowel contents in the small or large intestine.
  - Mechanical causes include obstruction tumors, strictures, adhesions, volvulus, impaction, or intussusception.
  - Functional causes include paralytic ileus, inflammatory disease, or prior intestinal surgeries that alter regular bowel function.
  - Other risk factors for obstruction include hypokalemia, peritonitis, sepsis, opiate or barium intake, hernia, and diverticulitis.
- Obstruction prevents the absorption of water, vitamin synthesis, and breakdown of bilirubin, in the large bowel, which can lead to further complications.

COMPLICATIONS

Strangulation leading to ischemic bowel is a major complication of bowel obstructions. Patients with ischemic bowel are at risk to develop tissue necrosis or bowel perforation, putting them at an increased risk for peritonitis and sepsis.

Signs and Symptoms

- Small bowel obstruction:
  - Abdominal pain
    - Intermittent
    - Sometimes described as colicky
    - Reported to have improvements in pain after vomiting
  - Bloating
  - Bowel sounds from hyperactive to absent, depending on severity of obstruction
  - Decreased appetite
  - Distended abdomen
  - Frequent bilious vomiting
  - Focal abdominal tenderness
  - Severe constipation
- Large bowel obstruction
  - Bowel sounds from hyperactive to absent, depending on severity of obstruction
  - Constant abdominal pain
  - Constipation
  - Diffuse abdominal tenderness
  - Distended abdomen
  - Decreased appetite
  - Intermittent feculent vomiting

Diagnosis

Labs

- BMP: May show hyperkalemia (K >5.0 mmol/L) in severe obstruction or bowel necrosis
- Blood cultures (if concern for peritonitis/sepsis)
- CBC:
  - WBCs may be elevated in infection.
  - H/H may be decreased with bleeding.
- Lactate: >2 mmol/L

 ALERT!

Patients with an ischemic or perforated bowel will have a markedly elevated lactate. This is due to decreased blood flow to the ischemic or perforated area resulting in anerobic metabolism, thus elevating lactate.

Diagnostic Testing

- Abdominal ultrasound with Doppler
- KUB
- Abdominal CT scan

Treatment

- Bowel rest
- Comorbid condition management
- Foley catheter for strict urinary output monitoring
- IV fluids (Table A.3) and electrolyte replacement (Table 8.4), if indicated
- NG tube for bowel decompression and emesis control
- NPO
- Pain control (Table A.2)
- Surgery consultation if:
  - Bowel obstruction caused by hernia (nonemergency surgery will reduce hernia)
  - Bowel obstruction caused by strangulated or nonreducible hernia (immediate surgical consult and emergency surgery indicated)

Nursing Interventions

- Assess airway, breathing, and circulation.
- Assess for signs of hypoperfusion and sepsis.
- Draw and monitor serial labs as ordered.
- Monitor for the presence of flatus.
- Maintain NG tube to low-intermittent wall suction as ordered.
- Maintain strict I/O.
- Monitor the volume of NG tube output.
- Note for any occurrence of bowel movements.
- Perform serial abdominal exams. Note for any of the following:
  - Firm or rigid abdomen
  - Increased size/distention
  - Increased abdominal pain
- Position patient with HOB at 30° or higher to prevent risk of aspiration.
- Provide therapeutic communication and support.

 NURSING PEARL

Strangulated or ischemic bowel that is unnoticed or untreated has nearly a 100% mortality rate. Detailed assessment and prompt communication of condition to the surgical team can decrease the mortality rate to <10% after timely intervention.

Patient Education

- Ambulate/change positions as ordered and tolerated to decrease risk of DVT and increase GI motility.
- Adhere to diet orders: NPO, clear liquids, and so on.

- Maintain DVT prevention/prophylaxis protocols.
  - Anticoagulation
  - SCDs
- Self-assess and identify potential lifestyle or dietary choices that may contribute to bowel obstruction. Diet or lifestyle modifications to prevent bowel obstructions include increasing daily fiber and water intake.
- Self-monitor for symptoms or worsening condition, if possible.
- Take laxatives as prescribed by provider to prevent recurrence of bowel obstruction and improve GI motility.

POP QUIZ 7.1

A patient is admitted to the PCU for a bowel obstruction with complaints of abdominal pain, constipation, and intermittent vomiting of feculent nature. Based on the patient's presentation, which type of bowel obstruction is suspected?

DIABETIC GASTROPARESIS

Overview

- Gastroparesis is delayed gastric emptying without evidence of obstruction.
- Gastroparesis is a common finding in poorly controlled diabetic patients, which results in dysfunction of the autonomic nervous system, neurons, pacemaker cells of the stomach, intestines, and smooth muscle of the GI tract.

COMPLICATIONS

Complications of diabetic gastroparesis include malnutrition, aspiration pneumonia, and worsening diabetes, which may progress to hypoglycemia, DKA, or a hyperosmolar hyperglycemic state. Prompt treatment is needed to prevent progression of the condition.

Signs and Symptoms

- Abdominal distention
- Bloating
- Early satiety
- Halitosis
- Neuropathy
- Postprandial fullness
- Poor glycemic control
- Vomiting: Often contains undigested, chewed food
- Weight changes

Diagnosis

Labs

- Labs are not diagnostic for diabetic gastroparesis; labs are to confirm poorly controlled diabetes:
  - Elevated point-of-care blood glucose values
  - HgbA1C >7%

Diagnostic Testing

- Abdominal CT scan
- Endoscopy
- Scintigraphy gastric emptying test

Treatment

- Lifestyle modifications
  - Avoiding carbonated beverages
  - Decreasing alcohol use

(continued)

Treatment *(continued)*

- Diet and exercise to achieve stricter glycemic control
- Small, frequent meals
- Smoking cessation
- Medications (Table 7.1*; Table 4.1 [for diabetes medications])
- Tube placement:
  - G-tube
  - G/J-tube
  - NG tube
- Surgery: Partial gastrectomy with Roux-en-Y, gastrojejunostomy, and gastric resection

ALERT!

Little data exist on surgical treatments for diabetic gastroparesis. Therefore, surgery to treat diabetic gastroparesis should be the last treatment option and should be recommended by a gastroenterologist.

Nursing Interventions

- Administer medications as ordered.
- Assess airway, breathing, and circulation.
- Assess for signs of worsening symptoms.
- Assess the skin, securement, and placement of tube site if present.
- Draw and monitor serial labs as ordered.
- If performing gastric decompression with an NG tube, assess color, quantity, and consistency of gastric contents.
- Measure gastric residuals prior to medication or tube feed administration. Re-instill gastric contents back to patient to not cause electrolyte imbalances.
- Check the patient's blood glucose before meals and at bedtime.
- Administer appropriate insulin dosages as directed by the provider based on the patient's blood glucose.
- Provide therapeutic communication and support.

Patient Education

- Achieve glycemic control as evidence by HbA1C <6%.
- Adhere to a low-carbohydrate diet and keep track of daily carbohydrate intake.
- Eat small, frequent meals. Do not rush while eating, and avoid large quantities of fluid at one time to decrease likelihood of developing nausea.
- Limit alcohol intake.
- Maintain daily physical activity of at least 30 minutes.
- Monitor blood glucose before meals, at bedtime, and when feeling symptomatic.
- Monitor for daily bowel movements.
- Pursue smoking cessation.
- Refer to social worker to ensure accessibility to medications and blood glucose monitoring supplies.
- Rotate insulin injection site, which may include the abdomen, upper arm, thigh, lower back, hips, or buttocks.
- Take medications as prescribed.
- Understand the signs of hyper- and hypoglycemic episodes and how to care for each.

POP QUIZ 7.2

A patient in the PCU has been admitted for diabetic gastroparesis. He has an NG tube and is receiving intermittent tube feedings, 200 mL every 3 hr as tolerated. What should the first step be prior to administering his tube feeding?

---

* Table 7.1 is located at the end of this chapter.

GASTROESOPHAGEAL REFLUX DISEASE

Overview

- GERD is the backwards flow of stomach contents into the esophagus.
- Although there is no clear cause for GERD, possible causes include:
  - Hiatal hernia
  - Impaired esophageal mucosal defense against gastric reflux
  - Impaired lower esophageal sphincter
  - Poor esophageal peristalsis

COMPLICATIONS

Complications of GERD include Barrett's esophagus (an erosive esophagitis), esophageal strictures, and esophageal adenocarcinoma. Early identification, treatment, and appropriate management can prevent these complications.

Signs and Symptoms

- Belching
- Dysphagia
- Epigastric pain
- Heartburn
- Nausea
- Regurgitation

Diagnosis

Diagnostic Testing

There are no diagnostic tests specific to diagnose GERD. However, the following may be helpful to rule out complications:

- EGD
- Barium swallow study

Treatment

- Weight loss and diet modification
  - Eliminate acidic foods.
  - Improve dietary choices to enable weight loss.
- Exercise
- Eating pattern and frequency
  - Avoid large meals.
  - Avoid spicy or fried foods, onions, garlic, caffeine, and carbonated beverages.
  - Eat small, frequent meals.
  - Eat at least 3 hr before bedtime.
- Medication (Table 7.1)
- Surgery
  - Bariatric surgery
  - Laparoscopic Nissen fundoplication

Nursing Interventions

- Assess airway, breathing, and circulation.
- Assess for worsening symptoms.
- Avoid foods that are high in fat, salts, or spices including fatty meats, processed snacks, cheese, greasy or fried foods, or spicy foods.

(continued)

Nursing Interventions *(continued)*

- Avoid acidic foods like tomato sauces, citrus, chocolate, peppermints, or carbonated beverages.
- Encourage ambulation and/or movement as tolerated.
- Encourage foods that are high in fiber (whole grains, root vegetables, or green vegetables), are alkaline (melons, cauliflowers, nuts, bananas, etc.), or have high water content (tea, celery, lettuce, broth-based soups, etc.).
- Maintain HOB 30° or greater at mealtimes and while sleeping.
- Promote exercise with PT.

Patient Education

- Engage in appropriate dietary modifications.
- Engage in physical activity.
- Keep up to date on current status and plan of care.
- Pursue a smoking and/or alcohol cessation program.
- Sleep with extra pillows or a wedge pillow under head or shoulders for elevation to decrease the risk of reflux.
- Take medications as prescribed (omeprazole, pantoprazole, or famotidine).

GASTROINTESTINAL BLEED

Overview

- GI bleed can be categorized as upper or lower, each with different symptoms and presentation.
- Causes for an upper GI bleed include peptic ulcer disease, varices, postsurgical bleeds, GI tumors, gastritis, duodenitis, and esophagitis.
- Causes for a lower GI bleed include diverticulosis, infectious or ischemic colitis, inflammatory bowel disease, hemorrhoids, colon cancer, anal fissures, and postsurgical bleeds.

Signs and Symptoms

- Upper GI bleed
  - Abdominal tenderness
  - Decreased pulse pressure
  - Epigastric pain
  - Hematemesis, bright red or coffee ground
  - Hyperactive bowel sounds
  - Hypotension
  - Melena
  - Nausea and vomiting
  - Orthostatic hypotension
  - Pale skin or mucous membranes
  - Presyncope/syncope
- Lower GI bleed
  - Abdominal cramping or discomfort
  - Diarrhea
  - Hematochezia: often bright or dark red; may pass clots with stool
  - Hypotension
  - Orthostatic hypotension
  - Pale skin or mucous membranes
  - Presyncope/syncope

COMPLICATIONS

GI bleed, regardless of upper or lower, can result in respiratory distress, MI, infection, hypovolemic shock, and death. Early identification and treatment are needed to prevent deterioration of condition.

ALERT!

Risk factors for GI bleeding include varices, portal hypertension, alcohol or tobacco use, ulcers, *Helicobacter pylori*, diverticulitis, hemorrhoids, inflammatory bowel disease, NSAIDs, and anticoagulation and antiplatelet agents. Complete a thorough physical and health history to identify potential risk factors.

Diagnosis

Labs

- Active type and screen
- CBC: Decreased hemoglobin (<13.5 g/dL in men and 12.0 g/dL in women) and hematocrit (<41% in men and 36% in women)
- Coagulation may be increased: PT >13.5 seconds/INR >1.1, PTT >35 seconds
- Guaiac test: GI contents and stool
- Helicobacter pylori test: May be positive
- Lactate (>2.2 mmol/L)
- LFTs: Elevated LFTs (AST >40 u/L and AST >56 u/L) may cause increased clotting times contributing to increased blood loss
- Stool culture: *Clostridium difficile* and *Escherichia coli* may be detected

Diagnostic Testing

- CT angiography
- Colonoscopy
- Endoscopy

Treatment

- Blood products as needed/ordered (Table 5.4)
- Balloon tamponade (requires transfer to higher level of care)
- *IV fluid resuscitation*: LR or NS (Table A.3)
- Medications as needed (Table 7.1)
- NPO
- Oxygen support
  - Avoid NIPPV with ongoing vomiting.
  - Prepare for intubation if patient's mental status becomes altered or they are unable to protect the airway.
- Placement of at least two large-bore peripheral IVs or central-line access
- Stop/reverse anticoagulation if indicated
- Treatment of underlying condition that may have caused the GI bleed

> **ALERT!**
>
> If patient is experiencing a massive GI bleed with hemodynamic instability, Blakemore or Minnesota tube placements may be inserted. Surgery should be consulted, and the patient should be considered for transfer to higher level of care.

Nursing Interventions

- Administer medications as ordered.
- Assess airway, breathing, and circulation.
- Assess hemodynamics and frequent vital signs.
- Ensure two large-bore IVs are appropriately placed and patent.
- Maintain calm and therapeutic communication with the patient.
- Monitor emesis and administer antiemetic as needed.
- Monitor patient's stool for color and consistency. Perform a guaiac test if ordered.
- Perform serial CBCs to monitor hemoglobin and hematocrit.
- Transfuse blood products as ordered (if consented by patient).

Patient Education

- Follow nutritional changes per provider recommendations.
- Follow up with resources for alcohol cessation, if indicated.
- Notify provider of any change in symptoms, pain, or sensation.
- Monitor for symptoms of bleeding, which include frank blood or black tarry stools.
- Self-assess for any changes or signs of worsening anemia including pallor, dizziness, fatigue, lightheadedness, palpitations, and shortness of breath.
- Stop anticoagulant medications if indicated by provider.
- Take medications as advised.

GASTROINTESTINAL INFECTIONS

Overview

- GI infections can be bacterial, viral, or parasitic.
  - Bacterial infections include *Salmonella, Listeria monocytogenes, E. coli, Shigella*, and most notably *C. difficile* (with recent antibiotic intake).
  - Parasitic infections include giardia.
  - Viral infections include norovirus and rotavirus.

Signs and Symptoms

- Abdominal pain
- Diarrhea (watery or bloody, three or more loose stools/d)
- Fever
- Nausea
- Vomiting

Diagnosis

Labs
- Stool culture: May be positive for pathogenic bacteria
- CBC: Will show elevated WBC
- Blood cultures: May be positive if GI Infection has spread
- BMP: May show hypokalemia (K <3.5 mmol/L)

Diagnostic Testing
- Abdominal x-ray
- CT scan of the abdomen
- Colonoscopy

Treatment

- Symptom management
- Oral or IV fluid (Table A.3) and electrolyte supplementation (Table 8.4)
- Antiemetics
- Antibiotic therapy
  - Ampicillin
  - Azithromycin
  - Fluoroquinolones
  - Tetracyclines
- *C. difficile*
  - Discontinue causative antibiotic
  - Vancomycin, fidaxomicin, or metronidazole
  - Fecal transplant

Nursing Interventions

- Administer medications and fluids as ordered/tolerated.
- Assess vital signs.
- Assess abdomen and GI tract frequently for changes.
- Assess I/Os to prevent dehydration.

COMPLICATIONS

GI infection can result in dehydration and electrolyte abnormalities from vomiting and diarrhea that usually accompany infection. Infections can further progress to irritable bowel syndrome, chronic fatigue syndrome (giardia), sepsis, toxic megacolon, intestinal perforation, and necrotizing colitis.

 ALERT!

If a patient abruptly begins having watery diarrhea more than three times in 1 day, especially while receiving antibiotics, the patient should be tested for *Clostridium difficile*.

- Draw and monitor serial labs as ordered.
- Monitor fever and provide cooling interventions if needed.
- Maintain skin integrity given increased stool output.
- Monitor stool output.

Patient Education

- Verbalize understanding of cause of GI infection and actions to prevent reinfection in the future.
  - Cook meat thoroughly based on type and cut.
  - Do not leave food out at room temperature.
  - Obtain access to safe and clean drinking water.
- Take medications as ordered.
- Stay up to date about current status and plan of care.
- Stay up to date of any upcoming tests or procedures.

GASTROINTESTINAL SURGERIES

Overview

- A GI surgery refers to an intervention performed on any organ or tissue housed within the abdominal space.
- Surgical interventions can be either open or laparoscopic and include adrenalectomy, appendectomy, bariatric surgery, cholecystectomy, colon and rectal surgery, hiatal hernia repair, Nissen fundoplication, nephrectomy, pancreatic surgery, retroperitoneal surgery, splenectomy, Roux-en-Y, and Whipple procedures.
- Many life-threatening or fatal complications can arise from GI surgery.

 COMPLICATIONS

Complications of GI surgery include perforation, biliary leak, postsurgical or retroperitoneal bleeding, infection, sepsis, and death. Close postoperative monitoring is needed to identify changes and deterioration of condition.

Signs and Symptoms

- Signs and symptoms of GI surgery complication:
  - Abdominal distention
  - Abdominal pain
  - Absent bowel sounds
  - Changes in abdominal assessment: increased firmness, distention, rigidity, or pain
  - Dyspnea
  - Dull back pain
  - Ecchymosis
  - Fever
  - Hemodynamic instability
    - Hypotension
    - Tachycardia
  - High volume of frank blood or output from the following:
    - Drains
    - NG tube
    - Surgical
    - Wound vac

 ALERT!

Postoperative complications resulting in severe hemodynamic instability may need immediate surgical consult with transfer back to the OR or to a higher level of care. Closely monitor changes to advocate for appropriate elevation in care as needed.

Diagnosis

Labs
- Blood cultures
- BMP
- CBC
- Lactate

Diagnostic Testing
- Chest, abdomen, and pelvis CT scan
- Endoscopy
- MRI
- X-ray (chest and abdomen)

Treatment

- Ambulation per postoperative orders, moving out of bed to chair as ordered
- Incentive spirometer hourly
- Bowel rest as ordered with NGT for gastric decompression
  - NPO
  - Slow progression and advancement of enteral nutrition as ordered by surgeon and tolerated by patient
- Pain control
- Medications as ordered (Table 7.1)
- Treatment of surgical complications:
  - Bleeding: Blood product administration and continuous hemodynamic monitoring
  - Hemodynamic instability: IV fluids (Table A.3), continuous EKG monitoring, vasopressors (Table 2.8), and ionotropic agents as necessary for MAP goal >65
  - Infection: Blood cultures; antibiotics specific to disease process
- Possible transfer to higher level of care if hemodynamically unstable and condition deteriorating

Nursing Interventions

- Assess airway, breathing, and circulation.
- Administer postoperative medications as ordered.
- Apply abdominal binder and/or splinting pillow postoperatively as ordered.
- Change wound vac cannisters when filled and record output, color, and consistency.
- Continuously assess vital signs and notify provider of any changes.
- Draw and monitor serial postoperative labs as ordered.
- Encourage use of incentive spirometry postoperatively (instructions for use in Patient Education section).
- Monitor I/O, including volume and characteristics of gastric tube output.
- Monitor for postoperative DVT, PE, or skin breakdown from positioning on the OR table.
- Perform detailed assessment of drain output volume, color, and consistency. Empty drains as ordered by surgeon.
- Perform detailed assessment of surgical incision site for drainage or oozing.
- Perform dressing change daily or as frequently as ordered by provider.
- Perform serial abdominal assessments for bleeding indications: Dehiscence, evisceration, or rigidity.
- Provide education to patient on PCA control.
  - PCA is programmed to deliver a certain dose when the button is pressed.
  - The button is on a timer based on the provider's order, and the PCA will only deliver one dose of pain medication per programmed time frame.
- Take special precautions with bariatric patients:
  - Monitor for signs of the following:
    - Anastomotic leak or dumping syndrome
    - Signs of OSA and the need for noninvasive positive pressure ventilation

- Provide the opportunity for small, frequent meals and wait 30 minutes after meals to drink fluids; do not drink fluids with meals (to avoid dumping syndrome).
- Utilize reverse Trendelenburg to optimize breathing mechanics. Positioning the bed steeply upright may limit normal diaphragmatic excursion.

Patient Education

- Brace the abdominal incision with a pillow when mobilizing to prevent pain and incision dehiscence.
- Take medications as advised, including completing antibiotic regimen as prescribed.
- Continue using incentive spirometry at home.
- To use incentive spirometer, exhale deeply and then make a tight seal around the mouthpiece. Inhale as deeply as possible to the targeted volume. Repeat this 10 times every 1 to 2 hr.
- In general, when caring for incisions after surgery:
  - Clean hands prior to and after touching the surgical site.
  - Assess the incision daily for any new redness, warmth around the site, foul or discolored drainage, edema, or bleeding.
  - If bleeding occurs from the incision site, hold firm manual pressure over the incision and contact provider immediately.
  - Obtain necessary materials to perform dressing changes once discharged home.
  - Change dressing daily as ordered by your provider, or if the dressing becomes soiled.
  - After cleaning hands, remove the old dressing, clean and rinse the incision site, pat dry, and apply new dressing as directed.
  - Avoid tight fitting clothes.
  - Itchiness is expected as wounds heal. Do not scratch or pick at wounds.
- For incisions with staples, stitches, or wound closure strip:
  - Wait 24 hr following surgery to shower and wash unless otherwise directed by provider.
  - Clean the incision with mild soap and water. Do not scrub.
  - Pat dry with a clean cloth once done bathing.
  - For wound closure strips, allow them to fall off on their own. Do not remove unless they do not fall off after 2 weeks.
- For incisions with tissue glue closure:
  - While skin glue is waterproof, avoid touching the glue for 24 hr and try to keep the wound dry for the first 5 days.
  - Have showers rather than baths, to avoid soaking the wound.
  - The glue will dry and fall away between 5 and 10 days. Do not pick or rub the glued area or put creams or lotions on the glue.
  - Avoid direct sunlight.

 POP QUIZ 7.3

A patient has been admitted to the PCU following an exploratory laparotomy for abdominal pain. During their admission assessment, they reported dull back and abdominal pain as a 2/10. An hr later, they are reporting the same back and abdominal pain as an 8/10. After completing a focused assessment, the nurse notes the surgical laparotomy sites are clean, dry, and intact; however, the abdomen is much firmer than when the patient was first admitted and is painful to palpation. Vital signs: HR 128, BP 90/54, RR 20, T 98.2 °F (36.8 °C), SpO$_2$ 93% on 4 L of oxygen via nasal cannula. What should the nurse suspect?

HEPATIC DISORDERS

Overview

- Hepatic disorders include viral infections (hepatitis A, B, C), autoimmune hepatitis, cirrhosis, hemochromatosis, biliary atresia, nonalcoholic fatty liver disease, and NASH.
- Some liver diseases can be reversed and treated, while others leave permanent scar tissue, resulting in cirrhosis or liver failure.

 COMPLICATIONS

The major complication of liver disease is acute and/or chronic liver failure. There currently is no medical cure for liver failure. Liver transplant is available to those who meet eligibility criteria.

Signs and Symptoms

- Liver disease may present with no symptoms.
- If present, symptoms may include the following:
  - Altered mental status/confusion
  - Abdominal pain in the right upper quadrant
  - Ascites
  - Darker colored urine
  - Edema
  - Encephalopathy
  - Ecchymosis
  - Fatigue
  - Itching
  - Jaundice
  - Nausea/vomiting
  - Poor appetite
  - Personality changes
  - Unexplained weight loss

Diagnosis

Labs
- Albumin: May be <3.4 g/dL
- Ammonia: May be >80 mcg/dL
- Bilirubin may be >1.2 mg/dL
- Blood and/or ascites fluid cultures
- CBC: May indicate elevated WBC in infection, decreased platelet count (<150,000/L)
- CMP: Will show elevated AST/ALTs (AST >40 u/L and AST >56 u/L)
- PT/INR (PT >13.5 seconds, INR >1.1)
- PTT >35 seconds
- Lactate: May be elevated (<2 mmol/L)
- Serum copper levels: May be elevated in Wilson's disease
- Toxicology screen: May be positive if illicit drugs are used
- Viral:
  - Hepatitis A antibody
  - Hepatitis B core antibody and surface antigen
  - Hepatitis C antibody (and/or PCR)
  - HSV PCR or serology tests

Diagnostic Testing
- Abdominal CT scan
- Abdominal ultrasound
- Chest x-ray
- ERCP
- Head CT scan (if hepatic encephalopathy is suspected and to rule out other neurologic causes)
- Liver biopsy
- MRI
- Upper endoscopy (if varices suspected)

Treatment

- Acute hepatic failure: Identify/reverse cause
- Alcohol cessation
- Coagulopathies possible: Treatment is blood products such as FFP and platelets
- Management of sequela of systemic effects of the disease

- Medication based on etiology (Table 7.1)
  - Lactulose
  - N-acetylcysteine and activated charcoal with acetaminophen toxicity
  - Rifaximin
- Lifestyle modifications:
  - Diet modifications
  - Physical activity
  - Weight loss
- Surgery:
  - Liver resection
  - Liver transplantation
  - TIPS procedure

Nursing Interventions

- Administer medications as ordered.
- Assess abdomen frequently for changes.
- Assess airway, breathing, and circulation.
- Assess neurologic status for evidence of worsening disease or encephalopathy.
- Assess the need for noninvasive oxygen or intubation in severe situations.
- Assess vital signs and hemodynamic stability.
- Draw and monitor serial labs as ordered.
- Monitor and record bowel movement frequency, consistency, and volume for all hepatic disorders, particularly if taking lactulose.
- Monitor for signs and symptoms of bleeding.
- Monitor I/Os daily.
- If the patient receives a liver transplant, monitor the following postoperatively:
  - Administer hemodynamic support with albumin, fluids, or vasopressors.
  - Assess and monitor all lines, drains, and tubes.
  - Assess vital signs.
  - Draw and monitor serial labs, tacrolimus levels, and blood glucoses.
  - Encourage working with PT and OT to regain functional ability postsurgery.
  - Transition to advanced diet as tolerated once extubated.

Patient Education

- Call provider for any new signs of bleeding, including increased bruising.
- Follow up with alcohol cessation or mental health resources, if indicated.
- If liver transplantation is received, take antirejection and immunosuppressive medications as prescribed.
- Self-monitor for worsening symptoms of disease (see Signs and Symptoms).
- Strictly adhere to follow-up office visits and testing.
- Take medications as prescribed.

ILEUS

Overview

- An ileus is the inability to tolerate oral intake due to the lack of GI propulsion with no sign of mechanical obstruction. There is an inability of the intestine to contract normally and move waste out of the body.

 ALERT!

While UNOS is the governing body for organ allocation in the United States, each hospital and health system is responsible for determining which patients meet eligibility criteria to be added to the solid organ transplant list. For alcoholic liver disease, some hospitals require 6 months of sobriety prior to being listed; however, others are moving away from this requirement. Check with your institution for the most current policy for liver transplantation eligibility.

POP QUIZ 7.4

A patient with alcoholic liver disease and associated cirrhosis has been without alcohol for 3 months. He has consistently been compliant with his treatment plan and medications and is ready to be listed for transplant. He was admitted to the PCU with hepatic encephalopathy. His wife asks if he will be listed for transplant because of his deteriorating condition. What is the most appropriate response?

 COMPLICATIONS

Complications of an ileus include aspiration due to vomiting and can result in a prolonged hospital stay with additional interventions.

(continued)

Overview *(continued)*

- The most common causes of ileus include surgery, medication, trauma, peritonitis, or severe illness. However, an ileus is often unavoidable after abdominal or retroperitoneal surgery and critical illness.

Signs and Symptoms

- Abdominal distention
- Absent or hypoactive bowel sounds
- Bloating
- Diffuse pain
- Inability to tolerate PO intake or pass gas
- Nausea and vomiting
- Slow onset of symptoms

Diagnosis

Labs
There are no labs specific to diagnose an ileus. However, the following may be helpful for an initial workup:
- Blood cultures
- BMP
- CBC

Diagnostic Testing
- Abdominal CT scan
- Abdominal x-ray

Treatment

- Bowel rest
- HOB at 30° or higher to prevent risk of aspiration
- IV fluids (Table A.3)
- NG tube insertion to assist with bowel decompression
- NPO
- Monitoring for presence of flatus
- Noting for any occurrence of bowel movements
- Treatment of underlying condition
- Physical activity

 NURSING PEARL

Early recovery after surgery protocols includes minimal fasting before surgery, returning to normal eating, drinking, and activities within 1 day of surgery, and using multimodal analgesia with appropriate opioid use if needed. If implemented, these protocols help increase speed of recovery, shorten hospital stays, and significantly reduce complications like postoperative ileus.

Nursing Interventions

- Administer medications and fluid and electrolyte replacement as ordered/needed.
- Assess for other signs of underlying disease or medication contributing to ileus.
- Assess for symptoms of hypovolemia.
- Assess patient for intolerance to PO intake and/or vomiting.
- Assess vitals continuously.
- Draw and monitor serial labs as ordered.
- Encourage physical activity. Assist patient out of bed to the chair daily.
- Provide a safe environment and engage in therapeutic communication.
- Monitor for return of bowel function (passing flatus, active bowel sounds).
- Monitor volume of NG tube output.

Patient Education

- Ambulate in room or in the hallways with therapy.
- Notify nurse of any return of bowel function (passing flatus, having a bowel movement).

IRRITABLE BOWEL SYNDROME

Overview

- IBS is defined as abdominal pain/discomfort with altered bowel habits without a diagnosable cause.
- This can result from impaired motility, visceral sensation, brain–gut interactions, and psychosocial distress.

Signs and Symptoms

- Abdominal pain or discomfort
- Altered bowel habits including constipation, diarrhea, or both
- Bloating
- Distention
- Pain location changes
- Stool changes
- Worsened symptoms with food intake

Diagnosis

Labs

There are no labs specific to diagnose IBS. However, the following are indicated if IBS is atypical, or if patient complains of alarming symptoms (weight loss, hematochezia, iron deficiency):
- CBC
- CMP
- Fecal tests
  - Leukocytes
  - *Clostridium difficile*
  - Giardia
  - Cryptosporidium
- Inflammatory markers
  - C-reactive protein
  - Erythrocyte sedimentation rate
- Thyroid-stimulating hormones

Diagnostic Testing

There are no diagnostic tests specific to diagnose IBS. However, the following are indicated if IBS is atypical, or if patient complains of alarming symptoms (weight loss, hematochezia, iron deficiency):
- Intestinal biopsy via colonoscopy
- Abdominal x-ray

Treatment

- Symptom management:
  - Constipation: Fiber supplements, laxatives
  - Diarrhea: Loperamide, probiotics

(continued)

Treatment *(continued)*

- Increased physical activity, which increases colonic transit time to improve symptoms
- Diet modifications:
  - Avoidance of foods that fall under the FODMAP category:
    - Dairy
    - Fruit
    - Highly fermentable carbohydrates
    - Onions
    - Sorbitol
    - Vegetables
    - Wheat
- Low-dose tricyclic antidepressant or SSRI (Table 11.1) if constant and chronic abdominal symptoms persist

Nursing Interventions

- Administer medications as ordered.
- Assess bowel movement frequency.
- Assess for changes in quality and sensation of pain.
- Assess for new or worsening symptoms of IBS.
- Assess quality and consistency of stool, if possible.
- Continuously assess vital signs.
- Perform frequent abdominal physical assessments.
- Provide safe space and engage in therapeutic communication to support the patient.

Patient Education

- Make note of any patterns in symptom presentation.
- Stay up to date on current status and plan of care.
- Work with a registered dietician or nutritionist to modify diet and avoid FODMAPs.
- Take medications as prescribed.

NURSING PEARL

FODMAP stands for fermentable oligosaccharides, disaccharides, monosaccharides, and polyols. It includes dairy, fruit, highly fermentable carbohydrates, onions, sorbitol, vegetables, and wheat. Adhering to a FODMAP-free diet may require additional assistance and support from a nutritionist or dietitian.

POP QUIZ 7.6

A patient diagnosed with IBS is trying to order a breakfast tray while avoiding foods that fall under the FODMAP category. The patient asks if they are able to have scrambled eggs for breakfast. What should the nurse's response be?

ISCHEMIC BOWEL

Overview

- Ischemic bowel occurs when there is a decrease in blood flow to the small or large intestine, resulting in cell and tissue death.
- The cause of decreased blood flow can be acute or chronic and result from atherosclerotic disease, mesenteric venous thrombosis, mesenteric arterial thrombosis, intestinal hypoperfusion during systemic shock, or mesenteric arterial embolism.

COMPLICATIONS

Complications of bowel ischemia include bowel infarction and perforation, necrotic bowel, MODS, toxic megacolon, fistula, colonic stricture, and sepsis. For severe bowel infarction, surgery may be indicated.

Signs and Symptoms

- Abdominal pain
- Bowel habit changes
- Guarding
- Rebound tenderness

- Sepsis
  - Chills or rigors
  - Diaphoresis
  - Elevated lactate and WBC counts
  - Fever
  - Hypotension
  - Tachycardia

Diagnosis

Labs

- Amylase >140 u/L
- BMP: May show hyperkalemia >5.0 mmol/L
- CBC: May show elevated WBCs in infection (>11,000/mcL)
- Lactate: May be elevated >2 mmol/L

Diagnostic Testing

- CT angiography
- Duplex ultrasound
- Invasive angiography
- MRI with angiography

Treatment

- Antibiotics
- Electrolyte replacement as needed
- Hemodynamics support
  - Blood products
  - Volume replacement
- Pain control
- Oxygen support
- Surgical intervention
  - Endovascular
    - Balloon angioplasty
    - Catheter-directed thrombolysis
    - Mechanical thrombectomy
  - Open surgery
    - Exploratory laparotomy
    - Resect infarcted intestine or necrotic bowel
    - Revascularization of affected bowel: Embolectomy or mesenteric bypass

Nursing Interventions

- Administer lactulose to ordered number of daily bowel movements or ammonia level as ordered.
- Administer medications as ordered.
- Assess airway, breathing, and circulation.
- Assess the need for noninvasive oxygen or intubation in severe situations.
- Assess neurologic status for evidence of worsening disease.
- Assess abdomen frequently for changes.
- Assess abdominal incisions each shift, monitor for signs of infection including redness, warmth to the touch, swelling or edema, bleeding, or foul-smelling or purulent drainage.
- Draw and monitor serial labs as ordered.
- Encourage pulmonary hygiene through ambulation, position changes, and incentive spirometry.
- Monitor for evidence of systemic infection including fever, hypotension, or tachycardia.
- Provide abdominal binder or splinting pillow.

Patient Education

- Continue using incentive spirometry at home. See Patient Education in Gastrointestinal Surgeries for instructions.
- Monitor for recurring symptoms of recurrent ischemia and/or infection, which include the following:
  - Abdominal pain
  - Changes in bowel habits
  - Fatigue or malaise
  - Fever
  - Increased heart rate
  - Low blood pressure
- Monitor for surgical site infection by assessing for new or worsening redness, warmth to the touch, swelling, foul-smelling or purulent drainage, or fever.
- Perform incision care until appropriately assessed by provider at follow-up appointment. See Patient Education in Gastrointestinal Surgeries instructions.
- Take medications as prescribed.

 POP QUIZ 7.7

Laboratory tests are nonspecific for diagnosing bowel ischemia. What imaging is critical for diagnosis?

MALNUTRITION

Overview

- Malnutrition is defined as insufficient total calorie intake, which can be chronic or acute.
- There are a variety of causes for malnutrition, including chronic or acute disease, mental health disorders, or physical access to food.

Signs and Symptoms

- Decreased muscle function and strength
- Decreased oral intake
- Dehydration
- Edema
- Electrolyte abnormalities
  - Hypokalemia
    - Muscle twitching or cramps
    - Palpitations or dysrhythmia
  - Hypomagnesemia
    - Anorexia
    - Fatigue
    - Nausea and vomiting
    - Tetany
    - Weakness
  - Hypocalcemia
    - Circumoral numbness
    - Cramps and spasms
    - Parathesis
    - Seizures
    - Tetany
  - Hypoglycemia
    - Anxiety
    - Hunger

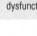 **COMPLICATIONS**

Malnutrition complications can result in electrolyte abnormalities and risk of developing refeeding syndrome, heart failure and/or dysrhythmia, impaired wound healing, UTI, sepsis, GI malabsorption, endocrinologic dysfunction, hypothermia, and death.

ALERT!

Thiamine plays a central role in carbohydrate metabolism. Thiamine deficiency can alter cellular energy production, especially in the brain, which requires glucose metabolism. Signs of thiamine deficiency include Wernicke's encephalopathy, cardiomyopathy, lactic acidosis, and peripheral neuropathy. Common etiologies of thiamine deficiency are alcoholism, hypermetabolic states, furosemide therapy, and magnesium depletion.

- ○ Irritability
- ○ Palpitations
- ○ Sweating
- Frequent infections
- Infections
- Mood changes
  - Apathy
  - Anxiety
  - Depression
  - Self-neglect
- Poor wound healing
- Weight loss

Diagnosis

Labs

- Albumin <3.5 g/dL/prealbumin <10 mg/dL
- CBC is drawn to rule out anemia
- CMP
- Lactate
- Osmolality >295 mosm/kg
- Thiamine <2.5 mcg/dL
- Vitamin D <20 mg/mL

Diagnostic Testing

- EKG to detect electrolyte abnormalities

Treatment

- Appetite stimulants in patients with malignancies, receiving chemotherapy, or those with poor oral intake
- Electrolyte replacement based on CMP results
- Enteral/parenteral nutrition:
  - Enteral nutrition via temporary (or permanent) tube feeding: NG, orogastric, gastrostomy, or jejunostomy
  - Parenteral nutrition, if unable to tolerate enteral feeds
- IV fluid replacement (Table A.3)
- Medication management dependent on condition for patients with malnourishment
- Nutritional supplementation, including necessary vitamins and protein, if not contraindicated
- Psychiatric consult if needed
- PO intake if able
- Treatment of associated infections

 ALERT!

In the first week of severe malnutrition, patients are most likely to develop refeeding syndrome. Patients should be slowly given between 60% and 80% of required calorie intake for age to prevent this complication.

Nursing Interventions

- Administer nutritional, electrolyte, and fluid replacement medications as ordered based on lab results.
- Assess vital signs for early indications of change in status.
- Consult dietary and nutrition as needed.
- Consult a social worker to be sure patient has adequate resources for food.
- Draw and monitor serial labs as ordered.
- Minimize interruptions in enteral and parenteral nutrition.
- Monitor I/O and nutritional intake.

(continued)

Nursing Interventions *(continued)*

- Monitor for signs of malnutrition, including routine skin assessment for wounds.
- Monitor for signs of respiratory distress or aspiration following NG or orogastric tube placement.
- Monitor securement and site marking for NG and orogastric tubes.
- Provide protein supplementation as indicated.
- Provide safe therapeutic environment.

Patient Education

- Adhere to dietary recommendations made by provider.
  - Choose high-protein, nutrient-dense foods if possible.
  - Consult a dietician or nutritionist to help establish improved dietary choices.
  - Consult a social worker to help getting resources to obtain food.
- Follow up with alcohol or drug cessation resources if indicated.
- Self-monitor for status or symptom changes if possible.
- Take medications as ordered.

PANCREATITIS

Overview

- *Pancreatitis* is an inflammatory condition related to autodigestion of the pancreas by proteases.
- This process can range from mild edema to pancreatic necrosis and hemorrhage.
- Pancreatitis can be classified as acute or chronic.
  - *Acute pancreatitis* is the result of pancreatic injury.
  - *Chronic pancreatitis* occurs when permanent damage is sustained to the structure and endocrine and exocrine functions of the pancreatitis.
- Both acute and chronic pancreatitides are commonly caused by alcohol abuse.

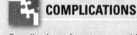 **COMPLICATIONS**

Complications of acute pancreatitis include pancreatic pseudocyst, necrosis, peripancreatic fluid collection, ARDS, compartment syndrome, AKI, DIC, and death. Complications of chronic pancreatitis include pseudocysts and pseudoaneurysms, diabetes, and pancreatic cancer.

Signs and Symptoms

- Altered mental status
- Dehydration
- Diaphoresis
- Diffuse visceral tenderness
- Distended abdomen
- Hemorrhagic signs
  - Cullen's sign
  - Grey Turner's sign
- Hypoactive or absent bowel sounds
- Low-grade fever
- Nausea/vomiting
- Rebound tenderness
- Steatorrhea
- Upper abdominal pain radiating to the back
- Weight loss

Diagnosis

Labs

- BMP: May show elevated BUN and creatinine
- CBC: May show elevated WBC with pancreatic inflammation or infection
- C-Reactive protein: May be elevated with increased inflammation
- Ionized calcium
- Lactate may be elevated >2.2 mmol/L
- Serum amylase >140 u/L
- Serum lipase >140 u/L
- Triglycerides >10 mmol/L
- Urine amylase >21.2 IU/h

Diagnostic Testing

- Abdominal CT scan
- MRI
- X-ray
- Ultrasound

Treatment

- Electrolyte replacement
- ERCP if biliary tract occlusion suspected
- Medications
  - Analgesics (Table A.2)
  - Antibiotics (Table A.1)
  - Antiemetics (Table 7.1)
  - Insulin (Table 4.1)
  - IV fluids (Table A.3)
  - Pancreatic enzyme replacement (Table 7.1)
  - Vasopressors (Table 2.8)
- Nutritional support
  - NPO initially
  - Enteral feeding below the duodenum
- Pain management
- Primary goals in the inpatient setting:
  - Blood sugar management
  - Fluid resuscitation and blood pressure support
  - GI prophylaxis
  - Pain and nausea management

Nursing Interventions

- Administer nutritional, electrolyte, and fluid replacement medications as ordered.
- Assess for signs of retroperitoneal bleeding.
- Assess respiratory status for early signs of atelectasis or effusions.
- Complete detailed frequent head to toe assessment to assess for systemic change.
- Continuously assess vital signs.
- Draw and monitor serial labs as ordered.
- Monitor and treat elevated blood glucose.
- Monitor urine output for signs of hypoperfusion or adequate resuscitation.
- Provide safe therapeutic environment.

Patient Education

- Follow dietary and lifestyle modification recommendations.
- Self-monitor for status or symptom changes if possible.
- Take medications as ordered.
- Participate in an alcohol cessation program.
- Modify daily diet. If assistance is needed, consider working with a nutritionist or dietitian to assist with lifestyle modifications.

Table 7.1 Gastrointestinal Medications

Indications	Mechanism of Action	Contraindications, Precautions, and Adverse Effects
Antibiotics: Rifamycins (rifaximin)		
• Hepatic encephalopathy	• Reduce ammonia-producing bacteria in the colon, thus reducing ammonia burden	• Monitor for signs of worsening hepatic disease. • Monitor for bleeding or worsening coagulation tests.
Anticonstipation: Contact/stimulant laxatives (sennosides)		
• Treatment of constipation	• Irritates the sensory nerve endings stimulating colonic motility • Reduces colonic water absorption to alleviate constipation	• Medication is contraindicated in patients with bowel or other GI obstruction. • Use caution in pregnancy. • Adverse effects include diarrhea, fecal urgency, abdominal pain, and flatulence.
Anticonstipation: Osmotic laxatives (lactulose)		
• Hepatic encephalopathy • Constipation	• Increases osmotic pressure to cause fluid accumulation that breaks down stool • Ionizes ammonia in the colon to the ammonium ion, preventing ammonia diffusion into the bloodstream, which can lower serum ammonia levels by 25%–50%	• Monitor for hypernatremia, hypokalemia, and metabolic acidosis.
Anticonstipation: Softeners, emollients, enemas for constipation (docusate sodium)		
• For the prevention or treatment of constipation	• Decreases surface tension to allow water and lipids to penetrate the stool, hydrating it and allowing it to be passed	• Use caution in patients experiencing abdominal pain of unknown origin, GI bleeding, or vomiting. • Adverse reactions include diarrhea.

(continued)

Table 7.1 Gastrointestinal Medications *(continued)*

Indications	Mechanism of Action	Contraindications, Precautions, and Adverse Effects
Antidiarrheal (loperamide)		
• Control diarrhea	• Interferes with peristalsis by direct action on the circular and longitudinal muscles of the intestinal wall to slow motility	• Contraindications include dysentery, fever, gastroenteritis, infection, pseudomembranous colitis, cardiac dysrhythmia, constipation, toxic megacolon, UC, and AIDS. • Use caution in hepatic disease. • Adverse effects include ileus, toxic megacolon, angioedema, lethal dysrhythmias and cardiac arrest, constipation, rash, respiratory depression, and QT prolongation.
H2 receptor antagonists (famotidine)		
• GI disorders such as peptic ulcers and GERD	• Inhibit binding of histamine to H2 receptors on gastric cells decreasing gastric acid secretions	• Use caution in gastric cancer, GI bleed, infection, hepatic disease, QT prolongation, renal impairment, PKU, vitamin B12 deficiency, and smoking. • Adverse effects include seizures, angioedema, dysrhythmia, agranulocytosis, pancytopenia, rhabdomyolysis, constipation, liver impairment, renal impairment, delirium, confusion, and hallucinations.
Propulsive (metoclopramide)		
• Diabetic gastroparesis	• Inhibits dopamine receptors in the chemoreceptor trigger zone • Decreases sensitivity of the visceral afferent nerves that transmit from the GI system to the vomiting center in the chemoreceptor trigger zone	• Medication is contraindicated in paraben and procainamide hypersensitivity. • Use caution in GI bleed, obstruction or perforation, Parkinson's disease, seizures or tardive dyskinesia, cardiac disease, heart failure, hypertension, hepatic disease, renal failure, breast cancer, and malignant hyperthermia. • Adverse effects include seizure, suicidal ideation, tardive dyskinesia, dysrhythmia, hepatotoxicity, angioedema, serotonin syndrome, depression, confusion, or hepatic and renal disease.
Pancreatic enzymes (pancrelipase)		
• Management of exocrine pancreatic insufficiency	• Release lipase, amylase, and protease at high levels, assisting with hydrolysis of fats, breakdown of starches into sugars, and breakdown of proteins into peptides	• Use caution in patients with porcine protein hypersensitivity, gout, renal impairment, and hyperuricemia. • Adverse effects include abdominal pain, elevated hepatic enzymes, hyperuricemia, nausea, and vomiting.

(continued)

Table 7.1 Gastrointestinal Medications *(continued)*

Indications	Mechanism of Action	Contraindications, Precautions, and Adverse Effects
Phenothiazine antiemetics (e.g., promethazine, Compazine)		
• Nausea	• Block H1 receptors causing anticholinergic actions, resulting in reduced CNS stimulation of nausea and motion sickness	• Monitor for oversedation. • Monitor IV side for extravasation and tissue necrosis. • Use caution in patients with hepatic disease.
Proton pump inhibitors (pantoprazole, omeprazole)		
• GERD; empirically used for upper GI bleeds	• Suppress gastric acid secretion by inhibiting gastric ATPase enzyme pump, decreasing acid	• Contraindications include interstitial nephritis. • Use caution in hepatic disease, gastric cancer, colitis, diarrhea, vitamin B12 and zinc deficiency, bone fractures, osteopenia/osteoporosis, hypomagnesemia, prolonged QT interval, and lupus. • Adverse reactions include GI bleeding, seizures, MI, dysrhythmias, elevated hepatic enzymes, interstitial nephritis, anemias, headache, nausea, and abdominal pain.
Serotonin receptor antagonists (ondansetron)		
• Diabetic gastroparesis • Nausea and vomiting	• Block the serotonin 5-HT3 receptors at the peripheral vagal nerve terminals in the intestines, blocking signal transmission to the CNS to antagonize the effect of serotonin and decrease the presence of nausea and vomiting	• Use caution with hepatic disease, PKU, GI obstruction or ileus, any cardiac dysrhythmia, electrolyte imbalance, malnutrition, MI, and thyroid disease. • Adverse effects include bradycardia, bronchospasm, hepatic failure, dysrhythmia, angioedema, laryngeal edema, laryngospasm, constipation, urinary retention, hypokalemia, and hypotension.
Vasoactive medications (somatostatin, octreotide)		
• Treating variceal bleeding by inhibiting vasodilatory hormone release	• Bind to somatostatin receptors • Lead to smooth muscle contraction in blood vessels	• Use caution in pancreatitis, hepatic or renal disease, DM, biliary obstruction, goiter, hypothyroidism, vitamin deficiency, alcoholism, and cardiac dysrhythmia and disease. • Adverse effects include bradycardia and dysrhythmia, GI bleeding or obstruction, hyperglycemia, constipation, goiter, edema, jaundice, ascites, nausea, abdominal pain, and rash.

RESOURCES

American Association of Critical Care Nurses. (2018). *The gastrointestinal system*. In T. Hartjes (Ed.), *Core curriculum for high acuity, progressive care, and critical-care nursing* (7th ed., pp. 552–598). Elsevier.

Cleveland Clinic. (2019, March 20). *Small bowel obstruction*. https://my.clevelandclinic.org/health/diseases/15850-small-bowel-obstruction

Gupta, E. (n.d). *Gerd diet: Foods that help with acid reflux (heartburn)*. Johns Hopkins Medicine. https://www.hopkinsmedicine.org/health/wellness-and-prevention/gerd-diet-foods-that-help-with-acid-reflux-heartburn

Mayo Clinic. (2017, June 6). *Over-the-counter laxatives for constipation: Use with caution*. https://www.mayoclinic.org/diseases-conditions/constipation/in-depth/laxatives/art-20045906

Mayo Clinic. (2020, October 15). *Irritable bowel syndrome*. https://www.mayoclinic.org/diseases-conditions/irritable-bowel-syndrome/symptoms-causes/syc-20360016

National Institute of Diabetes and Digestive and Kidney Diseases. (n.d.). *Acid reflux (GER & GERD) in adults*. U.S. Department of Health and Human Services, National Institute of Diabetes and Digestive and Kidney Diseases. https://www.niddk.nih.gov/health-information/digestive-diseases/acid-reflux-ger-gerd-adults

National Institute of Diabetes and Digestive and Kidney Diseases. (n.d.). *Liver disease*. U.S. Department of Health and Human Services, National Institute of Diabetes and Digestive and Kidney Diseases. https://www.niddk.nih.gov/health-information/liver-disease

National Institute of Diabetes and Digestive and Kidney Diseases. (n.d.). *Treatment for gastroparesis*. U.S. Department of Health and Human Services, National Institute of Diabetes and Digestive and Kidney Diseases. https://www.niddk.nih.gov/health-information/digestive-diseases/gastroparesis/treatment

Prescribers' Digital Reference. (n.d.). *Amitriptyline hydrochloride* [Drug information]. PDR Search. https://www.pdr.net/drug-summary/Amitriptyline-Hydrochloride-amitriptyline-hydrochloride-1001#11

Prescribers' Digital Reference. (n.d.). *Colace capsules (docusate sodium)*[Drug information]. PDR Search. https://www.pdr.net/drug-summary/Colace-Capsules-docusate-sodium-1023

Prescribers' Digital Reference. (n.d.). *Ledipasvir/Sofosbuvir* [Drug information]. PDR Search. https://www.pdr.net/drug-summary/Harvoni-ledipasvir-sofosbuvir-3630#11

Prescribers' Digital Reference. (n.d.). *Loperamide hydrochloride* [Drug information]. PDR Search. https://www.pdr.net/drug-summary/Loperamide-Hydrochloride-Capsules-loperamide-hydrochloride-2664#15

Prescribers' Digital Reference. (n.d.). *Metoclopramide* [Drug information]. PDR Search. https://www.pdr.net/drug-summary/Metoclopramide-Injection-metoclopramide-3898

Prescribers' Digital Reference. (n.d.). *Ondansetron hydrochloride* [Drug information]. PDR Search. https://www.pdr.net/drug-summary/Zofran-Injection-ondansetron-hydrochloride-243.2904

Prescribers' Digital Reference. (n.d.). *Pantoprazole sodium* [Drug information]. PDR Search. https://www.pdr.net/drug-summary/Protonix-I-V--pantoprazole-sodium-2096.5821

Prescribers' Digital Reference. (n.d.). *Potassium chloride* [Drug information]. PDR Search. https://www.pdr.net/drug-summary/Micro-K-10-potassium-chloride-770

Prescribers' Digital Reference. (n.d.). *Sennakot (Sennosides)* [Drug information]. PDR Search. https://www.pdr.net/drug-summary/Senokot-sennosides-3182#5

Saunders, J., & Smith, T. (2010). Malnutrition: Causes and consequences. *Clinical Medicine, 10*(6), 624–627. https://www.ncbi.nlm.nih.gov/pmc/articles/PMC4951875/

Weaver, K. R., Melkus, G. D. E., & Henderson, W. A. (2017). Irritable bowel syndrome. *The American Journal of Nursing, 117*, 48–55. https://www.ncbi.nlm.nih.gov/pmc/articles/PMC5453305/

8

RENAL SYSTEM

ACUTE KIDNEY INJURY

Overview

- AKI refers to the sudden decrease in kidney function, resulting in the retention of urea and other waste products and in the dysregulation of extracellular volume and electrolytes.
- While AKI can be associated with a high mortality rate, it can also be reversible in certain situations.
- Causes of AKI are divided into three categories: Prerenal, intrarenal, and postrenal.
  - Prerenal results from blood flow changes, including hypovolemia, hypotension, renal vasoconstriction, and glomerular efferent arteriolar vasodilation.
  - Intrarenal causes include acute tubular necrosis secondary to major surgery, shock, sepsis, blood transfusion reaction, rhabdomyolysis related to trauma, prolonged hypotension, and nephrotoxic drug administration (Table 8.1).
  - Postrenal causes result from mechanical obstruction in the outflow of urine including benign prostatic hyperplasia, prostate cancer, renal calculi, trauma, or extrarenal tumors.

COMPLICATIONS

Complications of AKI include electrolyte abnormalities (hyperkalemia, hyperphosphatemia, etc.), metabolic acidosis, pulmonary and peripheral edema, HF due to fluid overload, and CNS effects (lethargy, altered mental status, and encephalopathy) due to uremia. These complications contribute to the increased mortality rate associated with AKI. Prompt identification and treatment is necessary to prevent these complications; transfer to a higher level of care may be indicated.

Signs and Symptoms

- Asterixis
- Edema and fluid retention
- Flank pain
- Hypovolemia

(continued)

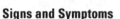

Table 8.1 Intrarenal Causes of AKI

Ischemic Causes	Nephrotoxic Causes
Burns	Contrast dye
Cardiac surgery	Drug use
HF	Medications
Hemorrhage	Rhabdomyolysis
Sepsis	

Signs and Symptoms *(continued)*

- Oliguria
- Metabolic acidosis
- Peaked T waves
- Metabolic acidosis
- Weakness
- Widening QRS complex

Diagnosis

Labs

- ABG
- BMP: Assess for an increased creatinine by ≥0.3 mg/dL (27 mcmol/L) relative to a known baseline value within 48 hr, or an increase to ≥1.5 times the known or presumed baseline value within 7 days
- CBC
- Creatinine clearance
- GFR
- Urinalysis
  - Protein
  - Osmolality
  - Albumin to creatinine ratios
  - Electrolytes
  - Urine sediment examination
- Urine specific gravity

> 🔊 **ALERT!**
>
> In addition to lab findings, a decrease in urine volume to <0.5 mL/kg over 6 hr also indicates a possible AKI.

Diagnostic Testing

- Abdominal CT scan
- Chest x-ray
- Fluid challenge (to determine if AKI is prerenal unless contraindicated)
- Intravenous pyelography
- KUB
- MRI
- Renal biopsy
- Renal ultrasound

> 🔊 **ALERT!**
>
> Medications are a common source of AKI. Dosages of drugs shown to cause nephrotoxicity may need to be adjusted or medications may need to be discontinued if AKI is suspected. Nephrotoxic agents that can cause kidney damage include heavy metals, certain medications, illicit drug use, rhabdomyolysis, and radiocontrast dye.

Treatment

- Identify cause/correct underlying problem
- Nephrotoxic agents: avoid if possible or administer renal dosage of certain medications
- Dialysis if needed: early initiation beneficial to prevent exacerbation of and currently manage acute and chronic renal failure
  - Hemodialysis
  - Peritoneal dialysis
  - Continuous RRT (may require transfer to higher level of care
- Electrolyte level monitoring and replacement (Table 8.2)
- Fluid volume maintenance:
  - Monitor for overload
  - Fluid restriction or IV hydration depending on patient clinical status

- Diuretics may be used to relieve hypervolemia among non-anuric patients with AKI (Table 8.4*)
- Nutritional therapy if able to tolerate PO:
  - High protein
    - Patients with AKI on RRT should receive a basic intake of at least 1.5 g/kg/day of protein with an additional 0.2 g/kg/day to compensate for amino acid/protein loss during RRT.
  - Restrict potassium, phosphate, and sodium

Nursing Interventions

- Administer medications as ordered.
- Assess and maintain sterility of dialysis sites and lines.
- Assess AV fistula, if applicable:
  - Auscultate for bruit.
  - Palpate for thrill.
  - Assess skin color, pulse, and capillary refill of distal extremity.
- Assess EKG tracings for signs of worsening condition, electrolyte imbalances, or respiratory compromise.
- Assess vital signs for signs of worsening condition or respiratory compromise.
- Maintain strict I/Os.
- Monitor and draw serial labs as ordered.
- Monitor fluid volume status:
  - Extra heart sounds (S3/S4, gallops, murmurs, and/or pericardial friction rubs)
  - Fluid intake from PO and/or IV fluids
  - JVD
  - Lung sounds
  - Mucous membranes
  - Peripheral edema
  - Skin turgor
  - Urine output
- Monitor neurologic status. Assess for altered mental status and decreased level of consciousness.
- Perform bladder scan, if needed.
- Provide therapeutic communication and support.

NURSING PEARL

Multiple medications have nephrotoxic properties. Antibiotics drug classes such as aminoglycosides, beta-lactams, quinolones, and sulfonamides are commonly used nephrotoxic medications. Make sure to monitor the patient's creatinine and BUN when administering these medications.

ALERT!

The National Kidney Foundation recommends that patients receiving dialysis avoid drinking more than 32 oz of fluid per day. When teaching both patients and family, provide education on the importance of this guideline and how exceeding this fluid intake may impact clinical status.

Patient Education

- Avoid nephrotoxic agents (certain antibiotics, diuretics, contrast dye, statins, antihypertensives, or benzodiazepines) unless directed by provider.
- Confirm understanding of renal diet modifications, including any diets with fluid restrictions, high protein, and low potassium, phosphate, and sodium.
- Follow up with scheduled outpatient appointments, dialysis appointments, and blood draws.
- Self-monitor for signs of fluid overload, worsening dyspnea, palpitations, or chest pain and call for help if indicated.

POP QUIZ 8.1

A patient with AKI is admitted to the PCU with a potassium value of 6.5 mmol/L. The patient has received calcium gluconate, regular insulin IV, and glucose with minimal improvement in potassium level. If this patient is unresponsive to medical therapy, what is the next step to lower potassium?

---

* Table 8.4 is located at the end of this chapter.

CHRONIC KIDNEY DISEASE

Overview

- Unlike AKI, CKD is the irreversible loss of kidney function that will progress to ESRD.
- *CKD* is defined as the presence of kidney damage or deceased kidney function, as evidenced by an estimated GFR of <60 mL/min/1.73 m², for 3 or more months, irrespective of the cause.

Signs and Symptoms

CKD affects every body system and has many symptoms of varying degree and severity depending on the stage. Signs and symptoms include any of the following:
- Urine output changes:
  - Oliguria
  - Anuria
- Cardiovascular abnormalities:
  - CAD
  - HF
  - HTN
  - Pericarditis
  - PAD
- GI disturbances:
  - Gastritis
  - GI bleed
  - Nausea and vomiting
- Endocrine disturbances:
  - Amenorrhea in women
  - Erectile dysfunction in men
  - Thyroid abnormalities
- Hematologic abnormalities:
  - Anemia
  - Bleeding
  - Infection
- Neurologic abnormalities:
  - Encephalopathy
  - Peripheral neuropathy
  - Restless leg syndrome
  - Sleep disturbances
- Pulmonary complications:
  - Pneumonia
  - Pulmonary edema
  - Uremic pleuritis
- Integumentary changes:
  - Dry, scaly skin
  - Ecchymosis
  - Pruritus
- Musculoskeletal:
  - *Calciphylaxis*: Buildup of calcium in the blood vessels, skin, and visceral fat that causes painful ulcers and infection
  - Soft tissue and vascular calcifications

 COMPLICATIONS

- Complications of CKD include electrolyte abnormalities (hyperkalemia, hyperphosphatemia), metabolic acidosis, HTN, anemia, ESRD, and death.
- Complications of ESRD include electrolyte and acid-base abnormalities, mineral and bone disorders, anemia, HTN, dysrhythmia, and death. Careful monitoring and compliance with dialysis appointments is essential to managing ESRD.

 ALERT!

Risk factors for chronic kidney disease include diabetes type 1 and type 2, HTN, glomerulonephritis, chronic tubulointerstitial nephritis, hereditary or polycystic disease, vasculitis, plasma dyscrasia or cancer, and sickle cell nephropathy. Minority populations including African and native Americans and Hispanic males are most likely to develop CKD. Dialysis and renal transplant are the only effective therapy options for ESRD.

 NURSING PEARL

Stages of CKD:
- *Stage 1:* Kidney damage with normal or slightly increased GFR (>90 mL/min/1.73 m²)
- *Stage 2:* Mild loss in GFR (60–89 mL/min/1.73 m²)
- *Stage 3:* Moderate loss in GFR (30–59 mL/min/1.73 m²)
- *Stage 4:* Severe loss in GFR (15–29 mL/min/1.73 m²)
- *Stage 5:* Kidney Failure (ESRD) requiring dialysis (GFR <15 mL/min/ 1.73 m²)

Diagnosis

Labs
- ABG
- Albumin
- BMP
- Glomerular filtration rate (see Nursing Pearl: Stages of CKD section for lab values of GFR)
- CBC
- Creatinine clearance
- Lipid profile
- Urinalysis

Diagnostic Testing
- Abdominal and pelvic CT scan
- MRI
- Renal biopsy
- Renal ultrasound

Treatment

- Dialysis:
  - Continuous RRT (requires transfer to higher level of care)
  - Hemodialysis
- Kidney transplant
- Medications to manage complications, including the following (Table 8.4):
  - Anemia (Table 5.6)
  - Dyslipidemia
  - HTN (Table 2.8)
  - Metabolic/electrolyte disorders
- Nutritional therapy:
  - Fluid restriction
  - Low-protein diet of 0.6 to 0.8 g/kg/d
  - Sodium, potassium, and phosphate restriction

Nursing Interventions

- Refer to AKI, Nursing Interventions.

Patient Education

- Refer to AKI, Patient Education.

ALERT!

Consider consulting a dietitian or nutritionist to assist with meal planning and food options when preparing for discharge.

POP QUIZ 8.2

A patient has been admitted to the PCU with the following lab values: creatinine of 3.4, estimated GFR <60, and potassium 5.8. Upon admission assessment, the patient reports that she typically eats a big bowl of fruit for breakfast. For lunch, she usually has milk with a peanut butter sandwich. For dinner, she has broccoli, beans, or potatoes with meat protein. What should the nurse's next action be?

ELECTROLYTE IMBALANCE

Overview

- It is important to maintain normal electrolyte levels for the body to function appropriately.
- Renal disease often impairs the natural electrolyte balance within the body (Table 8.2).

COMPLICATIONS

While many electrolyte imbalances can be asymptomatic, it is essential that electrolytes be closely monitored in patients with renal disease to prevent dangerous complications, such as lethal dysrhythmias.

Table 8.2 Electrolyte Imbalances

Electrolyte	Causes	Signs and Symptoms	Treatment
Calcium (normal value: 8.5–10.5 mmol/L)			
Hypercalcemia	• Cancer • Hyperparathyroidism	• Bone pain and fractures • Coma • Confusion • Depressed reflexes • Dehydration and polyuria • Dysrhythmias • EKG changes include shortened ST and QT segments/intervals • Fatigue • Heart blocks • Hypotonicity • Lethargy • Neurological changes including confusion, psychosis, personality changes, memory issues, stupor, and coma • Nephrolithiasis • Seizures • Ventricular dysrhythmias • Weakness	• Furosemide to promote diuresis • Calcitonin • Hemodialysis if patient cannot tolerate additional fluids • High-rate IV fluids. (0.9% NS)
Hypocalcemia	• Fluoride poisoning • Hypomagnesemia • Hypoparathyroidism • Pancreatitis • Thyroid surgery • Toxic shock syndrome • Tumor lysis syndrome	• EKG changes include prolonged ST and QT segment, ventricular tachycardia • Facial paralysis • Hyperreflexia • Laryngeal spasm • Muscle cramps • Neurological changes including anxiety, depression, or confusion • Numbness and tingling of the extremities and around the mouth • Positive Chvostek and Trousseau signs • Seizures • Tetany	• Replacement with either calcium gluconate or calcium chloride • Magnesium replacement • Vitamin D supplementation
Magnesium (normal value: 1.5–2.2 mg/dL)			
Hypermagnesemia	• Increased use of magnesium-containing medications such as laxatives and antacids • Renal failure	• Ataxia • Absent deep tendon reflexes • Bradydysrhythmia • Cardiac arrest • Confusion • Drowsiness • Fatigue • Flushing • Muscular weakness • Paralysis • Respiratory depression/arrest • Somnolence	• Calcium, which binds to and removes excessive magnesium • Dialysis • Diuresis with IVF 0.9% NS or furosemide

(continued)

Table 8.2 Electrolyte Imbalances *(continued)*

Electrolyte	Causes	Signs and Symptoms	Treatment
Magnesium (normal value: 1.5–2.2 mg/dL) (continued)			
Hypomagnesemia	• Alcoholism • DKA, HHS • GI abnormalities • Malnutrition • Thyroid dysfunction	• Altered mental state • Cardiac dysrhythmias • Coma • Concurrent electrolyte/ hormonal abnormalities (hypocalcemia, hypoparathyroidism, hypokalemia) • Delirium • EKG changes including widening QRS complex, peaked T wave, prolonged PR interval • Hyperreflexia • Muscle tremors • Ocular nystagmus • Positive Chvostek and Trousseau signs • Seizure • Tetany/tremors • Torsades de Pointes	• IV magnesium sulfate
Phosphate (normal value: 3–4.5 mg/dL)			
Hyperphosphatemia	• Renal failure	• Anxiety • Concurrent hypocalcemia • Deposition of calcium phosphate precipitates in skin, viscera, and blood vessels • Facial twitching • Irritability • Muscle dysfunction: tetany	• Aluminum hydroxide • Correct hypocalcemia with treatments in hypocalcemia section
Hypophosphatemia	• Alcoholism • TPN	• CNS depression including confusion and coma • Dysrhythmias • Decreased stroke volume • Fatigue • Lethargy • Muscle weakness including decreased respiratory drive • Osteomalacia • Rhabdomyolysis	• Replace with PO or IV sodium or potassium phosphate

(continued)

Table 8.2 Electrolyte Imbalances *(continued)*

Electrolyte	Causes	Signs and Symptoms	Treatment
Potassium (normal value: 3.5–5 mmol/L)			
Hyperkalemia	• Adrenal cortical insufficiency • Blood administration • Crush injuries • DKA • Potassium sparing diuretic use • Renal failure • Rhabdomyolysis	• Bradycardia • Cardiac arrest • EKG abnormalities including flattening or missing P waves, widening QRS complex, shortened QT interval, peaked T waves • Leg cramps • Paralysis of skeletal muscle • Respiratory failure • Weakness	• Calcium chloride, sodium bicarbonate, insulin, and glucose administration • Correct acidosis • Dialysis • Eliminate drugs that may be the cause • Furosemide • Kayexalate
Hypokalemia	• GI loss • Malnutrition • Renal failure	• Dysrhythmias • Cardiac arrest • Decreased GI motility • EKG findings: flattened T waves, emergence of the U wave, peaked P waves with increased amplitude • Fatigue • Hyperglycemia • Ileus • Muscle cramping • Paralysis • Respiratory failure • Weakness	• PO or IV potassium chloride replacement
Sodium (normal value: 135–145 mEq/L)			
Hypernatremia	• Water loss • Cushing's syndrome • Hyperaldosteronism • GI loss • DI • DKA • hyperosmolar hyperglycemic syndrome	• Agitation • Altered mental status • Coma • Dehydration • Irritability • Lethargy • Weakness • Seizures	• Replacement with free water via PO or through NG tube • IV D5 or D5 1/2 if unable to tolerate enteral administration • Gradual correction to prevent cerebral edema or neurologic complications

(continued)

Table 8.2 Electrolyte Imbalances *(continued)*

Electrolyte	Causes	Signs and Symptoms	Treatment
Sodium (normal value: 135–145 mEq/L) (continued)			
Hyponatremia	• CHF • Cirrhosis with ascites • Excess water intake • Fluid overload • Hypothyroidism • Renal failure • SIDAH • Thiazide diuretics	• Coma • Confusion • Nausea • Headache • Irritability • Lethargy • Seizures • Vomiting	• Sodium tablets and restrict free water • 3% NS intravenously • Gradual correction to prevent cerebral edema and osmotic demyelination

Diagnosis

Labs
- BMP
- Magnesium
- Parathyroid hormone
- Vitamin D levels

Diagnostic Testing
- EKG tracings help signal electrolyte abnormalities as evidenced by changes in cardiac conduction.

Nursing Interventions

- Administer medications to treat corresponding electrolyte imbalance as ordered (Tables 8.2 and 8.4).
- Assess musculoskeletal and neurologic status for changes or worsening condition.
- Draw and monitor serial labs as ordered.
- Ensure appropriate nutrition by adhering to fluid and electrolyte restrictions or supplementations.
- Monitor EKG tracings for electrolyte-related changes.

Patient Education

- Follow specific diet for corresponding electrolyte abnormality (Table 8.3).
- Follow up with lab draws to monitor levels of electrolytes.
- Self-monitor for worsening symptoms of corresponding electrolyte abnormality (Table 8.2), if possible.
- Take medications as prescribed to maintain regular electrolyte levels.

 ALERT!

Chvostek sign is a twitching of the facial muscles when tapping on the facial anterior nerve.

Trousseau sign is a carpopedal spasm that occurs while inflating a blood pressure cuff on the arm. Both are abnormal and can indicate an electrolyte abnormality.

 POP QUIZ 8.3

A patient diagnosed with hypokalemia is not responding appropriately to potassium supplementation. What additional labs should be checked?

Table 8.3 Electrolyte-Rich Foods

Electrolyte	Foods
High-potassium foods	<ul><li>Vegetables:<ul><li>Broccoli</li><li>Mushrooms</li><li>Leafy greens</li><li>Peas</li><li>Potatoes</li><li>Spinach</li><li>Sweet potatoes</li></ul></li><li>Dairy products: Milk, Yogurt</li><li>Fish: Tuna, cod, or halibut</li><li>Beans or legumes</li></ul>
High-sodium foods	<ul><li>Boxed or frozen meals</li><li>Canned foods</li><li>Cottage cheese</li><li>Deli meat</li><li>Ham</li><li>Hot dogs</li><li>Jerky or dried meats</li><li>Pickles</li><li>Pizza</li><li>Pork rinds</li><li>Shrimp</li><li>Salad dressing</li><li>Soups</li><li>Tortillas</li><li>Vegetable juice</li></ul>

Table 8.4 Renal Medications

Indications	Mechanism of Action	Contraindications, Precautions, and Adverse Effects
Alkalinizing agents (e.g., sodium bicarbonate)		
<ul><li>Management of metabolic acidosis, adjunct treatment of life-threatening hyperkalemia</li></ul>	<ul><li>Act as alkalinizing agent by releasing bicarbonate ions, thus correcting metabolic acidosis and shifting potassium intracellularly</li></ul>	<ul><li>Contraindications include metabolic or respiratory acidosis, hypocalcemia, and hypernatremia.</li><li>Use caution in CHF, renal failure, or concurrent use with corticosteroids.</li><li>Adverse effects include edema, metabolic alkalosis, hypernatremia, hypocalcemia, hypokalemia, sodium and water retention, tetany, and cerebral hemorrhage.</li></ul>

(continued)

Table 8.4 Renal Medications *(continued)*

Indications	Mechanism of Action	Contraindications, Precautions, and Adverse Effects
Calcium supplementation (e.g., calcium gluconate, calcium chloride)		
• Treatment and prevention of hypocalcemia, emergency treatment of hyperkalemia, hypermagnesemia, and adjunct treatment in cardiac arrest	• Replaces calcium in deficiency and helps maintain cell membrane and capillary permeability • Assists with contractility of cardiac, skeletal, and smooth muscle	• Medication is contraindicated in hypercalcemia, renal calculi, and ventricular fibrillation. • Use caution in patients receiving digoxin, patients with severe respiratory compromise, and patients with renal or cardiac disease. • Adverse effects include cardiac arrest, syncope, dysrhythmias, phlebitis, and calculi.
Cation exchanger (e.g., patiromer, zirconium cyclosilicate)		
• Treatment of hyperkalemia	• Binds potassium in GI lumen to increase fecal potassium excretion, thus decreasing serum potassium	• Use caution in patients with constipation, fecal impaction, GI obstruction, or a history of hypomagnesemia. • Do not give with other medications. Administer either 3 hr before or after any other medication. • Adverse effects include hypomagnesemia, constipation, hypokalemia, edema, diarrhea, and abdominal pain.
Diuretics: Loop (furosemide)		
• Fluid overload • Renal dysfunction	• Secretion of electrolytes and water by preventing resorption and increasing urine output	• Contraindications include hypersensitivity and cross sensitivity with sulfonamides (thiazide diuretics). • Use caution in hypokalemia, digoxin therapy, cardiac disease, and dysrhythmia. • Adverse effects include hypokalemia, dehydration, hypomagnesemia, and hyponatremia.
Dextrose (D50)		
• Hypoglycemia related to regular IV insulin administration to treat hyperkalemia	• Glucose replacement and supplementation	• Contraindications include hyperglycemia. • Adverse effects include hyperglycemia.
Electrolytes (magnesium sulfate)		
• Hypomagnesemia	• Increase magnesium levels to maintain acid-base balance, electrolyte balance, and homeostasis	• Contraindications include hypermagnesemia, hypocalcemia, anuria, and heart block. • Use caution in renal insufficiency. • Adverse effects include decreased respiratory drive, dysrhythmia, hypotension, drowsiness, diarrhea, and muscle weakness.

(continued)

Table 8.4 Renal Medications *(continued)*

Indications	Mechanism of Action	Contraindications, Precautions, and Adverse Effects
Electrolytes, phosphorous supplements (e.g., sodium phosphate, potassium phosphate)		
• Hypophosphatemia	• Increase serum phosphorous levels to maintain electrolyte balance	• Contraindications include hyperkalemia, hyperphosphatemia, infected phosphate stones, and severe renal impairment. • Use caution in patients with HTN, CHF, severe hepatic disease, renal insufficiency, and dehydration. • Adverse effects include dysrhythmia, abdominal discomfort, nausea, vomiting, diarrhea, and arthralgia.
Electrolytes (potassium chloride)		
• Hypokalemia	• Maintain acid-base balance and homeostasis	• Contraindications include hyperkalemia, hypermagnesemia, and severe renal disease. • Use caution in cardiac disease and/or dysrhythmia, renal impairment, or patients using potassium-sparing diuretics. • Adverse effects include dysrhythmia, confusion, restlessness, abdominal pain, flatulence, and IV site pain/burning.
Mineral binding agents (e.g., sodium polystyrene)		
• Treatment of life-threatening hyperkalemia	• Exchange sodium ions for potassium ions in the intestines, allowing for excretion of excessive potassium from the GI tract	• Medication is only used in rare settings. • Medication may be used *only* in a patient who meets *all* the following criteria: (a) potentially life-threatening hyperkalemia, (b) dialysis is not readily available, (c) new cation exchangers are not available, and (d) other therapies to remove potassium have failed or are not possible. • Do not give to the following patients due to the high risk for intestinal necrosis: postoperative patients, patients with an ileus or who are receiving opiates, patients with a large or small bowel obstruction, patients with underlying bowel disease. • Adverse effects include constipation, fecal impaction, nausea and vomiting, hypocalcemia, hypokalemia, sodium retention/hypernatremia, hypomagnesemia, and intestinal necrosis.
Polypeptide hormones (calcitonin)		
• Treatment of hypercalcemia	• Inhibit osteoclastic bone resorption and promote renal excretion of calcium-lowering serum calcium levels	• Contraindications include hypersensitivity to salmon protein or gelatin diluent. • Adverse effects include nausea and vomiting, facial flushing, and anaphylaxis.

(continued)

Table 8.4 Renal Medications *(continued)*

Indications	Mechanism of Action	Contraindications, Precautions, and Adverse Effects
Short-acting human insulin (regular insulin)		
• Hyperkalemia	• Forces potassium to move intracellularly	• Medication is given intravenously. • Contraindications include hypoglycemia. • Use caution in infection, stress, and changes in diet. • Adverse effects include hypoglycemia.
Vitamin D (vitamin D3: calcitriol, cholecalciferol, etc.)		
• Management of hypocalcemia in chronic renal disease or hypoparathyroidism	• Activation in the liver to promote the absorption of calcium and decrease PTH concentration to improve calcium and phosphorous homeostasis in patients with deficiency with or without CKD	• Contraindications include hypercalcemia, vitamin D toxicity, and malabsorption problems. • Use caution in patients receiving concurrent digoxin therapy. • Adverse effects include dizziness, dyspnea, pancreatitis, dysrhythmias, and edema.

RESOURCES

American Heart Association. (2005). Part 10.1: Life-threatening electrolyte abnormalities. *Circulation, 112*(24), IV-121–IV-125. https://www.ahajournals.org/doi/10.1161/CIRCULATIONAHA.105.166563

Griffin, B. R., Liu, K. D., & Teixeira, J. P. (2020, March). Critical care nephrology: Core curriculum 2020. *American Journal of Kidney Diseases, 75*, 435–452. https://www.ncbi.nlm.nih.gov/pmc/articles/PMC7333544/

National Kidney Foundation. (2019, May 31). *Sodium and your CKD diet: How to spice up your cooking*.https://www.kidney.org/atoz/content/sodiumckd

National Kidney Foundation. (2020, June 15). *Potassium and your CKD diet*. https://www.kidney.org/atoz/content/potassium

Prescribers' Digital Reference. (n.d.). *Calcitonin-salmon rDNA origin* [Drug information]. PDR Search. https://www.pdr.net/drug-summary/Fortical-calcitonin-salmon--rDNA-origin--1939

Prescribers' Digital Reference. (n.d.). *Calcium chloride* [Drug information]. PDR Search. https://www.pdr.net/drug-summary/10--Calcium-Chloride-calcium-chloride-3148

Prescribers' Digital Reference. (n.d.). *Potassium chloride* [Drug information]. PDR Search. https://www.pdr.net/drug-summary/K-Tab-potassium-chloride-1073

Prescribers' Digital Reference. (n.d.). *Regular, human insulin rDNA origin* [Drug information]. PDR Search. https://www.pdr.net/drug-summary/Humulin-R-regular--human-insulin--rDNA-origin--2912.3423

Prescribers' Digital Reference. (n.d.). *Sodium polystyrene sulfonate* [Drug information]. PDR Search. https://www.pdr.net/drug-summary/Kayexalate-sodium-polystyrene-sulfonate-2925.1687#14

Prescribers' Digital Reference. (n.d.). *Veltassa (patiromer)* [Drug information]. PDR Search. https://www.pdr.net/drug-summary/Veltassa-patiromer-3812

MUSCULOSKELETAL SYSTEM

FALLS

Overview

- A *fall* can result from a multitude of physical or environmental factors (Table 9.1).
- Patients can experience falls inside or outside of the hospital due to acute illness, medications, delirium, or overestimation of one's strength or functional ability.
- Falls increase morbidity and mortality and can lead to decreased functioning in all patients.

COMPLICATIONS

Falls can result in an acute fracture, TBI, subdural hematoma, pain, surgical intervention, decreased functioning ability, fear of additional falls, decreased quality of life, and/or transfer to an assisted living facility.

Table 9.1 Physical and Environmental Fall Risk Factors

Cognitive risk factors	• Acute or chronic memory impairments related to intellectual disabilities, dementia, or TBIs
Environmental risk factors	• Patients who live alone • Poor lighting in residence • Slippery floors • Tripping hazards (rugs, small animals, poor footwear, etc.) • Uneven surfaces
Psychological risk factors	• Fear of falling
Physical risk factors	• Female gender • History of previous falls • Increased age • Patients with comorbidities including: electrolyte or metabolic abnormalities, dysrhythmias or syncopal episodes, MI, stroke, infection, arthritis, vascular disease, thyroid dysfunction, diabetes, depression, COPD, incontinence, vertigo, and orthostatic hypotension or altered mental status • Patients with immobility, deconditioning, and/or gait impairments • Polypharmacy (benzodiazepines, antiarrhythmics, digoxin, diuretics, sedatives, and psychotropics) • Poor nutrition
Sensory risk factors	• Hearing impairments • Patients with neuropathy or poor circulation to the lower extremities • Vision impairment

Signs and Symptoms

Patients who have fallen may present with any of the following:

- Altered mental status
- Bruising
- Confusion
- Cuts or scrapes
- Fractures
- Head or facial trauma
- Lacerations
- Memory loss

> **NURSING PEARL**
>
> Patients who take certain medications such as benzodiazepines, antiarrhythmics, digoxin, diuretics, sedatives, and psychotropics have been found to be at higher risk for falls.

Diagnosis

Labs

There are no labs specific to diagnose falls. However, the following may be helpful to clarify the etiology, cause, and extent of sustained injury:

- BMP: assess electrolyte abnormalities to rule out anemia
- CBC: determine if fall is related to infectious process (WBC may be elevated) or anemia (low hemoglobin and hematocrit)
- Coagulation panel: determine coagulation status if patient on blood thinners (may be elevated)
- Glucose point of care: assess for hyper- or hypoglycemia or autonomic neuropathy related to diabetes
- Serum 25-hydroxyvitamin D levels: identify individuals with vitamin D deficiency who may benefit from vitamin D supplementation

Diagnostic Testing

There are no diagnostic tests specific to diagnose falls. However, the following may be helpful to clarify the etiology, cause, and extent of sustained injury:

- CT scan of the head, chest, and/or abdomen
- MRI
- TTE
- Ultrasound
- X-rays of the chest, pelvis, spine, or extremities

Treatment

- Address/treat secondary injuries resulting from the fall:
  - If a fracture was sustained, consult ortho/trauma for evaluation and possible surgery.
  - If a neurological injury was sustained, see Chapter 6.
- Extremity examination to uncover possible deformities of the feet contributing to risk of falling (bunions, calloused, and arthritic deformities)
- Full work-up to determine any underlying causes; for example, a syncopal episode may require a full cardiac work-up (Chapter 2)
- PT/OT consult
- Review/discontinue unnecessary medications contributing to polypharmacy
- Visual acuity, hearing, and muscle function assessment
- Vitamin D supplements as needed (Table 9.2*)

> **ALERT!**
>
> Be alert to older adult patients taking anticoagulants who have experienced a fall with head trauma, as they are at increased risk for intracranial bleeding.

Nursing Interventions

- Assist patient to the bathroom if not using Foley catheter/bedpan.
- Consult social work to perform in-home assessment.

---

* Table 9.2 is located at the end of this chapter.

- Discuss mobility orders with the patient (bedrest, with assistance, with assistive device, etc.).
- Instruct patient on fall risk precautions.
- Maintain fall precautions as ordered.
  - Adjust bed rails as ordered.
  - Keep call bell and personal belongings within reach.
  - Lower bed to lowest setting.
  - Place appropriate signage on door.
  - Place appropriate falls wrist band on patient.
  - Use antislip socks in the fall color corresponding to hospital policy (e.g., yellow).
- Obtain postural vital signs to rule out orthostatic hypotension.
- Perform serial neurological assessments if patient sustained a head bleed from the fall or shows any signs of deterioration in neurological status.
- Provide assistive devices (walker, cane) and personal support (gait belt) to maintain patient safety while ambulating.
- Provide a safe environment free of tripping hazards if patient is ambulatory. Remove or secure:
  - Clutter on floor
  - IV lines/tubes
  - Medical devices
  - SCDs
- Provide therapeutic communication.

Patient Education

- Engage in exercise programs that encourage balance, endurance, flexibility, and resistance:
  - Tai chi
  - Yoga
- Collaborate with caregivers on home modifications to decrease environmental risk for falls.
- Encourage proper nutrition.
- Use call bell for needs outside of reach. (e.g., lunch tray, book and personal belongings)
- Home assessment:
  - Add nonslip surfaces/mats
  - Add rails
  - Fall alert system, if appropriate
  - Flatten uneven surfaces; place ramps over steps
  - Remove rugs
  - Shower chairs

 POP QUIZ 9.1

A patient is admitted to the PCU after an unwitnessed fall at home. During your intake assessment, you learn that the patient has a past medical history of diabetes, A-fib, and GERD. The patient also wears glasses. He lives alone, but his daughter visits daily. She is currently working to fall proof his house by removing loose rugs and installing handrails on the stairwells. Which of the five types of risk factors for falls does this patient currently present with?

GAIT DISTURBANCES

Overview

- A *gait disturbance* is any deviation from a normal walking pattern that results in an increased risk for an injury or fall.
- Gait disturbances can occur due to a multitude of conditions, including degenerative disk or bone disease, Parkinson disease, multiple sclerosis, kyphosis, muscle atrophy, or any condition that causes exercise intolerance and decreased mobility.
- Neurological and musculoskeletal abnormalities are the most common cause of gait abnormalities and disturbances.

 COMPLICATIONS

Patients with gait abnormalities are at increased risk for falls, paralysis, syncope, skeletal fractures, epidural/subdural trauma, and psychosocial stigma. Those who do experience a fall are at increased risk for morbidity, mortality, and reduced functioning.

Signs and Symptoms

- Symptoms of gait disturbances may include abnormalities in any of the following:
  - Arm swing
  - Posture
  - Running pattern
  - Speed
  - Stance
  - Standing
  - Step length
  - Walking pattern
- Additionally, gait disturbances may manifest as:
  - Freezing
  - Heels walking
  - Positive Romberg's test
  - Tandem gait
  - Toes walking
  - Turning

Diagnosis

Labs
There are no labs specific to diagnose gait disturbances.

Diagnostic Testing
Imaging dependent on findings obtained during history and physical:
- CT scan
- MRI
- X-rays

Treatment

Treatment dependent on etiology of the gait disturbance:
- Aerobic exercise
- Electrical stimulator
- Low resistance strength training
- Medications (Table 9.2)
  - Dopamine agonist/Antiparkinson agents
  - Vitamin B12
- Muscle strengthening
- Shoe lifts
- Solid or hinged ankle foot orthosis
- Surgery

 ALERT!

Gait abnormalities resulting from Parkinson disease are best treated with a combination of medication therapy, deep brain stimulation, and allied health support including treadmill walking, cognitive training, and home-based exercise programs.

Nursing Interventions

Maintain fall precautions as ordered (see Falls section for additional details).

Patient Education

- Follow treatment guidelines for specific etiology causing gait disturbances.
- Use assistive devices as ordered.
- See the Falls section for additional patient education.

 POP QUIZ 9.2

Patients with gait abnormalities resulting from Parkinson disease would benefit from which therapies to improve stability?

IMMOBILITY

Overview

- Immobility can result from critical illness, lack of motivation, or a combination of both.
- For patients admitted to the PCU, immobility may complicate primary illness and result in an increased length of stay due to a range of both short- and long-term effects.

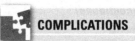

COMPLICATIONS

Immobility can result in pressure ulcers, deformities, joint pain, loss of muscle and bone mass, DVT, PE, atelectasis, pneumonia, and decreased functioning in cardiovascular, endocrine, immune, GI, excretory, vestibular, cognitive, and psychological systems. These can impact morbidity and mortality rates.

Signs and Symptoms

- Flaccid extremities
- Lack of motivation
- Lack of movement/inability to mobilize any part of the body
- Muscle atrophy

Diagnosis

Labs

There are no labs specific to diagnose immobility. However, the following may be helpful in the initial workup to understand causes for immobility.

- BMP
- CBC
- Coagulation panel

Diagnostic Testing

- Imaging to rule out underlying etiology:
  - CT scans
  - MRI
  - X-ray
- Musculoskeletal assessment (e.g., the timed up and go test)
- Neurological assessment
  - Cognitive functioning
  - Gait assessment
  - Motor strength

Treatment

- Identification and correction of underlying cause of functional disability as possible
- Participation in PT and OT sessions
  - Scheduled activity sessions to encourage mobility
  - Repetition of skills practiced with PT, which may include sitting at the side of the bed, standing, pivoting to a chair, and ambulating
  - Activity as often as safely possible, being mindful of potential removal of drains, lines, or tubes
  - Can be completed in a bed or chair (e.g., arm raises, calf pumps, and leg raises)
- Administration of corresponding treatments and medications to assist in correcting underlying cause of functional disability
- Identification and treatment of any complications of prolonged immobility if present:
  - Clot prevention:
    - Anticoagulants (Table 3.1)
    - Interior vena cava filter
    - SCDs

(continued)

Treatment *(continued)*

- Pneumonia
  - ○ Chest PT
  - ○ Medications (Table A.1)
- Pressure ulcer prevention

Nursing Interventions

 NURSING PEARL

While immobility may be due to critical illness, sometimes it may be due to a lack of personal patient motivation. To help encourage and motivate the patient, develop a therapeutic relationship and seek to understand motivations. Motivating factors could be family (kids, grandkids, spouse), pets, work, or hobbies. Encourage the patient and establish achievable goals both in and out of the hospital.

- Administer anticoagulation medications as ordered.
- Coordinate mobilization or ambulation attempts with additional support staff as needed (e.g., respiratory therapy and PT).
- Communicate directions and plan for mobilization effectively.
  - Secure all devices, drains, lines, and tubes prior to mobilization or ambulation.
  - Place call bell within reach if mobilizing patient out of bed to chair.
- Encourage patient to perform daily care as much as independently possible (e.g., brushing teeth, washing face, and brushing hair).
- Monitor vital signs changes during activity.
- Prevent pressure ulcers.
  - Change pads, dressings, diapers, or sheets if wet or soiled.
  - Keep skin clean and dry.
  - Offload pressure on bony prominences by turning patient with pillows and elevating heels.
  - Reposition frequently to alleviate pressure on bony prominences and redistribute weight.
  - Monitor for new areas of skin breakdown.
  - Pad bony prominences and skin that comes into contact with lines, drains, or tubes to prevent skin breakdown.
  - Perform skin assessment each shift and document changes as noted.
  - Turn every 2 hr as ordered.
  - Elevate heels to prevent skin breakdown.
  - Encourage appropriate nutrition to decrease risk of pressure ulcers.
- Provide emotional and therapeutic support for patients engaging in physical activity during or shortly following critical illness.
  - Create and encourage attainable goals.
  - Celebrate accomplishments and improvements.
  - Encourage and motivate patient, if possible, to perform physical activity and regain mobility to achieve postdischarge goal.

Patient Education

 POP QUIZ 9.3

Promoting physical activity and preventing immobility is essential to prevent which three major pulmonary, integumentary, and circulatory complications?

- Identify personal motivating factors.
  - Create future goals to help motivate patient to remain as active as possible.
  - Performing physical activity with others at a gym, with family members, or with support groups.
- If patient is completely immobile or requires total care, family might consider obtaining a home lift to assist with mobility and turning or consult home healthcare assistance.
- Offload pressure on bony prominences at home by elevating extremities, turning, and repositioning.

● Perform as much activity as physically able to prevent additional loss of mobility.
  ● Start slow and increase pace as able and indicated by provider.
  ● Set appropriate and attainable goals.

Table 9.2 Musculoskeletal Medications

Indications	Mechanism of Action	Contraindications, Precautions, and Adverse Effects
Antiparkinson agents (levodopa/carbidopa)		
● Treatment of motor fluctuations in patients with advanced Parkinson disease	● Cross the blood-brain barrier to increase dopamine levels within the corpus striatum to improve nerve impulse and decrease motor symptoms	● Contraindications include concurrent use with MAOIs. ● Do not abruptly discontinue. ● Use caution with cardiac disease, MI, hypotension, behavioral changes, depression, psychosis, coadministration with other CNS depressants, GI disease, diabetes mellitus, melanoma, pheochromocytoma, pulmonary, hepatic and renal disease, peripheral neuropathy, HF, and electrolyte imbalances. ● Adverse effects include akinesia, seizures, GI bleeding, GI obstruction, MI, new primary malignancy, angioedema, hypotension, depression, confusion, hallucinations, increased hepatic enzymes, urinary incontinence, edema, blurred vision, nausea, anxiety, and vomiting.
Vitamin D supplement (ergocalciferol)		
● Vitamin D deficiency	● Metabolize vitamin D into calcitriol, which promotes renal reabsorption of calcium, increases intestinal absorption of calcium and phosphorus, and increases calcium mobilization from bone to plasma, which promotes skeletal strength and increases muscle fiber growth to help with balance	● Vitamin D supplements are contraindicated in hypercalcemia and malabsorption syndrome. ● Use caution in renal failure, renal disease, and pregnancy. ● Adverse effects include fatigue, headache, nausea, increased thirst, and increased urinary frequency.
Vitamin B12 supplements (cyanocobalamin)		
● Vitamin B12 deficiency	● Assist in metabolic processes, such as fat and carbohydrate metabolism, protein synthesis, cell production, and hematopoiesis	● Vitamin B12 is contraindicated in cobalt hypersensitivity. ● Use caution in renal impairment, myelosuppression, uremia, infection, iron or folate deficiency, and polycythemia. ● Adverse effects include headache, nausea, anxiety, ataxia, diarrhea, itching, swelling, infection, thrombocytosis, or hypokalemia.

RESOURCES

Alaparthi, G. K., Gatty, A., Samuel, S. R., & Amaravadi, S. K. (2020, November 26). Effectiveness, safety, and barriers to early mobilization in the intensive care unit. *Critical Care Research and Practice*. https://www.ncbi. nlm.nih.gov/pmc/articles/PMC7714600/

AHRQ. (2021). *Tool 3H: Morse fall scale for identifying fall risk factors*. https://www.ahrq.gov/patient-safety/settings/ hospital/fall-prevention/toolkit/morse-fall-scale.html

Deglin, J. H., Vallerand, A. H., & Sanoski, C. A. (2011). *Davis's drug guide for nurses*. F.A. Davis.

Epocrates. (n.d). *Cyanocobalamin (vitamin B12) adult dosing* [Drug information]. *Epocrates Web*. https://online. epocrates.com/drugs/1877/cyanocobalamin-vitamin-B12?MultiBrandAlert=true

Huether, S. E., & McCance, K. L. (2012). *Understanding pathophysiology*. Elsevier/Mosby.

InformedHealth.org. (2018, November 15). *Pressure ulcers: Overview*. Institute for Quality and Efficiency in Health Care. https://www.ncbi.nlm.nih.gov/books/NBK326428/

Lewis, S. M. (2011). *Medical-surgical nursing: Assessment and management of clinical problems*. Mosby.

Lupescu, O., Nagea, M., Patru, C., Vasilache, C., & Popescu, G. I. (2015, June). *Treatment options for distal femoral fractures. Maedica*. https://www.ncbi.nlm.nih.gov/pmc/articles/PMC5327816/

National Institute on Aging. (n.d.). *Prevent falls and fractures*. U.S. Department of Health and Human Services, National Institute on Aging. https://www.nia.nih.gov/health/prevent-falls-and-fractures

Parida, S., & Mishra, S. K. (2013, November). Urinary tract infections in the critical care unit: A brief review. *Indian Journal of Critical Care Medicine*, *17*(6), 370–374. https://www.ncbi.nlm.nih.gov/pmc/articles/PMC3902573/

Prescribers' Digital Reference. (n.d.). *Sinemet* [Drug information]. PDR Search. https://www.pdr.net/drug-summary/Sinemet-carbidopa-levodopa-388#11

Prescribers' Digital Reference. (n.d.). *Ergocalciferol* [Drug information]. PDR Search. https://www.pdr.net/drug-summary/Ergocalciferol-ergocalciferol-24306#10

Wu, X., Li, Z., Cao, J., Jiao, J., Wang, Y., Liu, G., Liu, Y., Li, F., Song, B., Jin, J., Liu, Y., Wen, X., Cheng, S., & Wan, X. (2018). The association between major complications of immobility during hospitalization and quality of life among bedridden patients: A 3 month prospective multi-center study. *PLoS One*, *13*(10), e0205729. https:// www.ncbi.nlm.nih.gov/pmc/articles/PMC6185860/#:~:text=Immobility%20is%20independently%20 associated%20with,(UTI)%20%5B4%5D

ACUTE AND CHRONIC PAIN

Overview

- Acute and/or chronic pain exacerbations are common causes for hospital admissions.
  - *Acute pain* is sudden, often resulting from acute injury, trauma, or disease process.
  - *Chronic pain* persists for 6 or more months.
- In the hospital setting, pain can be caused by:
  - Devices such as drains, endotracheal tubes, Foley catheters, or invasive monitoring lines
  - Immobility
  - Invasive procedures
  - Suctioning
  - Surgical incisions
  - Trauma
  - Wound care
- It is important to identify the cause of pain to appropriately treat the pain. The pain or discomfort can often be relieved by nonpharmacologic intervention and assessing for and treating complications from above causes.

COMPLICATIONS

If pain is not treated, delayed wound healing, hyperglycemia, atelectasis, delirium, depression, and PTSD may occur.

Signs and Symptoms

- Agitation
- Anxiety
- Crying
- Dependence/substance abuse (chronic pain)
- Depression (chronic pain)
- Facial grimacing
- Feelings of discomfort that can be described as:
  - Burning
  - Dull
  - Pressure
  - Ripping
  - Sharp
  - Stabbing
  - Tearing
  - Tingling
- HTN
- Muscle tension
- Tachycardia
- Vocalization of distress: yelling or screaming

NURSING PEARL

Physiologic reactions to pain such as tachycardia should be monitored, as this can exacerbate or worsen clinical condition.

Diagnosis

Labs

There are no labs specific to the diagnosis of acute and chronic pain. However, the following may be indicated based on the patient's clinical status:

- ABG
- CBC
- CMP

Diagnostic Testing

Further work-up may be indicated if pain is suspected in a specific area on the body:

- CT scan
- MRI
- Ultrasound
- X-ray

Treatment

- Analgesics (Table A.2)
- Identification and treatment of cause of the pain
- Methods to prevent pain from occurring:
  - Avoidance of triggers (if known)
  - Frequent assessment
  - Timely medication administration
- Nerve blocks if appropriate
- Nonpharmacologic intervention, including:
  - Elevation of effected extremity
  - Hot/cold compress
  - Rest
- Possible need for sedation if analgesics alone cannot treat pain; may require transfer to higher level of care

Nursing Interventions

- Assess pain as the sixth vital sign. Use appropriate pain scale for patient (e.g., 0–10, Faces, and pain assessment in advanced dementia scale).
- Collaborate with interdisciplinary team for a pain management plan.
- Ensure analgesic reversal medications are easily available in the event of accidental oversedation.
- Ensure pain assessment accuracy by utilizing the appropriate pain scale for the patient.
- Provide nonpharmacologic methods to reduce pain, such as repositioning, cold or heat, range of motion, relaxation techniques, and providing a calm environment.

Patient Education

- Avoid self-medicating with illicit drugs, unprescribed medications, or alcohol.
- Consult with a pain clinic for outpatient follow-up and maintenance of medication regimens.
- Ensure family or caregiver is involved in pain management plan.
- Ensure realistic pain score goals.
- Ensure understanding of pain management plan at discharge.

 POP QUIZ 10.1

A patient returns from surgery, where they had a laparoscopic hysterectomy. They received pain medication in the PACU and were returned to the PCU. On first assessment, the patient's abdomen is soft to palpitation and lap sites are clean, dry and intact. The patient, however, reports pain 6/10 in the lower abdomen that she describes as stabbing or cramping. The patient is only verbally responsive to touch and can keep her eyes open only for a few seconds. Vital signs are as follows: HR 91, BP 105/74, RR 8, SPO₂ 92% on 4LNC, and temperature 97.8 °F (36.6 °C). Given the patient's clinical presentation and pain rating, what should the nurse's next action be?

- Follow up with outpatient appointments as scheduled.
- If applicable, seek extra support through or continue to attend AA and/or NA meetings.
- If pain is worsening or the prescribed regimen is no longer working, contact the provider, pain management service, or clinic for further work-up.
- Take prescribed medications as ordered.
- Utilize nonpharmacologic interventions to manage pain.
- Utilize pain prevention methods.
- Utilize the minimum dosage of analgesics necessary to relieve pain.
- Wean pain medications as indicated per physician order.

END-OF-LIFE CARE

Overview

- Goals of care at the transition of end-of-life range from curing disease to improving comfort and quality of life.
- Care at the end-of-life requires collaboration between healthcare providers, patients, and families to provide care that focuses on comfort and minimal pain or suffering.

Signs and Symptoms

- Alterations in breathing
  - Apnea
  - Cheyne–Stokes breathing
  - "Death rattle"
- Cognitive changes
- Delirium
- Fatigue
- Lethargy
- Increased oral secretions
- Immobility
- Loss of interest in food or drink

Treatment

- Palliative care/hospice (see Palliative Care section for additional information).
- Medications to relieve pain and suffering:
  - Antiemetics (Table 7.1)
  - Anxiolytics (Table 11.1)
  - Opioid analgesics (Table A.2)
- Psychosocial and spiritual support

Nursing Interventions

- Administer medications as ordered for pain relief and symptom management.
- Assess for respiratory distress.
- Collaborate with patient, family, and all members of interdisciplinary care.
- Consider consult to spiritual care, palliative care, and/or hospice.
- Encourage nutrition as possible.
- Establish relationship and rapport with patient and family.
- Identify any cultural considerations the patient and family may have.
- Mobilize patient per patient request.
- Monitor family and patient behavior for signs of physical or emotional distress.
- Monitor lung sounds.

(continued)

Nursing Interventions *(continued)*

- Monitor sleep patterns.
- Provide oxygen if necessary (as determined by plan of care).
- Provide non pharmacologic interventions to promote a calm and comfortable environment.

Patient Education

- Family:
  - Learn what to expect in the final stages of death.
  - Understand interventions to alleviate and reduce pain or suffering.
- Learn the importance of legal documents such as advanced directives and power of attorney and share with family.

HEALTHCARE-ACQUIRED INFECTIONS
Overview

- *Healthcare-acquired infections* are infections that were not present on admission but are acquired through the course of a hospital stay.
- Common health-acquired infections are: CAUTIs, CLABSIs, and SSIs (see Surgical Wound section).
  - *CAUTIs* are urinary tract infects that result from a bladder catheter.
  - *CLABSIs* are bloodstream infections that result from any type of central line insertion.
  - Both CLABSIs and CAUTIs are preventable infections that can lead to severe complications in the acutely ill patient population.
- Healthcare staff should maintain a high standard for infection control and be vigilant in assessing for these infections to protect their patients.

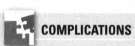 **COMPLICATIONS**

Healthcare-associated infections can complicate a patient's condition, lead to prolonged hospitalization, and cause bacteremia, sepsis, septic shock, and death. Infection protocols should be enforced in all areas of the hospital to prevent these complications.

Signs and Symptoms

- CAUTI
  - Abdominal, flank, or suprapubic pain
  - AMS or delirium
  - Burning with urination
  - Fever or chills
  - Foul-smelling urine
  - Positive urinary culture
  - Pus or drainage around insertion site
  - Urine color or consistency changes (cloudy, dark, etc.)
- CLABSI
  - AMS or delirium
  - Central line insertion site:
    - Drainage or pus
    - Pain
    - Red or feel warmth to touch
    - Swollen
  - Fever or chills
- SSI
  - Fever or chills
  - Surgical incision site incision:
    - Pain
    - Poor wound healing

- Pus or foul-smelling drainage
- Redness or warm to the touch
- Swollen

Diagnosis

Labs
- BMP
- CBC: WBC likely elevated with an infectious process
- Cultures:
  - Blood culture likely positive in patients with CLABSI
  - Urine culture likely positive in patients with CAUTI
- Lactate: likely elevated in septic patients

Diagnostic Testing
- CT scan
- Ultrasound
- X-ray

Treatment

- Antibiotics (Table A.1)
- Fluid resuscitation
- Removal of infected line or tube; possible replacement of central line in new location as indicated per institutional protocol and patient clinical status
- Possible for SSI:
  - Drains
  - Exploration and debridement
  - Negative pressure wound therapy
  - See Wounds: Surgical Wounds section

ALERT!

Closely monitor wound drainage on either the dressing or surgically placed drain for changes in output, color, volume, or consistency. This may indicate postsurgical infection and require prompt assessment and intervention.

Nursing Interventions

- Administer medications as ordered.
- Assess airway, breathing, and circulation.
- Assess lines, drains, tubes, and wounds for signs of infection.
- Assess vital signs for symptoms of infection.
  - Fever
  - Hypotension
  - Tachycardia
- CAUTI prevention:
  - Assess urinary output for color, consistency, and odor as frequently as recommended per institutional protocol.
  - Perform peri-care and Foley care every shift with institutionally recommended hygiene solutions.
  - Remove or exchange Foley as recommended per institutional protocol.
- CLABSI prevention:
  - Assess central line site every shift.
  - Assess each port for patency each shift.
  - Change central line dressing per institutional protocol or if dirty/soiled.
  - Change IV tubing for all medications per institutional protocol.
  - Make sure dressing remains occlusive.
  - Scrub the central line hubs for at least 15 seconds before use.

(continued)

Nursing Interventions *(continued)*

- SSI prevention:
  - Assess the surgical site each shift.
  - Keep surgical site clean and change dressing, as ordered.
  - See the Surgical Wounds section for more information.
- Initiate appropriate isolation precautions.
- Provide medication management.
- Remove lines when no longer necessary
- Perform frequent hand hygiene and don gloves. If a patient is on contact precautions, wear gown before entering room.

Patient Education

- If going home with a chronic indwelling urinary catheter, make sure to clean around the catheter at least daily and when soiled.
- Notify the nurse or healthcare team for any changes at the catheter, central line, or surgical site.
- Practice good infection prevention practices and frequent hand hygiene.

 POP QUIZ 10.2

A 55-year-old female is admitted to the PCU with a suspected CAUTI. The provider ordered broad-spectrum antibiotics to be given now and every 8 hr for the next week. The nurse removes the antibiotics from the medication dispensing system but, before administering, notices that blood cultures were never collected in the emergency room. What should the nurse's next action be?

INFLUENZA

Overview

- *Influenza* (commonly called the flu) is a contagious viral disease that affects the upper and lower respiratory tract.
- While influenza can affect people of all ages, it is especially dangerous for young children, pregnant women, or patients who are elderly or immunocompromised.

 COMPLICATIONS

Complications of influenza include secondary bacterial pneumonia, ARDs, myositis, myocarditis, respiratory and multiorgan failure, and death. Prevention, early identification, and treatment are key to preventing these dangerous complications.

Signs and Symptoms

- Congestion
- Cough
- Cyanosis
- Dyspnea
- Fever
- Fatigue
- Headache
- Hypotension
- Myalgia
- Respiratory distress
- Rhinorrhea
- Sore throat
- Tachycardia
- Weakness

Diagnosis

Labs
- ABG
- CBC

- Influenza swab for antigen or PCR testing
- Respiratory viral panel
- Sputum cultures

Diagnostic Testing
- Chest x-ray

Treatment

- Antiviral therapy (e.g., oseltamivir) (Table 10.3*)
- Symptom management
  - Acetaminophen for fever
  - Cough suppressants
- Support oxygenation
  - Oxygen therapy as needed
  - Respiratory therapy consult as needed
  - Acid–base balance and CO_2 monitoring to avoid complications
  - Regular chest x-rays to monitor for worsening infection, new infection, or lung damage

Nursing Interventions

- Administer fluids to prevent dehydration.
- Assess airway, breathing, and circulation.
- Assess respiratory status and vital signs.
  - Administer oxygen if needed.
  - Administer antipyretics as needed.
- Initiate droplet precautions.
- Encourage pulmonary hygiene (turn cough and deep breath).
- Encourage use of incentive spirometry.
- If status continues to worsen despite escalation of oxygenation therapy, notify the provider and prepare for transport to higher level of care. Patient may require pressors, ventilation, and/or ECMO support depending on clinical status.
- Update patient on current status, such as improving labs or vital signs.

Patient Education

- Get seasonal influenza vaccine in future influenza seasons.
- Infection control: Stay home until fever free for at least 24 hr (without the use of antipyretics) before returning to normal activities.
- Take OTC medications to manage symptoms.

MULTIDRUG-RESISTANT ORGANISMS

Overview

- Multidrug resistance develops when bacteria evolve and become resistant to certain antibiotics.
- MDROs render many pharmacologic treatments ineffective, as these antibiotics can no longer be used to control or kill the bacteria.

COMPLICATIONS

Organisms resistant to pharmacologic treatment can result in deterioration of condition, sepsis, and death, especially in acutely ill or immunocompromised patients.

Signs and Symptoms

- Bacterial infections and organisms unresponsive to standard antibiotic therapy
- Deteriorating condition despite treatment:

(continued)

---

* Table 10.3 is located at the end of this chapter.

Signs and Symptoms *(continued)*

- Acid-base imbalances
- Altered mental status
- Cyanosis/hypoxia
- Fever or hypothermia
- Hypotension
- Irritability
- Lethargy
- Normal or decreased BP
- Oliguria
- Pallor
- Shortness of breath
- Skin warmth
- Tachycardia
- Tachypnea

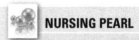 **NURSING PEARL**

When treating an MDRO, collaboration between nursing, pharmacy, and medicine is necessary to implement an effective course of treatment.

Diagnosis

Labs

- Positive cultures from any of the following, based on suspected location or type of infection:
  - Blood
  - Fecal
  - Sputum
  - Urine
- Sensitivity studies to determine which medications MDROs are susceptible

Treatment

- Collaboration with pharmacy to devise appropriate pharmacologic combination therapy based on cultures
- Appropriate antimicrobial therapy based on susceptibilities from culture results

 ALERT!

Patients with MDRO infections should be placed on the appropriate contact, respiratory, or airborne precautions to prevent further spread to other patients on the unit.

Nursing Interventions

- Administer medications as ordered.
- Assess airway, breathing, and circulation.
- Draw and monitor labs as ordered.
- Don institutionally required PPE to enter contact precaution room. This may include a disposable gown and gloves to reduce transmission to other patients and reduce contact with bodily fluids.
- Perform a complete head-to-toe assessment.
- Perform hand hygiene before entering and after leaving room.

Patient Education

- Finish all the antimicrobial therapy prescribed as indicated, even if feeling better.
- Notify future providers of history of MDRO infection.
- Once discharged from the hospital, frequently wash hands, towels, bed sheets, kitchen, and bathroom countertops to prevent transmission to others.
- Stay up-to-date on infection status.

- Understand contact precautions if infected with MDRO.
- Understand and stay up-to-date on plan of care.

PALLIATIVE CARE

Overview

- Palliative care prioritizes quality of life by anticipating, treating, and preventing suffering for patients with terminal or serious illness.
- In addition to the physical and psychosocial aspects of care, palliative care also focuses on the emotional and spiritual needs of the patient.

Signs and Symptoms

Patients progressing toward palliative care may exhibit any of the following symptoms:
- Bowel habit changes
- Cognitive changes
- Delirium
- Difficulty sleeping/changes to sleep–wake cycles
- Fatigue
- Lethargy
- Increased oral secretions
- Immobility
- Loss of interest in food or drink

Treatment

- Consult to palliative care/hospice services
- Medications to relieve pain and suffering:
  - Antiemetics (Table 7.1)
  - Anxiolytics (Table 11.1)
  - Opioid analgesics (Table A.2)
- Psychosocial and spiritual support
- Transfer to home or an outpatient hospice facility if applicable

Nursing Interventions

- Assess for acute changes in breathing and respiration.
- Assist frequently with peri-care and anticipate an increasing loss of bowel/bladder control.
- Collaborate with patient, family, and all members of interdisciplinary team.
- Consider consult to spiritual care, social work, home care, and/or hospice.
- Provide small, frequent meals with foods the patient enjoys, as tolerated.
- Provide non pharmacologic interventions to promote a calm and comfortable environment.
- Provide oxygen and IV hydration, if necessary, as determined by plan of care.

Patient Education

- Consult social work to provide information on how to set up legal documents such as an advanced directive and power of attorney.
- Learn what to expect in the stages of death and ensure family understands.
- Understand and ensure family understands what to expect moving into palliative care:
  - Palliative care, unlike hospice care, has no deadline/timeline.
  - Quality of life is emphasized over duration of life.

RHABDOMYOLYSIS

Overview

- *Rhabdomyolysis* is the rapid breakdown of muscle and release of intracellular muscle constituents into the bloodstream.
- Rhabdomyolysis has many causes including trauma, drugs, infection, excessive muscular contraction, DKA, heatstroke, and severe electrolyte disorders.

Signs and Symptoms

- Abdominal pain
- Dark-colored urine (cola/coffee colored)
- Fever
- Malaise
- Muscle pain
- Nausea and vomiting
- Tachycardia
- Weakness

Diagnosis

Labs

- BMP:
  - Elevated BUN and creatinine
  - Hyperkalemia
  - Hyperphosphatemia
  - Hypocalcemia
  - Metabolic acidosis common, and increased anion gap possible
  - Severe hyperuricemia
- CBC: May indicate elevated WBC with infection and crush injuries
- Elevated serum CK levels:
  - At presentation: usually at least five times upper limit of normal, but range from approximately 1,500 to over 100,000 international units/L
  - Begins to rise within 2 to 12 hr following onset of muscle injury and reaches maximum within 24 to 72 hr
- ESR and CRP: Likely elevated with infection and crush injuries
- Toxicology screen: May be positive
- Urinalysis: Possible evidence of myoglobinuria from urine sample

Diagnostic Testing

There are no diagnostic tests specific to diagnose rhabdomyolysis. However, the following may be helpful in the overall workup:

- CT scan
- EMG
- MRI
- Muscle biopsy

Treatment

- Major therapy: Early and aggressive fluid resuscitation (Table A.3)
  - No formal treatment guideline or protocol available
  - Follow institutional guidelines.

COMPLICATIONS

Rhabdomyolysis can result in acute kidney injury, chronic renal failure, electrolyte abnormalities (potassium, phosphate, calcium), and DIC. It is essential to identify and treat rhabdomyolysis before the kidneys become compromised.

ALERT!

Hyperkalemia can develop in patients with rhabdomyolysis as a result from decreased renal clearance from acute kidney injury and additionally from potassium release from damaged muscle. Standard hyperkalemia treatments can help manage this complication.

- Dialysis: Management of hyperkalemia, correction of acidosis, or for the treatment of volume overload
- Possible fasciotomy if complicated by compartment syndrome; pressure relief in compartment to increase muscle perfusion and prevent muscle breakdown and death
- Treatment of metabolic abnormalities possibly required, including:
  - Hypocalcemia: calcium gluconate
  - Hyperkalemia: regular insulin, dextrose, nebulized beta 2 agonists, furosemide, sodium polystyrene, and so forth.
  - Hyperuricemia: allopurinol
  - In patients with DIC, possible FFP

ursing Interventions

- Administer IV fluids as ordered. Ensure peripheral IV access site is patent or deliver high volume fluid resuscitation through central line if available.
- Assess and draw CK and BMPs as ordered to treat renal function, electrolyte changes, and assess whether patient is responding to fluid resuscitation.
- Maintain plasma pH <7.5.
- Monitor hourly urine output and labs for the following:
  - Urine output goal of 200 mL/hr
  - Urine pH >6.5
- Monitor vital signs for EKG changes related to electrolyte abnormalities.
- Perform neurovascular checks if there is a concern for compartment syndrome.
- Treat electrolyte abnormalities as ordered.

atient Education

- Stay up to date on current status, changes to condition, and/or plan of care (e.g., initiation of dialysis).
- Notify the nurse of status changes:
  - Dizziness
  - New or worsening tremor
  - Palpitations
  - Worsening weakness
  - Worsening pain
- Pursue drug and alcohol cessation as appropriate based on presenting condition.

POP QUIZ 10.3

A patient with rhabdomyolysis is admitted to the PCU. They have received medical treatment for the resulting hyperkalemia; however, the most recent potassium on the BMP was 6.2. Urine output was 15 mL/hr over the last 2 hr. What should the next intervention be?

SEPSIS

Overview

- *Sepsis* refers to systemic inflammatory response syndrome with an accompanying infectious source.
- Sepsis has a high morbidity and mortality rate; early identification and treatment is essential to prevent complications.

COMPLICATIONS

Complications of sepsis include septic shock, multiorgan failure, and death.

Signs and Symptoms

- Changes in mentation
  - Altered mental status
  - Confusion
  - Delirium

(continued)

Signs and Symptoms *(continued)*

- Cyanosis
- Dyspnea
- Pain
- Skin changes
  - Cold and clammy
  - Warm and flushed
- Vital sign changes
  - Fever or hypothermia (>100.4 °F (38 °C) or <96.8 °F (36 °C)
  - Hypotension
  - Tachycardia
  - Tachypnea

Diagnosis

Labs

- ABG: may indicate acidosis, hypoxemia, or hypercarbia
- Blood cultures: likely positive
- Blood glucose
- CBC: elevated WBC
- CMP
- Coagulation panel
- CRP: likely elevated
- Lactate level: likely >2 mmol/L if septic shock
- Mixed venous ScvO$_2$
- Troponins
- Urinalysis
- Urine cultures

Diagnostic Testing

- Chest x-ray
- CT scan
- Ultrasound

Treatment

- Antibiotics (Table A.1)
- Corticosteroids (Table A.4)
- Fever control
- Identification and treatment of cause of infection
- If possible, removal of infectious source
- IV fluid resuscitation (Table A.3)
- Organ support
  - Dialysis
  - Ventilation
- Vasopressors—patient may require higher level of care (Table 2.8)

Nursing Interventions

- Administer medications as prescribed.
- Assess mental status.

 NURSING PEARL

Use the following criteria for grading sepsis and septic shock:

- *Systemic inflammatory response syndrome* is a systemic response to infection with at least two of the following symptoms:
  - Temperature outside of range 96.8 °F–100.4 °F (36 °C–38 °C)
  - HR >90
  - RR >20
  - PaCO$_2$ >32 mmHg
  - WBC outside of range 4,000 to 12,000
- *Sepsis* is an identified infection in combination with at least two criteria for systemic inflammatory response syndrome.
- *Severe sepsis* is sepsis with evidence of end organ dysfunction.
- *Septic shock* is severe sepsis with both of the following:
  - Persisting hypotension with vasopressor use to maintain MAP ≥65 mmHg
  - Lactate >2 mmol/L despite fluid resuscitation

 NURSING PEARL

Positive blood cultures are helpful for individualized treatment; however, they are not a prerequisite for diagnosis. Up to 33% of sepsis patients have negative blood cultures due to intermittent bacteremia.

- Collect and monitor serial labs and blood cultures.
- Follow infection prevention procedures:
  - Assess bladder catheters for signs of infection.
  - Assess central line and IV insertion areas for signs of infection.
  - Change IV tubing and IV/central line dressings per institutional protocol.
  - Don gloves.
  - Perform frequent peri-care, at least once a shift.
  - Scrub IV hubs with alcohol for 15 seconds before use.
  - Wash hands.
- Increase nutrition as possible.
- Monitor urine output.
- Monitor vital signs hourly.
- Perform head-to-toe assessment frequently to assess for changes.
- Provide nutritional support.
- Transfer to higher level of care if condition continues to deteriorate.
- Utilize cooling devices as allowed per institution/unit to control fever.

Patient Education

- Ensure blood glucose control if diabetic.
- Ensure early mobilization; ambulate as often as possible.
- Ensure pulmonary hygiene using incentive spirometry.
- Follow infection precaution practices while at home, including:
  - Avoid others who are sick.
  - Avoid touching eyes, face, and mouth.
  - If diabetic, be especially cautious of infection development, and assess feet daily.
  - If performing other wound care, dress wound as ordered and monitor for signs or symptoms of infection.
  - Wash cuts or abrasions with antimicrobial soap and dress with clean dressing.
  - Wash hands frequently.
- Maintain infection prevention strategies.
- Take medications, especially antibiotics, as prescribed.

SHOCK STATES

Overview

- *Shock* occurs when the body is unable to function properly as a result of inadequate oxygenation. This can be due to either decreased perfusion in the body or the cells being unable to utilize the oxygen delivered.

 COMPLICATIONS

Shock states can progress rapidly and result in multiorgan failure and death. Early identification and treatment are needed to prevent further decompensation.

- Shock can be broken down into three stages:
  - *Compensatory stage:* The sympathetic nervous system produces adrenalin to compensate for the body's loss of oxygen, resulting in tachycardia, peripheral vasoconstriction, and normalized BP.
  - *Progressive stage:* The compensatory mechanisms are no longer sufficient enough to maintain hemodynamic stability and early organ dysfunction is starting.
  - *Refractory stage:* The final stage of shock, leading to end or multiorgan damage and patient no longer responding to intervention.
- There are several different types of shock. The exam focuses on distributive and hypovolemic shock.
  - *Distributive shock* occurs from profound peripheral vasodilation. Septic, anaphylactic, and neurogenic shock are classified as distributive shock.
  - *Hypovolemic shock* occurs when there is decreased intravascular volume and perfusion to the body. It can be classified as either hemorrhagic and non hemorrhagic

Signs and Symptoms

- Anaphylactic shock
  - Hypotension
  - Hypotonia
  - Incontinence
  - Syncope
  - Respiratory symptoms
    - Dyspnea
    - Hypoxemia
    - Inability to protect airway
    - Persistent cough/throat clearing
    - Stridor
    - Wheezing
- Hypovolemic shock
  - Agitation
  - Confusion
  - Dry mucous membranes
  - Hypotension
  - Lethargy
  - Muscle cramps
  - Orthostatic hypotension
  - Tachycardia
  - Thirst

Diagnosis

Labs
Possible work-up for a patient presenting with shock:
- ABG
- BMP
- Blood cultures
- Cardiac biomarkers
- CBC
- CMP
- Coagulation panel
- Lactate level
- Plasma histamine
- Serum or plasma total tryptase
- Type and screen
- Urinalysis

Diagnostic Testing
Imaging as indicated per patient status:
- Chest x-ray
- CT scan
- Transthoracic echocardiogram
- Ultrasound

Treatment

- Anaphylactic shock
  - Airway management
  - Antihistamines (Table 5.6)

- Bronchodilators (Table 3.1)
- Causative agent removal, if known
- Corticosteroids (Table A.4)
- Epinephrine (Table 2.8)
- IV fluids (Table A.3)
- Vasopressors (Table 2.8)
- Hypovolemic shock
  - Administration of blood products if severe blood loss and hemoglobin <7 g/dL
  - IV fluids if volume down and under resuscitated
  - Stop/control bleeding
  - Surgery consult if hypovolemia due to rapid blood loss or suspected trauma

Nursing Interventions

- Administer antibiotics, fluids, blood products, and other medications as needed.
- Collect and monitor serial labs and blood cultures.
- Educate patient on plan of care and possible OR procedures as needed.
- Monitor airway and breathing; administer oxygen as needed. Communicate as needed with respiratory therapy for additional respiratory support.
- Monitor intake and output hourly and labs as ordered.
- Monitor vital signs hourly.
- Perform head-to-toe assessment frequently to assess for changes.
- Transfer to higher level of care if condition continues to deteriorate.

Patient Education

- Ensure infection prevention.
- Ensure pulmonary hygiene
- Identify and have rescue medications on hand for anaphylactic triggers.
- Once discharged after an anaphylactic reaction:
  - Carry an epinephrine auto-injector as needed.
  - Consider wearing a medical alert bracelet or necklace.
  - Drink adequate fluids.
  - Follow up with allergist for thorough allergy testing.
  - Notify all other healthcare providers of history of anaphylaxis.
  - Once possible allergy is identified, avoid as best as possible.
- Take medications, especially antibiotics, as prescribed.

TOXICITY

Overview

Medication toxicity from both prescribed and non prescribed medications is a common reason for admission to the PCU.

- The ingestion of toxins may be intentional or accidental.

It is important to identify the ingested toxin and administer the antidote as soon as possible (Table 10.1).

- Toxins that cause complications when ingested include illicit drugs, prescription medications, alcohol, chemicals, or illegally obtained analgesics or benzodiazepines.

 COMPLICATIONS

Complications of toxicity or overdose include electrolyte abnormalities, cardiac dysrhythmia, altered mental status, seizures, respiratory depression, renal or hepatic failure, cardiac or respiratory arrest, and death.

Table 10.1 Toxins and Antidotes	
Toxin	**Antidote**
Acetaminophen	N-Acetylcysteine
Benzodiazepine	Flumazenil
Opioid	Naloxone

Signs and Symptoms

- Altered mental status
- Bradycardia
- Bradypnea
- Confusion
- Hallucinations
- Hypotension
- Lethargy
- Respiratory depression
- Seizure
- Sweating
- Vomiting

Diagnosis

Labs
- Acetaminophen overdose: increased acetaminophen level >200 mcg/mL 4 hr or more after ingestion
- CMP may indicate:
  - Electrolyte abnormalities
  - Elevated AST/ALT
  - Elevated creatinine and BUN
- ETOH level
- Salicylate level: elevated with aspirin overdose ≥50 mg/dL
- Urine drug screen

Diagnostic Testing
There are no diagnostic tests specific to diagnose toxicity. However, the following may confirm complications:
- Chest x-ray to identify aspiration
- ECG to identify potential arrythmias
- Head CT to identify head trauma

Treatment

- Antidote if applicable (Table 10.1)
- Activated charcoal if within 4 hr of a known or suspected acetaminophen ingestion
- Hemodialysis
- IV fluid resuscitation (Table A.3)
- Respiratory support with CPAP, BiPAP, or intubation (requiring transfer to higher level of care)

Nursing Interventions

- Assess psychologic status.
  - Ask the patient about any suicidal ideations.
  - Initiate suicide or psychologic precautions if intentional, per institutional protocol.
  - Maintain a sitter with 1:1 observation if indicated.
- Consult social worker for support resources at discharge.
- If naloxone given, prepare to address pain, discomfort, or aggressive behaviors.
  Insert NG/OG tube for gastric lavage.
- Maintain patient airway.
- Monitor for arrythmias.
- Monitor intake and output.
- Monitor vital signs. Depending on agent ingested, vital signs may show:
  - Tachypnea or bradypnea
  - Hypotension or HTN
  - Tachycardia or bradycardia
- Notify poison control.
- Provide supplemental oxygen, if indicated.

Patient Education

- Do not abruptly stop taking benzodiazepine or opioid medications, as it may cause withdrawal.
- Ensure effective pain management strategies.
- Follow appropriate guidelines for OTC medications.
  - Acetaminophen can be taken every 4 to 6 hr, up to four times in a 24-hr period. Do not exceed more than 4,000 mg of acetaminophen in a 24-hr period.
  - Aspirin should be taken at the recommended dose and time. For example, 81 mg of aspirin should be taken once daily. If taken for pain, one to two tablets of 325 mg can be taken every 4 to 6 hr with a daily limit of no more than 12 tablets in 24 hr. Extra strength aspirin (500 mg) can be taken every 4 to 6 hr with a daily limit of eight tablets in 24 hr.

WOUNDS

- Wounds in the PCU frequently occur from surgery, traumatic events, pressure injuries, or infectious sources.
- See Table 10.2 for the stages of wound healing.

Table 10.2 Stages of Wound Healing

Inflammatory phase	• Occurs between days 0 and 3 • Hemostasis is achieved • Inflammation and phagocytosis occur
Proliferation phase	• Occurs between days 3 and 21 • Angiogenesis and collagen synthesis occurs • Granulation and epithelization occur
Maturation phase	• 21 days–2 years • Reorganization of collagen

Source: Data from Hopkins Medicine.

PRESSURE INJURY

Overview

- *Pressure injuries*, also referred to as pressure ulcers, decubitus ulcers, or bed sores, are injuries to the skin and underlying tissue from prolonged pressure on the body's bony prominences.
- The most common site is the sacrum; however, pressure injuries can occur on the heels, hips, back of the head, shoulder blades, and elbows.
- Older adult and bed-bound patients are more prone to pressure injuries.
- Pressure injuries can also be device-related and can occur in relation to a nasal cannula, urinary catheter, endotracheal tube, or NG tube.
- Fragile skin, decreased blood flow, muscle volume loss, increased moisture, and nutritional deficits can contribute to increased risk of pressure injury.

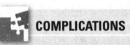 **COMPLICATIONS**

Pressure injuries can lead to the development of infection, osteomyelitis, bacteremia, sepsis, septic shock, and death. Frequent skin assessment and treatment is needed to prevent these complications.

Signs and Symptoms

- Changes in skin color (non blanchable redness)
- Drainage from an open wound
- Erythema
- Open wound on a bony prominence area
- Pain or tenderness
- Skin loss, exposing deeper layers of skin
- Skin swelling

Diagnosis

Labs

There are no labs specific to diagnose pressure injuries. However, the following may be included as work-up for a wound infection:

- Blood or wound culture: likely to indicate an organism
- BMP
- CBC: may indicate elevated WBC
- Lactate: may be elevated with severe infection

 NURSING PEARL

Pressure injuries can be staged according to severity.

- *Stage 1:* Non blanchable erythema of the skin
- *Stage 2:* Erythema with partial-thickness skin loss
- *Stage 3:* Full thickness ulcer involving subcutaneous fat
- *Stage 4:* Full thickness ulcer with muscle or bone involvement
- *Unstageable:* Unable to visualize wound bed due to eschar or tissue covering the wound bed

Diagnostic Testing

There are no diagnostic tests specific to diagnose pressure injuries. However, the following may confirm the depth of injury and infection of bone/surrounding tissue:

- CT scan
- X-ray

Treatment

- Antibiotics if an infected ulcer has caused a serious infection (Table A.1)
- Changing position
- Consult to wound therapy, as needed
- Mepilex/padded sacral dressing
- Surgical debridement to remove dead tissue, if necessary
- Topical barrier creams or ointments
- Topical medications (Table 10.3)
- Wound care

Nursing Interventions

- Administer nutritional support.
  - Administer liquid dietary supplements.
  - Increase protein intake.
  - An NG tube may be needed to provide additional nutritional support for wound healing.
  - Obtain nutrition consult.
- Change pads as soon as soiling is noted.
- Clean wounds with gentle cleanser and pat dry; do not scrub.
- Deeper wounds may require wet-to-dry dressings with normal saline-dampened gauze.
- Elevate heels off bed or utilize heel protector boots.
- Establish turning schedule.
  - Perform Q2H turns to relieve pressure on bony prominences.
  - Utilize positioning wedge and pillows.
- Perform frequent perineal hygiene.
- Perform frequent wound assessments.
  - Apply moisture barrier product.
  - Apply protective foam/adhesive dressing.
- Place on a pressure redistribution surface, such as a low air loss mattress or pressure relief overlay.
- Premedicate prior to wound changes as needed.
- Provide support surfaces and special cushions when sitting in the chair. Reposition at regular intervals while in the chair.
- Reposition movable devices.
- Utilize specialty pillows to prevent breakdown on the back of the patient's head.

Patient Education

- Learn and understand the importance of the following:
  - Change pads, dressings, diapers, or sheets if wet or soiled.
  - Keep skin clean and dry.
  - Maintain incontinence care at home. Consider using wicking materials to help reduce moisture or assistive devices like bedside urinals or female external suction catheters.
  - Reposition frequently to alleviate pressure on bony prominences and redistribute weight. If completely immobile or requiring total care, consider obtaining a home lift to assist with mobility and turning or consult home healthcare assistance.
- Perform wound care as needed.
  - For patient with diabetes, this includes daily skin checks, especially to the feet and heels. Diabetic neuropathy decreases the feelings and sensations to the feet, thus increasing the risk for pressure ulcer or wound development.
  - In general, when caring for pressure ulcers:
    - Assess incision daily for any new redness, warmth around the site, foul or discolored drainage, edema, or bleeding.
    - Avoid tight-fitting clothes.
    - Change dressing daily as ordered by provider, or if the dressing becomes soiled. After cleaning hands, remove the old dressing, clean and rinse the incision site, pat dry, and apply new dressing as directed.
    - Clean hands prior to and after touching the wound.
    - If possible, measure the wound to assess for any growth in width or depth.
    - Itchiness is expected as wounds heal. Do not scratch or pick at wounds.
    - Obtain necessary materials, if needed, to perform dressing changes once discharged home.
      - If ordered, apply prescribed ointment or barrier cream and dress with gauze or bandage dressing.
      - If wet-to-dry dressings are prescribed, they are generally applied with a normal saline-moistened gauze pad(s), a larger absorbent dressing, and tape to secure.

(continued)

Patient Education *(continued)*

■ If pressure ulcer wounds are severe, a wound VAC may be used prior to leaving the hospital. Assess the wound VAC frequently to ensure pressure is holding. If pressure is not being held, the wound VAC alarm will sound. Reinforce with transparent dressing and contact provider.

SURGICAL WOUNDS

Overview

- Surgical wounds result from a surgical incision, which may be superficial or involve all of the layers of the skin.
- Wound size can also vary greatly depending on the type of procedure and may be closed completely with sutures, staples, or glue, or left open to heal with wet-to-dry dressings or negative pressure wound therapy.

COMPLICATIONS

Surgical wounds are at increased risk for developing infection. Signs of infection include worsening swelling or edema, redness, warmth to touch, purulent or foul-smelling drainage, increased pain, fever, chills, or diaphoresis. This infection can progress to sepsis, septic shock, and even death. Frequent assessment and monitoring are required to identify potential infection early to decrease the risk for developing further complications.

Signs and Symptoms

- Erythema around incision site
- Mild swelling
- Pain
- Possible signs of infection:
  - Discharge
  - Drainage
  - Foul odor
  - Pain
  - Redness
- Serous, serosanguineous, or sanguineous bloody drainage

Diagnosis

Labs

There are no labs specific to diagnose surgical wounds. However, the following may be helpful as work-up for a wound infection:
- Blood or wound culture: likely indicates an organism
- BMP
- CBC: may indicate an elevated WBC
- Lactate: may be elevated with severe infection

Diagnostic Testing

- CT scan
- Ultrasound
- X-ray

Treatment

- Additional surgical debridement if needed
- Antibiotics (Table A.1)
- Surgical drains: drainage via suction or gravity to remove excess fluid
- Negative pressure wound therapy provides increased negative pressure to promote epithelization, increase blood flow, and continuously remove drainage
- Wound therapy consult as needed

Nursing Interventions

- Administer nutritional support with increased protein to promote wound healing.
- Apply abdominal binder as ordered.
- Empty and perform drain care as ordered.
  - Ensure drain tubing is free of clots or obstructions and remains patent.
  - Monitor surgical drains for increasing output, frank bleeding, or purulent drainage.
- Monitor site for signs of infection which include new or worsening swelling or edema, redness, warmth to the touch, pain, and foul-smelling or purulent drainage.
- Monitor vital signs for additional signs/symptoms of infection including new or worsening fever, tachycardia, and hypotension.
- Perform dressing changes as ordered and if soiled. Ordered dressing changes may be daily, every shift, or more frequently depending on situation.
- Perform frequent neurologic assessments to identify altered mental status or confusion, which may indicate infection.
- Perform wound care as ordered.
  - Wet-to-dry dressing: Apply gauze moistened with sterile water. Support with ABD pad and tape.
  - Manage wound VAC if applied to wound.
    - Assess machine to ensure occlusive and patent. Reinforce with other adhesive materials if seal is compromised. Notify the provider.
    - Change canister when full and document volume, consistency, and color.
- Provide splinting pillow or support to brace when coughing, bearing down, or repositioning in bed.

Patient Education

- Follow up as scheduled with all outpatient appointments.
- Include family and caregiver in education for at home management if assistance in changing dressing is needed.
- Maintain a healthy, high-protein diet to promote wound healing.
- Monitor for new or worsening systemic infection including fever, tachycardia, hypotension, or confusion.
- Perform dressing changes as needed. In general, when caring for wounds after discharge:
  - Assess incision daily for any new redness, warmth around the site, foul or discolored drainage, edema, or bleeding.
  - Change dressing daily as ordered by provider, or if the dressing becomes soiled. After washing hands, remove the old dressing, clean and rinse the incision site, pat dry, and apply new dressing as directed.
  - Itchiness is expected as wounds heal. Do not scratch or pick at wounds.
  - Obtain necessary materials, if needed, to perform dressing changes once discharged home.
  - Wash hands prior to and after touching the surgical site.
- Pursue smoking cessation as needed.
- Perform site inspection daily, assessing for new or worsening redness, swelling, warmth to touch, or purulent, foul-smelling drainage.
- Immunocompromised patients and those with diabetes or peripheral vascular disease may have impaired wound healing due to these comorbid conditions. Diligently monitor wound healing.
- Take medications as prescribed, especially full dose of antibiotics.

TRAUMATIC WOUNDS

Overview

- Traumatic wounds result from a sudden, unplanned injury.
- The size and damage sustained can also vary greatly but generally depends on the velocity, force, and item that caused the damage.

(continued)

Overview *(continued)*

- Anatomical location of traumatic wound injury also impacts severity of the wound.
- Traumatic wounds, if involving an artery or major organ, can quickly progress to a medical emergency and require prompt treatment and intervention.

Signs and Symptoms

- Entry or exit wound
- Lacerations caused by blunt or sharp mechanism
- Sanguineous, serosanguinous, or sanguineous drainage
- Swelling or edema
- Pain
- Possible signs of infection:
  - Discharge
  - Drainage
  - Foul odor
  - Pain
  - Redness

 COMPLICATIONS

Complications of traumatic wounds include bleeding, hemorrhage, secondary injury to surrounding tissue, vasculature and organs, and infection. Depending on the type of secondary injury, a wide variety of complications can result. Most commonly, widespread traumatic wounds like those experienced in a crush injury can result in rhabdomyolysis and AKI. Other complications include infection which can progress to sepsis, septic shock, or death. Diligent monitoring is required to identify and treat wound complications early.

Diagnosis

Labs

Lab work-up for a trauma patient may include:
- ABG
- CBC: May indicate a low hemoglobin and hematocrit if traumatic wound
- CMP
- Coagulation panel
- Type and screen

Diagnostic Testing

- CT scan
- Ultrasound
- X-rays

Treatment

- Antibiotics (Table A.1)
- Consultation of involved service (e.g., ENT or neurosurgery for head/facial trauma, orthopedics for injuries involving bones)
- Manual or surgical removal of objects if fully or partially retained (bullet(s), shrapnel, or other debris)
- Surgical intervention:
  - May involve debridement (burns, retained gravel, etc.) or closure of traumatic wound
  - Surgical drains: via suction or gravity to remove drainage
- Negative pressure wound therapy provides increased negative pressure to promote epithelization, increase blood flow, and continuously remove drainage

Nursing Interventions

See Surgical Wounds, Nursing Interventions.

Patient Education

See Surgical Wounds, Patient Education.

Table 10.3 Multisystem Medications

Indications	Mechanism of Action	Contraindications, Precautions, and Adverse Effects
Antidote, other (activated charcoal)		
• Emergency use following toxic ingestion/ poisoning	• Absorb ingested toxin, preventing it from being systemically absorbed in the stomach	• Use cautiously in intestinal bleeding, blockage or perforation, decreased level of consciousness, dehydration, slow digestion, and recent surgery. • Adverse effects include diarrhea, black stools, or vomiting.
Benzodiazepine antagonist, systemic antidotes (flumazenil)		
• Antidote for benzodiazepines • Overdose or toxicity	• Bind to GABA receptors to reverse the effects of benzodiazepine on the body	• Medication is contraindicated in patients who have received benzodiazepines to correct life-threatening conditions such as status epilepticus or increased ICP, or cyclic antidepressant overdose. • Monitor patient's level of consciousness, as re-sedation may occur following administration due to short half-life of drug. • Adverse effects include anxiety, vomiting, nausea, shivering, tremors, insomnia, headache, and agitation.
Mucolytics, systemic antidotes (N-acetylcysteine)		
• Antidote for acetaminophen	• Bind to oxygen free radicals to excrete them out of the body without causing cellular and organ damage	• Use cautiously in patients with history of asthma or bronchospasm. • Use cautiously in patients with esophageal ulcers, as it may induce vomiting and potentiates risk for GI bleed. • Adverse effects include flushing, rash, itching, nausea, and vomiting.
Neuraminidase inhibitor antivirals (oseltamivir)		
• Management of influenza A	• Competitively inhibit enzyme from influenza virus	• Medication is contraindicated in bacterial infections and immunosuppression. • Use cautiously in cardiac and pulmonary diseases, hepatic disease, renal failure, and psychosis. • Adverse effects include seizures, angioedema, hallucinations and confusion, headache, rash, emotional lability, anxiety, and agitation.
Opiate antagonist (naloxone)		
• Antidote for opioid toxicity or overdose	• Antagonizes pain receptors in the body to inhibit the effects of opioids on the body	• Monitor patient frequently, as respiratory depression may occur after initial improvement of symptoms. • Use cautiously in patients with cardiovascular conditions, as it may cause hypotension or ventricular dysrhythmias. • Adverse reactions include tremor, agitation, pain, headache, and vomiting.

(continued)

Table 10.3 Multisystem Medications *(continued)*

Indications	Mechanism of Action	Contraindications, Precautions, and Adverse Effects
Topical sulfonamides (silver sulfadiazine)		
• Gram positive and negative bacterial infection (topical)	• Disrupt bacteria and break down cell membrane to fight infection	• Do not give to patients with sulfa hypersensitivity. • Use cautiously in patients with hepatic and renal impairment or hematologic disease.

RESOURCES

Centers for Disease Control and Prevention. (2021, August 20). *Get ahead of sepsis – Know the risks. Spot the signs. Act fast.* U.S. Department of Health and Human Services, Centers for Disease Control and Prevention. https://www.cdc.gov/patientsafety/features/get-ahead-of-sepsis.html

DeMarco, S. (n.d.). *Wound and pressure ulcer management.* Johns Hopkins Medicine. https://www.hopkinsmedicine.org/gec/series/wound_care.html#wound_healing

Mayo Clinic Laboratories. (n.d.). *Test ID: SALCA.* https://www.mayocliniclabs.com/test-catalog/Clinical+and+Interpretive/37061

Mayo Foundation for Medical Education and Research. (2021, September 1). *Charcoal, activated (Oral route) side effects.* https://www.mayoclinic.org/drugs-supplements/charcoal-activated-oral-route/side-effects/drg-20070087

National Institute on Aging. (n.d.). *Providing care and comfort at the end of life.* U.S. Department of Health and Human Services, National Institute on Aging. https://www.nia.nih.gov/health/providing-comfort-end-life

Prescribers' Digital Reference. (n.d.). *N-Acetylcysteine* [Drug information]. PDR Search. https://pdr.net/drug-summary/Acetylcysteine-acetylcysteine-668

Prescribers' Digital Reference. (n.d.). *Flumazenil* [Drug information]. PDR Search. https://pdr.net/drug-summary/Flumazenil-flumazenil-1729

Prescribers' Digital Reference. (n.d.). *Naloxone hydrochloride* [Drug information]. PDR Search. https://pdr.net/drug-summary/Naloxone-Hydrochloride-Injection--1-mg-mL--naloxone-hydrochloride-23987

Prescribers' Digital Reference. (n.d.). *Oseltamivir* [Drug information]. PDR Search. https://www.pdr.net/drug-summary/Tamiflu-oseltamivir-phosphate-2099.8269#14

Prescribers' Digital Reference. (n.d.). *Silver sufadiazine* [Drug information]. PDR Search. https://pdr.net/drug-summary/Silvadene-silver-sulfadiazine-2781

Schroeder, K., & Lorenz, K. (2018). Nursing and the future of palliative care. *Asia-Pacific Journal of Oncology Nursing, 5*(1), 4–8. https://www.ncbi.nlm.nih.gov/pmc/articles/PMC5763437/

Singer, M., Deutschman, C. S., Seymour, C. W., Shankar-Hari, M., Annane, D., Bauer, M., Bellomo, R., Bernard, G. R., Chiche, J.-D., Coopersmith, C. M., Hotchkiss, R. S., Levy, M. M., Marshall, J. C., Martin, G. S., Opal, S. M., Rubenfeld, G. D., van der Poll, T., Vincent, J.-L., & Angus, D. C. (2016, February 23). The third international consensus definitions for sepsis and septic Shock (sepsis-3. *Journal of the American Medical Association, 315*(8), 801–810. https://www.ncbi.nlm.nih.gov/pmc/articles/PMC4968574/

Torres, P. A., Helmstetter, J. A., Kaye, A. M., & Kaye, A. D. (2015). Rhabdomyolysis: Pathogenesis, diagnosis, and treatment. *The Ochsner Journal, 15*(1), 58–69. https://www.ncbi.nlm.nih.gov/pmc/articles/PMC4365849/

University of Rochester Medical Center. (n.d.). *Acetaminophen drug level.* https://www.urmc.rochester.edu/encyclopedia/content.aspx?contenttypeid=167&contentid=acetaminophen_drug_level#:~:text=The%20results%20of%20the%20acetaminophen,is%20risk%20for%20liver%20damage

11

BEHAVIORAL AND PSYCHOSOCIAL CONDITIONS

AGGRESSIVE/DISRUPTIVE/VIOLENT BEHAVIOR

Overview

- Acute agitation may be a symptom of many emergent health conditions. As such, a thorough investigation and assessment is needed to rule out physiological causes.
- Agitation that is caused by a variety of medical or psychiatric conditions can escalate into aggressive/violent behavior.
- The PCU team should assess all patients for risk for violence and attempt to facilitate therapeutic communication, provide diversionary activities, and utilize de-escalation techniques before a situation results in violence. The use of physical or chemical restraints should be a last resort.

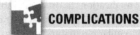

COMPLICATIONS

Violent behavior places patients and caregivers at risk for injury. Agitation and threats of violence should be addressed proactively, and de-escalation of the agitated patient should be prioritized to reduce incidences of violence in the PCU.

Signs and Symptoms

- Compromised reality checking (such as with patients experiencing dementia and delirium, hallucinations and/or delusions, de-realization, and/or de-personalization)
- Restlessness, pacing, increased vocalization/volume and use of profanity or threatening language, aggressive gestures, and erratic or impulsive behavior
- Signs of intoxication or substance use
- Violent or threatening statements or actions toward self or others

Diagnosis

Labs

There are no labs specific to diagnose aggressive/disruptive/violent behavior. However, the following may be indicated based on the patient's clinical status:

- CBC
- CMP
- ETOH level
- Urine drug screen
- Urinalysis

Diagnostic Testing

- Head CT scan to rule out underlying emergent medical condition
- X-rays as indicated for related injuries

Treatment

- De-escalation through diversionary techniques, limiting external stimuli, and facilitating therapeutic communication
- Isolation of violent patients in an area where potential hazards can be removed to maintain patient/staff safety
- Medical or physical restraints if the patient does not respond to prior interventions and patient or staff harm is imminent
- Psychiatry consult as inpatient admission may be indicated once medically cleared
- Thorough evaluation to rule out possible emergent medical causes of behaviors
- Threats taken seriously
- Visualization of the patient utilizing 1:1 observation, if indicated

Nursing Interventions

- Administer medications as ordered (Table 11.1*).
- Apply and monitor use of physical restraints as indicated by institutional protocols, as a last resort.
  - Perform regular circulatory and neurovascular checks to restrained extremities.
  - Provide assistance with oral intake and toileting as needed.
  - Assess skin integrity per facility protocol to decrease the risk of complications related to restraint use or immobility.
  - The patient may require a 1:1 sitter depending on facility protocol with the type of restraints required to maintain patient safety.
- Attempt to establish a therapeutic relationship.
- Continuously monitor for changes in vital signs.
- Facilitate de-escalation of the patient's behavior.
  - Remain calm.
  - Use simple language.
  - Establish therapeutic communication if possible.
  - Engage family members who may be present in de-escalation techniques if possible.
- Maintain an environment of safety.
  - Remove items that could become weapons.
  - Reinforce/protect dressings, lines, and tubes as much as possible.
  - Obtain an order for restraint if needed.
- Maintain visual and situational awareness of the patient at all times.
- Remain calm and speak to the patient using simple language.
- Remove the patient to an appropriate location to maintain patient and staff safety.

 ALERT!

De-escalating a potentially violent patient can take time but is frequently successful if approached in the correct manner.

- First, ensure the environment is safe for the patient and staff involved.
- Speak calmly and objectively to the patient.
- Encourage conversation and attempt to form an alliance.
- Listen to what the patient has to say and respond in a respectful manner.
- Incorporate active listening into the conversation; use reflection to help the patient identify underlying feelings. Nonverbal communication can help establish a therapeutic relationship.
- If possible, stand next to the patient to appear less threatening.
- Remember, safety comes first. Do not attempt de-escalation alone, and always stand between the patient and the door.

Patient Education

- Identify ways to manage anger and stress, which may include physical exercise and relaxation techniques (deep breathing, meditation, yoga, etc.).
- If agitation or aggression is not the result of acute critical illness, consider following up with a counselor or therapist to address aggressive behavior.
- Limit alcohol and other substance use.

---

* Table 11.1 is located at the end of this chapter.

- Some medications have adverse reactions and may cause aggression or agitation. Alert all future providers to avoid administering this medication if it contributed to aggression.

ALTERED MENTAL STATUS

Overview

- *AMS* can be described as an acute or chronic change in consciousness, arousal, self-awareness, expression, language, or emotions.
- AMS has a wide variety of causes ranging from metabolic derangements (e.g., alcohol withdrawal) to acute focal brain lesions (e.g., stroke) to chronic neurodegenerative diseases (e.g., Alzheimer dementia).
- Often, AMS is the primary reason for admittance to the PCU.

Signs and Symptoms

- Anxiety
- Attention impairment
- CNS depression and coma
- Cognitive impairment
- Confusion
- Emotional withdrawal or emotional outbursts
- Intermittent periods of lucidity
- Irritability
- Motor functioning changes
- Slowed, slurred speech
- Psychomotor agitation

Diagnosis

Labs

- Possible indication based on patient's clinical status:
  - ABG: May indicate acidosis, hypercarbia, or hypoxia
  - CMP:
    - May indicate electrolyte abnormalities
    - Elevated BUN/Cr indicating impaired renal function
    - Elevated ALT/AST indicating altered hepatic function
  - CBC: May indicate an elevated WBC count if AMS is the result of an infection
  - Point of care glucose testing to assess for hypo- or hyperglycemia
  - Toxicology screening: If AMS caused by drug or alcohol use
  - Urinalysis (UTI may cause confusion in an older adult)

Diagnostic Testing

- Glasgow Coma Scale
- Head CT scan to rule out a neurological abnormality
- Mini-mental status exam
- X-ray, if indicated

POP QUIZ 11.1

What is the first step the nurse should take to respond to an agitated patient who is shouting and hitting the side of the bed?

COMPLICATIONS

Complications of AMS include impaired cognitive, behavioral, and physical functioning, which may lead to combative or agitated behavior and place the patient at risk for accidental self-harm (accidental removal of lines, drains, or tubes, falls, etc.). Alternately, it may lead to further CNS depression, coma, or respiratory arrest.

Treatment

Treatment of altered mental status dependent on cause. This may include, but is not limited to:

- Airway management with:
  - BiPAP
  - Intubation
- Treatment of hypoglycemia (Chapter 4)
- Treatment of intracranial hemorrhage or encephalopathy with appropriate neurological intervention (Chapter 6)
- Treatment of infection or septic shock with:
  - Antibiotics (Table A.1)
  - Fluid resuscitation
  - Vasopressors (Table 2.8)
- Management of AMS if no clear etiology:
  - Antipsychotics if indicated (Table 11.1)
  - Delirium precautions
  - Maintaining sleep–wake cycles

 ALERT!

AMS could signal serious cerebral disease or illness including hemorrhage, tumors, abscesses, hematomas, or lesions. Any change in mental status should be thoroughly investigated.

 ALERT!

Sundowning is a condition of late-day confusion in which a patient who is otherwise alert and oriented during the day becomes disoriented as the sun sets.

Nursing Interventions

- Administer medications as ordered to treat underlying condition, pain/discomfort, and/or agitation.
- Assess vital signs for changes in hemodynamic stability.
  - Hypotension
  - Tachycardia
  - Tachypnea
- Build trusting relationship.
- Consult psychiatry as needed.
- Create a safe environment.
  - Consider using a bed or chair alarm to alert staff of unexpected ambulation or movement.
  - If patient is at risk of self-harm or harm to someone else:
    - Consider utilizing a sitter to maintain patient safety and prevent unwitnessed ambulation.
    - Place objects that can be used as projectiles or to harm self or someone else out of room.
  - Lower the bed to decrease risk of falls.
  - Position call bell, telephone, and other personal items of importance near the patient.
  - Protect or cover lines or tubes if patient is attempting to pull at them.
- Engage in therapeutic communication.
- Maintain sleep hygiene and promote a regular sleep–wake cycle.
  - Decrease environmental disruptions using sleep masks and do not disturb orders.
  - Reschedule medications and lab draws to reduce sleep interruption, if possible.
- Perform neurological assessment frequently. Regularly orient patient to current day and time with each interaction.
- Promote use of eyeglasses and hearing aids as needed.
- Provide urinal or assist to bedpan as needed.

Patient Education

- Depending on level of mental status alteration, patient may be unable to comprehend education provided by healthcare providers. However, make every effort to:
  - Answer questions appropriately.
  - Communicate effectively.

- Provide reassurance and therapeutically communicate.
- Reorient patient to person, place, time, and situation as needed/appropriate.
- If caregiver or family notices a sudden change in mental status, seek care through emergency services.
- If possible, avoid polypharmacy and taking unnecessary medications, especially if elderly.
- Follow a regular sleep-wake cycle. Get at least 8 hr of undisturbed sleep.
- Limit alcohol consumption.

ANXIETY

Overview

- Anxiety involves fear and worry accompanied by a heightened physiologic response with symptoms ranging from mild to severe.
- Hospitalized patients often experience acute anxiety due to a threat to life or physical health, loss of control, and foreign environment.
- Pain, poor sleep quality, mobility changes, medical equipment/devices, and nightly interruptions have also been found to increase anxiety among hospitalized patients.
- Chronic anxiety may also be exacerbated by hospital admission.

 COMPLICATIONS

Anxiety in acute illness can result in irrational behavior and impaired cognition, leading to aggression, agitation, and inadvertent removal of important lines, drains, or tubes. Physiologic complications of anxiety also include vital sign changes including tachycardia and tachypnea. These changes can worsen health status while hospitalized.

Signs and Symptoms

- Behavioral:
  - Avoidance of triggers
  - Impatient
  - Fearful
  - Frustrated
  - Quiet
- Cognitive:
  - Confusion
  - Difficulty speaking
  - Hyper vigilance for threat
  - Fear of loss of control
  - Fear of physical injury or death
  - Frightening mental thoughts or images
  - Poor concentration
- Physiologic:
  - Chest pain or pressure
  - Diaphoresis
  - Diarrhea
  - Dizziness
  - Dry mouth
  - Dyspnea
  - Nausea
  - Numbness and tingling
  - Palpitations
  - Shaking
  - Tachycardia
  - Weakness

 NURSING PEARL

Family members or caregivers can bring in pictures or familiar and comforting items to the patient to decrease anxiety in the hospital setting.

Diagnosis

Labs

There are no labs specific to diagnose anxiety. However, the following may be indicated based on the patient's clinical status:

- ABG
- Blood cultures
- BMP
- CBC
- Thyroid function test
- Toxicology screen
- Urinalysis

Diagnostic Testing

- Anxiety screening tools:
  - GAD-7
  - Hospital anxiety and depression screening tool
- Diagnostics to rule out physiologic causes:
  - Chest x-ray
  - EKG
  - Head CT scan

Treatment

- Medications (Table 11.1)
  - Antipsychotics
  - Benzodiazepines
  - Beta blockers (Table 2.8)
  - Buspirone
  - SSRIs
  - SNRIs
  - Tricyclic antidepressants
- Nonpharmacologic interventions:
  - Distraction through use of conversation, television, or music
  - Pet therapy
  - Therapeutic touch
- Psychotherapy if appropriate during the patient's PCU stay (may be deferred until transferred out of the unit)
- Ruling out underlying medical cause of anxiety symptoms
- Supplemental oxygen as needed for tachypnea or dyspnea

 ALERT!

Use extreme caution when treating older adult patients with benzodiazepines. Use another pharmacological agent if possible. Benzodiazepine use in older adult patients can impair mobility and cognition, increase the risk of falls, and enhance the risk of developing dementia and Alzheimer disease.

Nursing Interventions

- Administer scheduled antianxiety medications and assess the need for PRN dosages as ordered. Notify the provider if the schedule and PRN dosage has not alleviated symptoms of anxiety.
- Assess for suicidal or homicidal ideation.
- Engage in therapeutic communication; listen to the patient and allow them to voice their fears and concerns.
- Establish rapport with the patient and build a trusting relationship.
- Monitor vital signs for anxiety-induced changes including tachycardia, tachypnea, and decreased oxygen saturation.
- Provide a safe, familiar environment.

Patient Education

- Consider following up with a therapist or psychologist following discharge.
- Practice good health habits: get adequate sleep, eat a variety of foods, and exercise.
- Self-assess and identify what anxiety triggers may be. Remove or reduce triggers (if possible).
- Use nonpharmacologic anxiety-reducing techniques as needed, which include:
  - Aromatherapy
  - Guided imagery
  - Meditation
  - Music
  - Slowed breathing
  - Yoga

DELIRIUM

Overview

- *Delirium* is an alteration in mental status that is characterized by acute onset, fluctuating course, impaired attention, and either a disturbance in the level of consciousness or disorganized thinking.
- Delirium can manifest as hyperactive, hypoactive, or mixed.
- Patients experiencing critical illness and hospitalizations are at high risk for developing delirium, which manifests as an acute change in awareness or attention that appears over a short period of time.

 COMPLICATIONS

Complications of delirium include aspiration pneumonia, decreased mobility and functioning, falls, combative behavior leading to accidental self-harm, malnutrition, fluid and electrolyte imbalance, pressure ulcers, and long-term cognitive impairment. Additionally, delirium increases the risk of medical complications, prolonged hospitalizations, functional decline, and dementia.

Signs and Symptoms

- Alterations in sleep–wake cycle
- Behavioral changes
  - Emotional lability
  - Hallucinations or delusions
  - Irritability
  - Psychomotor agitation
  - Unsafe behavior
- Cognitive impairment
  - Anxiety
  - Disorganized thinking
  - Disorientation of consciousness
  - Emotional liability
  - Fluctuating changes in awareness

NURSING PEARL

Delirium coinciding with acute illness will often resolve with the treatment of underlying illness.

Diagnosis

Labs

There are no labs specific to diagnose delirium. Lab work-up may be similar for patients with AMS as noted in the previous section.

Diagnostic Testing

- Head CT scan to rule out underlying etiology
- Glasgow Coma Scale
- Mini-mental status exam

Treatment

- Underlying etiology treatment if known cause of delirium, including:
  - Glucose imbalances
  - Hypoxia or hypercarbia respiratory issues
  - Infection
- See Altered Mental Status Treatment section for more information.

Nursing Interventions

See Altered Mental Status, Nursing Interventions.

Patient Education

See Altered Mental Status, Patient Education.

DEMENTIA

Overview

- Dementia is characterized by a slow and chronic deterioration in cognition and decline in functional activities.
- Patients with dementia will have memory difficulties in addition to personality changes and difficulty with abstract thinking, word recall, executive functioning, and social and special skills.
- Patients with dementia are at high risk to develop a concomitant delirium, especially in the PCU setting.

COMPLICATIONS

Dementia complications include increased risk for infections (e.g., pneumonia or UTI), falls, fractures, inadequate nutrition and dehydration, depression, hallucinations, delusions, and death. Dementia is a progressive disease with high mortality rate.

Signs and Symptoms

- Behavioral changes
  - Aggression
  - Mood changes
  - Self-neglect
  - Social withdrawal
- Cognitive impairments
  - Communication difficulty
  - Difficulty performing tasks
  - Forgetfulness
  - Hallucinations
  - Memory loss

Diagnosis

Labs

- CBC to rule out anemia
- Serum B_{12} level to rule out vitamin B_{12} deficiency
- TSH to rule out hypothyroidism
- Additional routine labs to rule out other physiologic conditions if there is a specific suspicion for abnormality

Diagnostic Testing

- Autopsy examination of brain tissue to confirm Alzheimer/dementia diagnosis
- Head CT or MRI in the routine initial evaluation of patients with dementia

Treatment

- No cure available
  - Treatments alleviate some symptoms
  - The disease inevitably progresses in all patients.
- Interventions to manage and maintain baseline functioning:
  - Avoidance of stimulants
    - Alcohol
    - Caffeine
  - Daily exercise
  - Medications (Table 11.1)
    - Antidepressants
    - Anxiolytics
    - Antipsychotics
  - Pain control
  - Sleep hygiene
- In advanced dementia:
  - Hospice and palliative care consult
  - Management of infection/fever as needed

 ALERT!

Behavior changes exhibited as a result of dementia can manifest as depression, anxiety, or psychosis. Treatment of these manifestations remains the same independent of a dementia diagnosis.

Nursing Interventions

- Alleviate physical discomfort.
  - Administer medications as ordered.
  - Ambulate and mobilize as possible.
  - Reposition frequently.
- Assist with frequent toileting and/or perineal care.
- Encourage safe PO intake.
- Engage in therapeutic communication.
- Provide nutritional support. Assist patient with meals and/or administer tube feedings as ordered/scheduled.
- Provide safe environment for patient.
- Provide support with decision-making and advance care planning.
- Provide symptom management relief.
- Reorient patient as needed.

Patient Education

- Consider respite care support or alternative care setting.
- Improve oral intake with finger foods, smaller portions, nutritional supplements, and alternating textures of food.
- Stay updated on current status, plan of care, advanced health directives, and healthcare proxy prior to end-stage dementia.
- Update family members on clinical course of delirium, treatments, and clinical course. Understand what to expect at the end stage of the disease.

DEPRESSION

Overview

- Depression is common among patients with chronic illness. Often, depression from a hospital admission or acute disease can lead to anxiety and PTSD.
- Depressive disorders are characterized by prolonged periods of a depressed mood most often related to a chemical imbalance.
- It can be difficult to diagnose as a patient can have mild symptoms resulting from a specific situation or trigger or severe symptoms consistent with a mood disorder.
- Major depression has a high morbidity and mortality rate. Identification and treatment of depression is essential to preventing complications.

COMPLICATIONS

Depressed patients are at risk for impaired self-care, which can exacerbate preexisting physical conditions or lead to drug and alcohol abuse, self-harm, or suicide.

Signs and Symptoms

- Appetite/weight changes
- Decreased or loss of interest in usual activities
- Decreased energy/fatigue
- Depressed mood
- Difficulty concentrating
- Fatigue
- Feelings of worthlessness
- Psychomotor disturbances
- Sleep disturbances
- Suicidal or recurrent thoughts of death

NURSING PEARL

Any verbalization of depression or suicidal thoughts in a critically ill patient should be taken seriously. A psychiatric consult and mood-stabilizing medications may be indicated.

Diagnosis

Labs
There are no labs specific to diagnose depression. However, the following may be helpful to rule out physiological causes:
- CBC
- CMP
- ETOH level
- Rapid plasma region to rule out syphilis
- TSH to rule out hypothyroidism
- Toxicology screen to rule out illicit drug use
- Vitamin B_{12} to rule out vitamin B_{12} deficiency

Diagnostic Testing
There are no diagnostic tests specific to diagnose depression. However, the following may be indicated to rule out a neurological mass or abnormality if physiologic pathology is a suspected cause:
- CT scan
- MRI

Treatment

- Assessment/treatment: suicidal ideations or attempts assessment and treatment
- Assessment/treatment: any electrolyte abnormalities and nutritional deficits
- Medications to manage symptoms (e.g., anxiety, depression, and insomnia) (Table 11.1):
  - Atypical antidepressants
  - MAOIs

- SSRIs
- SNRIs
- Tricyclic antidepressants
- Ruling out underlying medical condition
- Consult to social work and case management to ensure referrals and resources are in place for continued outpatient treatment
- Possibly indicated once patient is clinically stable:
  - ECT: If antidepressant medications have not worked
  - Psychotherapy: Help treat depressive health problems by talking with a psychiatrist or other mental health provider
  - Psychiatric unit

 ALERT!

Use caution when starting depression treatments in the hospital setting. Often, these drugs take time to reach effectiveness, have multiple interactions with other medications, and should not be abruptly stopped. Request a psychiatric consult for a more in-depth evaluation.

Nursing Interventions

- Administer crystalloid fluids or nutritional supplements as indicated if underweight or malnourished.
- Administer medications as ordered.
- Arrange for a psychiatry consult.
- Assess for alcohol or drug use.
- Build a trusting relationship.
- Engage in therapeutic communication.
- Monitor vital signs continuously.
- Perform a focused psychological assessment.
- Provide a safe and familiar environment for the patient.

Patient Education

- If suicidal thoughts or feelings occur, reach out to:
  - Close family or friends for support
  - Support groups
  - Therapists or counselors
  - 911
- Maintain a healthy lifestyle with exercise, a proper diet, and good sleep hygiene.
- Pursue interventions to improve appetite if underweight, as well as weight loss programs if overweight.
- Take medications as ordered, even if feeling better.
- Understand the risk of abruptly stopping medication.
- Understand the importance of follow-up care in an outpatient setting.

 POP QUIZ 11.2

A patient is admitted to the PCU with hypertension due to medication noncompliance stemming from an untreated major depressive disorder. The provider starts the patient on an MAOI for his depression. The patient asks what other interventions are available to help treat his depression. What should the nurse's response be?

SUBSTANCE ABUSE

Overview

- *Substance abuse* is the excessive use of alcohol or other drugs that activate the brain's reward system to reinforce behavior.
  - This can include chronic drug or alcohol abuse or drug-seeking behavior, in addition to drug or alcohol withdrawal.

(continued)

Overview *(continued)*

- It may lead to significant problems or distress, such as substance-related legal problems and impaired relationships with friends and family.
- Patients in the PCU can be admitted as a direct result of their substance abuse (intoxication, withdrawal, etc.) or have a history of substance abuse. Acknowledgment of a substance abuse disorder is important to provide appropriate care.

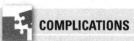 **COMPLICATIONS**

Patients with substance or alcohol addiction are at risk for developing cardiovascular disease, cancer, stroke, lung disease, or mental disorders, land liver failure, or for contracting HIV/AIDS or hepatitis B and/or C. Additionally, patients are also at risk for seizure and death from withdrawal of certain substances.

Signs and Symptoms

- Drug-seeking behavior:
  - Aggressively complaining about the need for a specific drug
  - Anger/irritability over detailed questioning about pain
  - Asking for a specific drug by name/brand name at specific time
  - Constant request for increased dose
  - Claiming multiple allergies to alternate drugs
  - Inappropriate self-medicating
  - Inappropriate use of general practice
  - Manipulative or illegal behavior
    - History of buying or selling drugs
    - History of theft
    - Pattern of lost or stolen prescriptions
  - Resistant behavior
    - Refusing to sign controlled substance agreement
    - Unwilling to consider other medications or nonpharmacologic treatments
- Varied signs and symptoms depending on the type of substance used, but may include:
  - Depressants
    - Ataxia
    - CNS depression
    - Coma
    - Multiorgan failure
    - Slurred speech
  - Stimulants
    - Anxiety
    - Hypertension
    - Psychosis
    - Tachycardia
    - Tachypnea
- Withdrawal signs may include:
  - Alcohol withdrawal
    - Agitation
    - Anxiety
    - Auditory disturbances
    - Difficulty thinking
    - Diaphoresis
    - Headache
    - Nausea and vomiting
    - Tactile disturbances
    - Tremor
    - Visual disturbances

 ALERT!

Alcohol withdrawal typically occurs 1–3 days following the patient's last drink. If possible, determine the date and time of last drink on admission. If date and time of last drink is unable to be determined and alcohol withdrawal is suspected, frequently monitor for condition changes consistent with alcohol withdraw withdrawal. Notify the provider and treat per institutional protocol.

- Drug withdrawal
  - Barbiturates and benzodiazepines
    - Psychotic symptoms
    - Seizure
    - Rhabdomyolysis
  - Opiates
    - Diarrhea
    - Dilated pupils
    - Nausea
    - Sneezing
    - Rhinorrhea
    - Vomiting
    - Yawning
  - Cocaine and amphetamines
    - Depression
    - Dysphoria
    - Excessive sleep
    - Hunger
    - Psychomotor slowing
    - Sleep disturbances

Diagnosis

Labs
There are no labs specific to diagnose substance abuse disorder. However, the following may be indicated based on the patient's clinical status.
- ABG to show acidosis, hypoxia, or hypercarbia
- CBC
- CMP to show abnormal electrolytes or altered renal or hepatic functioning, depending on substance abused
- Toxicology screen

Diagnostic Testing
There are no diagnostic tests specific to diagnose substance abuse. However, the following may be helpful to determine medical conditions as a result of substance toxicity, route of administration, and high-risk behaviors (needle sharing, unprotected sexual encounters, poor hygiene, etc.):
- Screening tools specific to institution, such as:
  - AUDIT
  - ASI
  - CAGE
    - Have you ever felt like you should Cut back on your drinking?
    - Have people Annoyed you by criticizing your drinking?
    - Have you ever felt Guilty about your drinking?
    - Have you ever had a drink first thing in the morning as an Eye-opener?
  - CIWA
  - COWS
  - T-ACE questions
    - How may drinks does it take to make you feel high (Tolerance)?
    - Have people Annoyed you by criticizing your drinking?
    - Have you ever felt you should Cut down on your drinking?
    - Have you ever had a drink first thing in the morning to steady your nerves or get rid of a hangover (Eye-opener)?

NURSING PEARL

Understanding the timing of the patient's last drink is essential to monitor and treat symptoms of alcohol withdrawal. Typically, patients can experience alcohol withdrawal 24 to 72 hr following their last drink.

Treatment

- Cognitive behavioral therapy
- Comprehensive mental health history
- Consult to psychiatry
- De-escalation techniques as first-line treatment for aggression:
  - Active listening
  - Diversionary techniques
  - Limiting external stimuli
  - Therapeutic communication
- Drug or addiction counseling, as indicated
- Medications as indicated (Table 11.1):
  - Antipsychotics: Supportive therapy for behavior changes related to drug or alcohol withdrawal
  - Benzodiazepines: Alcohol withdrawal
  - Methadone: Drug withdrawal
  - Naloxone: Opioid overdose
  - Thiamine: Alcohol abuse
- Motivational interviewing/motivational enhancement
- Mutual health and support groups
- Ruling out organic causes for signs and symptoms
- Thorough substance abuse history, physical examination, family history, and review of social factors

 ALERT!

Mental health issues often accompany addiction. Psychiatry involvement in care is often essential to provide the most comprehensive and holistic care possible.

Nursing Interventions

- Assess for suicidal or homicidal ideations.
- Administer medications as prescribed by provider to manage symptoms (e.g., anxiety, depression, and insomnia).
- Build a trusting relationship.
- Collaborate with social work to arrange resources at discharge.
- Engage in therapeutic communication.
- Frequently assess for symptoms of withdrawal (CIWA) and the potential for seizures.
  - Check for nausea or vomiting.
  - Check for signs of anxiety.
  - Monitor for visual, tactile, or auditory disturbances.
  - Look for tremors.
  - Observe for signs of diaphoresis.
- If aggressive:
  - Maintain visual and situational awareness of the patient utilizing 1:1 observation, if indicated.
  - Facilitate de-escalation of the patient's behavior.
  - Use medical and physical restraints if the patient does not respond to prior interventions and harm to the patient and/or staff is imminent.
- Instruct on measures to decrease/manage addiction and/or anxiety. Refer to online or in-person counseling or treatment options.
- Manage any underlying symptoms.
- Monitor vital signs to identify any hemodynamic changes requiring additional support.
- Notify provider of new or worsening psychological conditions, including:
  - Acts of self-harm.
  - Anxiety or depression.
  - Delusions or hallucinations.
  - Irrational or erratic behavior.
  - Self-destructive behavior including pulling at lines with intent to remove the lines despite education on importance to leave device intact (e.g., ripping at peripheral IVs, central lines, dialysis lines, and catheters).
  - Verbalization or intent to harm themselves or others.

- Perform frequent physical assessments and a focused psychological assessment.
- Perform frequent screening assessments per institutional protocol.
- Provide a safe environment for the patient by removing any potentially harmful objects from the room.
- Offer nourishment as indicated for patient's condition.
  - Manic symptoms: Feed high-calorie finger foods to meet the body's elevated caloric requirements.
  - Depressive symptoms: Encourage PO intake if patient's appetite is decreased. Supplement with NG tube feeding if needed.

POP QUIZ 11.3

What is the timeframe in which alcohol withdrawal symptoms typically manifest?

Patient Education

- Exercise regularly to help manage symptoms of depression.
- Follow up long term with outpatient providers and appointments to prevent relapse.
- Maintain good sleep hygiene practices.
- Obtain psychosocial support information.
  - AA/NA support group resources
  - Cognitive behavioral therapy resources
- Report any disabling side effects so that medications can be adjusted. Do not stop taking the medications unless advised by provider.
- Take all medications as prescribed, even if symptoms improve.

POP QUIZ 11.4

A patient with a substance abuse disorder asks the nurse what resources he has for long-term support to stay sober. What resources could the nurse discuss with the patient?

Table 11.1 Psychiatric Medications

Indications	Mechanism of Action	Contraindications, Precautions, and Adverse Effects
Antidepressants, atypical (bupropion hydrochloride)		
• Major depression	• Dopamine norepinephrine reuptake inhibitor, inhibit presynaptic reuptake of dopamine, and norepinephrine (with a greater effect upon dopamine)	• Medication is contraindicated in seizure disorders or concurrent use with MAOIs. • Use caution in Tourette's (can cause worsening tics), major hepatic, renal or cardiac disease, operating heavy machinery, or pregnancy. • Do not abruptly discontinue. • Adverse effects include anxiety, dry mouth, palpitations, restlessness, and difficulty sleeping.
Antidepressants: MAOIs (isocarboxazid)		
• Multiple psychiatric disorders, including treatment-resistant major depression	• Inhibit MAO through irreversible binding	• Medication is contraindicated in severe renal or liver impairments, concurrent use of medications known to interact with MAOIs, hypertension, or pheochromocytoma. • Use caution in concurrent use with contrast dye, procedures requiring general anesthesia, hyperthyroidism, diabetes, asthma, or seizure disorders. • Adverse effects include dry mouth, skin irritation/reactions, insomnia, increased risk for suicidal thoughts or actions following dosage change, and serotonin syndrome.

(continued)

Table 11.1 Psychiatric Medications *(continued)*

Indications	Mechanism of Action	Contraindications, Precautions, and Adverse Effects
Antidepressants: SSRIs (citalopram, escitalopram, fluoxetine, paroxetine, and sertraline)		
• Moderate-to-severe depression • Anxiety disorders	• Increase levels of serotonin in the brain by blocking the reuptake of serotonin in neurons making more available for transmitting signals	• Do not abruptly discontinue. • Adverse effects include nausea/vomiting, diarrhea, nervousness, agitation, restlessness, insomnia, weight loss or weight gain, sexual dysfunction, dry mouth, headache, serotonin syndrome, or suicidal thoughts or behaviors. • Use caution in pregnancy, heart, liver, and kidney disease and bleeding disorders.
Antidepressants: SNRIs (duloxetine and venlafaxine)		
• Primarily as treatment for depression • Can be effective in treating anxiety disorders and chronic or nerve pain	• Block reuptake of serotonin and norepinephrine in the brain	• Taper gradually to discontinue. • Do not administer with MAOIs. • Adverse effects include headache, nausea, dizziness, increased perspiration, fatigue, constipation, insomnia, decreased appetite, sexual dysfunction, increased suicidal thoughts or behaviors, hypertension, decreased liver functioning, and serotonin syndrome. • Use caution taking with blood thinners, if considering getting pregnant, or if pregnant.
Antidepressants: tricyclic (amitriptyline)		
• Fibromyalgia • Insomnia • Major depression • Painful diabetic neuropathy • Social phobia	• Mechanism of action not fully understood; thought to result from the decreased reuptake of norepinephrine and serotonin	• Medication is contraindicated in concurrent use with MAOIs or for patients in the acute recovery phase following acute MI. • Use caution in bipolar or mania, schizophrenia, alcoholism or CNS depression, seizure disorders, DM, geriatric populations, and pregnancy. • Do not abruptly discontinue. • Adverse effects include drowsiness, dry mouth, blurred vision, difficulty urinating or stooling, weight gain, or dizziness.
Antipsychotics: first generation (haloperidol)		
• Schizophrenia • Psychosis • Severe behavioral problems	• Mechanism of action not currently known; believed to block dopamine receptors	• Medication is contraindicated in coma or severe toxic CNS depression, Parkinson disease, and Lewy body dementia. • Use caution in cardiac, renal, liver, or pulmonary disorders, QT prolongation, seizure disorders, stroke, urinary retention, and pregnancy. • Do not abruptly discontinue. • Adverse effects include tremor, dyskinesias, anxiety, agitation, restlessness, diaphoresis, nausea, or vomiting. • IM formulary can be used for emergency treatment.

(continued)

Table 11.1 Psychiatric Medications *(continued)*

Indications	Mechanism of Action	Contraindications, Precautions, and Adverse Effects
Antipsychotics: second generation (e.g.,risperidone)		
• Schizophrenia • Psychosis • Severe behavioral problems	• Exhibit effects through some dopamine blockade, but more from blockade of serotonin receptors	• Use caution in CNS depression, hematologic disease, tardive dyskinesia, cardiac, renal, or hepatic disease, seizure disorders, Parkinson disease, dementia, PKU, DM, and in older adult patients. • Do not abruptly discontinue. • Adverse effects include nausea, vomiting, diarrhea or constipation, weight gain, anxiety, dry or discolored skin, decreased sexual function.
Anxiolytics: benzodiazepines (e.g.,alprazolam, chlordiazepoxide, clonazepam, diazepam, lorazepam, and midazolam)		
• Anxiety • Mood disorders	• Potentiate the effect of GABA, which increases the inhibition of the RAS system	• Do not abruptly discontinue. • Adverse effects include fatigue, nausea/vomiting, weight changes (loss or gain), sexual dysfunction, agitation, unsteady gait, slurred speech, or sedation. • Use caution in use with active suicidal ideation, psychosis or bipolar disorder, CNS depression, pulmonary disease, alcoholism or substance abuse, liver or renal disease, and geriatric populations.
Anxiolytics (buspirone)		
• Anxiety disorders	• Suppress serotonin while enhancing noradrenergic and dopaminergic cell firing to improve neurotransmission	• Medication is contraindicated in concurrent use with MAOIs. • Use caution in benzodiazepine dependence, renal or liver impairments, geriatric populations, or pregnancy. • Adverse effects include dizziness, headache, confusion, fatigue, nervousness, insomnia, mood changes, headache, palpitations, blurred vision, hives, or itching.
Opioid agonist (methadone)		
• Opioid withdrawal	• Bind to opiate receptor sites in CNS to alter perceptions of and response to painful stimuli, decreasing symptoms of withdrawal to opioids	• Medication is contraindicated in alcohol intolerance and concurrent use of MAOIs. • Use caution in heart disease, diuretic use, hypokalemia, hypomagnesemia, history of dysrhythmia, concurrent use with drugs that prolong QT interval, severe renal, hepatic, or pulmonary disease, and head trauma. • Adverse effects include confusion, sedation, hypotension, and constipation.

(continued)

Table 11.1 Psychiatric Medications *(continued)*

Indications	Mechanism of Action	Contraindications, Precautions, and Adverse Effects
Opioid antagonist (naloxone)		
• Suspected opioid overdose • Opioid induced respiratory depression	• Antagonize opioid effects by competing for the same receptor sites	• Use caution in patients with cardiovascular disease. • Adverse effects include ventricular dysrhythmias, hypertension, hypotension, nausea, and vomiting.
Vitamin B₁ supplements (thiamine)		
• Treatment of Wernicke–Korsakoff syndrome resulting from alcohol abuse • Vitamin B₁ deficiency	• Combine with ATP in the liver and kidneys to produce thiamine diphosphate, which acts as a coenzyme in carbohydrate metabolism allowing pyruvic acid to convert and enter the Krebs cycle	• Use caution in pregnancy. • Adverse effects include nausea, weakness, sweating, restlessness, or itching.

RESOURCES

James, J. (2016). Dealing with drug-seeking behaviour. *Australian Prescriber, 39*(3), 96–100. https://www.ncbi. nlm.nih.gov/pmc/articles/PMC4919169/

Jesse, S., Bråthen, G., Ferrara, M., Keindl, M., Ben-Menachem, E., Tanasescu, R., Brodtkorb, E., Hillbom, M., Leone, M. A., & Ludolph, A. C. (2017). Alcohol withdrawal syndrome: Mechanisms, manifestations, and management. *Acta Neurologica Scandinavica, 135*(1), 4–16. https://www.ncbi.nlm.nih.gov/pmc/articles/PMC6084325/

National Institute of Mental Health. (2018). *Anxiety disorders.* U.S. Department of Health and Human Services, National Institute of Mental Health. https://www.nimh.nih.gov/health/topics/anxiety-disorders

Prescribers' Digital Reference. (n.d.). *Amitriptyline hydrochloride (amitriptyline hydrochloride).* PDR Search. https:// www.pdr.net/drug-summary/Amitriptyline-Hydrochloride-amitriptyline-hydrochloride-1001

Prescribers' Digital Reference. (n.d.). *Buspirone hydrochloride tablets* [Drug information]. PDR Search. https://www. pdr.net/drug-summary/Buspirone-Hydrochloride-Tablets--USP--7-5-mg-buspirone-hydrochloride-1523#5

Prescribers' Digital Reference. (n.d.). *Duloxetine* [Drug information]. PDR Search. https://pdr.net/drug-summary/ Cymbalta-duloxetine-288

Prescribers' Digital Reference. (n.d.). *Haldol (haloperidol)* [Drug information]. PDR Search. https://www.pdr.net/ drug-summary/Haldol-haloperidol-942

Prescribers' Digital Reference. (n.d.). *Marplan (isocarboxazid)* [Drug information]. PDR Search. https://www.pdr. net/drug-summary/Marplan-isocarboxazid-1355

Prescribers' Digital Reference. (n.d.). *Methadone hydrochloride* [Drug information]. PDR Search. https://www.pdr. net/drug-summary/Dolophine-methadone-hydrochloride-727

Prescribers' Digital Reference. (n.d.). *Naloxone hydrochloride* [Drug information]. PDR Search. https://pdr.net/ drug-summary/Naloxone-Hydrochloride-Injection--1-mg-mL--naloxone-hydrochloride-23987

Prescribers' Digital Reference. (n.d.). *Risperidone* [Drug information]. PDR Search. https://pdr.net/drug-summary/ Risperidone-risperidone-3120

Prescribers' Digital Reference. (n.d.). *Thiamine (thiamine hydrochloride)* [Drug information]. PDR Search. https://www.pdr.net/drug-summary/Thiamine-thiamine-hydrochloride-2546#13

Prescribers' Digital Reference. (n.d.). *Wellbutrin (bupropion hydrochloride)* [Drug information]. PDR Search. https://www.pdr.net/drug-summary/Wellbutrin-bupropion-hydrochloride-237

Prescribers' Digital Reference. (n.d.). *Xanax (alprazolam)* [Drug information]. PDR Search. https://www.pdr.net/ drug-summary/Xanax-alprazolam-1873#6

Wilber, S. T., & Ondrejka, J. E. (2016). Altered mental status and delirium. *Emergency Medicine Clinics of North America, 34*(3), 649–665. https://doi.org/10.1016/j.emc.2016.04.012

12

PROFESSIONAL CARING AND ETHICAL PRACTICE

THE SYNERGY MODEL

Overview

- Nursing care should be implemented using the AACN's *Synergy Model for Patient Care.*
  - This patient-centered model focuses on the needs of the patient, the competencies of the nurse, and the synergy created when those needs and competencies match.
  - This model ensures that nurses with appropriate ability and competency levels are paired with patients who require these skills and competencies in their care.
- Nursing competencies can evolve with increasing knowledge, skill, experience, and a nurse's desire for change. This includes advocacy and moral agency, caring practices, diversity and the nursing response, learning facilitation, collaboration, systems thinking, and clinical inquiry.
- Following the AACN's *Synergy Model for Patient Care* allows the nurse to provide high quality professional and ethically appropriate care to any patient.

ADVOCACY AND MORAL AGENCY

Overview

- *Advocacy* is the support of another individual to promote their wellbeing, such as speaking on behalf of a patient whose voice is not represented.
  - Advocacy is key in the PCU, as these patients are vulnerable and often need help speaking up on their own behalf.
  - The nurse's continuous presence at the bedside with the patient and family, as well as the ability to collaborate with the other members of the healthcare team, puts them in an ideal position to advocate for the patient.

 NURSING PEARL

Both advocacy and moral agency are essential aspects to the ANA's code of ethics. Provision 3 states, "The nurse promotes, advocates for, and protects the rights, health and safety of the patient."

- When the patient's family or nurse advocates on behalf of the patient, the nurse or family communicates the patient's ethical or clinical concerns related to their care, when they cannot.
  - Hospitalization of a close family member may be a stressful and challenging time for families.
  - In these situations, families may feel vulnerable or helpless if the patient cannot participate or if they are unsure of what decisions to make/what the patient would want at certain points in their care (e.g., code status).
  - Families are always encouraged to act as the patient's advocate, similar to the nurse, speaking on their behalf.
- *Moral agency* is the ability to continue to provide quality care despite obstacles. These obstacles may be physical, emotional, psychological, or related to the healthcare system or unit status and/or access to resources (staffing, supplies, or technology).

(continued)

Overview *(continued)*

- Moral agency occurs in the healthcare setting when the nurse helps to resolve potential ethical or clinical conflicts for the patient, regardless of the nurse's personal beliefs.
- To be an effective advocate and moral agent, the nurse needs to identify the patient's personal beliefs, values, and morals, as well as their own.
- Overall awareness influences how the nurse cares for their patients and ensures that the nurse is capable of incorporating ethical decision-making into their practice.
- Accepting differences allows the nurse to identify potential ethical conflicts that may affect their care so that they may advocate on behalf of the patient.

Ethical Principles

Nurses provide safe and compassionate care to the patient by incorporating four ethical principles of nursing into daily practice.
- *Nonmaleficence*: Taking actions that do not cause harm
  - Nonmaleficence in nursing occurs when the nurse makes a choice or performs an action that prevents harm. One example of this can occur when holding a medication which may be causing adverse effects, discussing this with the provider, and finding an alternative treatment.
- *Beneficence*: Taking actions that are in the best interest of the patient, "doing good"
  - Beneficence in nursing occurs when the nurse makes a choice that is moral and in the best interest of the patient. One example of this occurs when the nurse assists a patient with basic hygiene.
- *Autonomy*: Respecting a patient and their right to choose
  - Autonomy in nursing occurs when the nurse supports a patient's choice, regardless of the nurses' personal beliefs. One example of this is accepting a patient's choice to decline blood transfusions for religious reasons with a low hemoglobin.
- *Justice*: Caring for patients equally, in modern terms: acting in ways to reduce health disparity
  - Justice in nursing occurs when the nurse provides the same high level of care to all patients. One example of this is providing the same level of care to all patients admitted to the hospital.

Nursing Considerations

To promote advocacy and moral agency, the nurse must:
- Identify and discuss advanced directives.
- Identify and support code status wishes.
- Identify and reconfirm goals of care.
- Promote informed decision-making.
- Promote patient and family centered care.

Advanced Directives

- *Advanced directives* are legal documents that can be used as a framework to make choices or appoint another to make choices on behalf of the patient. These include the durable power of attorney and living wills. All patients do not have advanced directives. If a patient wants to develop an advanced directive, a social worker or case management can help them create one during their hospital stay.
- *Durable power of attorney* is a legal document indicating a person to be appointed to make decisions on behalf of the patient and utilized in the event that patient is unable to make their own decisions.
- *Living wills* are another written legal document that is written by the patient. This document states their wishes should they find themselves unable to make their own decisions.
- Both advanced directive and living wills are typically completed before hospital admission (or critical illness) to verify legality of the document; however, the patient can create one during a hospital admission. Patients should consult with legal counsel or may fill out a form independently. Notarization of forms ensures that they are legally completed.

Code Status

- Code status should be identified and documented at time of admission. If code status is unknown, and no patient or next of kin is available to determine code status, assume patient is a full code.
- Code status includes the following:
  - *Full Code* status indicates that in the event of cardiac or respiratory arrest, the patient has determined that they would like all interventions performed to resuscitate them. This includes CPR, intubation, defibrillation, emergency medication administration, central line insertion, NG/OGT insertion, and possible emergency interventional procedure (cardiac catheterization lab, vascular interventional radiology, etc.).
  - *DNR* orders indicate that in the event of a cardiac or respiratory arrest, the patient has determined that they do *NOT* want any resuscitation protocols or procedures to be performed on them. All other aggressive treatments aside from CPR/ACLS protocols will be performed.
  - *DNI* orders indicate that in the event of increasing oxygenation requirements or respiratory arrest, the patient does not want to be intubated. All other resuscitation protocols will be administered.
  - *Comfort Care* indicates that in the event of cardiac or respiratory arrest, the patient has determined that they want to pass without any aggressive treatment or intervention. This is typically ordered with a DNR but more accurately describes goals of care.

Goals of Care

- Conversations regarding goals of care should occur at the time of admission to the facility or unit and throughout hospital stay.
- To advocate appropriately for the patient, understanding desired goals of care is essential.
- Follow up and revisit goals of care with the patient as appropriate, especially if dealing with critical or chronic illness.
  - These conversations can be difficult; however, it is important to remain impartial and nonjudgmental during these conversations.
  - By doing this, the patient's autonomy and right to choose is supported.
  - The patient should be aware of their right to choose their treatment path (curative versus hospice/comfort).
    - Curative treatment approaches will include all possible interventions to cure disease or achieve the highest level of functioning possible.
    - Palliative treatment approaches shift the focus from curing to promoting quality of life. This may mean making choices that improve quality of life and comfort but accelerate illness or ultimate demise.
- Per the patient/family request, consult the palliative and hospice care team to provide more information to the patient and families.
  - *Palliative care* is a branch of specialized medicine which prioritizes optimizing quality of life and alleviating patient suffering.
    - Palliative care requires an interdisciplinary team approach to appropriately manage symptoms and support the patient and their families in mind, body, and spirit.
    - Palliative care can be initiated at the time of diagnosis and coexist with curative treatment, unlike hospice or end of life care.
    - Be mindful that palliative care is not an act of "giving up," but an act of improving quality of life before, during, and after the end of life for patients and their families.
  - Hospice care and end-of-life care share common goals.
    - *Hospice care* is also a branch of specialized medicine which prioritizes optimizing quality of life, alleviating patient suffering at the end of life, and allowing patient wishes of comfort to be met.
    - Hospice care is limited to patients with a terminal illness with a life expectancy of less than 6 months.

(continued)

Goals of Care (continued)

- ○ If the patient or family desire to be transferred to hospice care, the nurse should make every effort to advocate and facilitate transfer to a hospice facility or inpatient unit by involving the primary team and consulting both case management and social work.
- End-of-life or comfort care can occur for patients in the PCU setting and often coincides with removal of invasive respiratory or hemodynamic support.
  - While end of life care occurs in the inpatient setting, the goals remain consistent with palliative and hospice care to alleviate suffering and allow for a peaceful death.
  - In the inpatient setting, the nurse is responsible for:
    - ○ Administering continuous IV infusion of analgesic medication (commonly morphine, Table A.2)
    - ○ Pushing IV anxiolytics (Table 11.1) and analgesics for breakthrough pain and anxiety
    - ○ Preparing to administer an anticholinergic to help alleviate oral secretions and prepare to provide oral care and suctioning as needed
  - Be mindful of the signs and symptoms of death, which include:
    - ○ Decreased alertness and mental status
    - ○ Decreased appetite
    - ○ Vital sign changes
    - ○ Increase in respiratory and oral secretions
    - ○ Audible respiratory sounds (commonly referred to as the death rattle)
    - ○ Loss of bowel and urinary control
  - Communicate with the family to understand their support needs during this time and consult additional services as appropriate.

Informed and Ethical Decision-Making

- While it is the advanced practice provider's role to initiate a goals of care conversation with patients and family, the PCU nurse should be mindful and aware of the patient or family's understanding surrounding the goals of care.
- Similar to informed consent for procedures, it is the provider's responsibility to explain and review all pertinent information, such as treatment modalities, possible interventions/options, and the variations of goals of care and code status.
- The PCU nurse should be ready to reinforce education provided by the physician and provide additional opportunities for discussion as needed for the patient and family to feel comfortable in their decision. If possible, direct patients and family to community resources or appropriate online community resources to help supplement their understanding.

Patient and Family Rights

- The nurse should be aware of the Patient's Bill of Rights when providing care and advocating for them. Patients have the right to:
  - Safe, considerate, and respectful care, consistent with their beliefs.
  - Confidential communications pertaining to records and plan of care.
  - Know and meet their coordinating physician.
  - Receive all information and education about their health status presented at their level of medical literacy.
  - Have a legally appointed representative when unable to receive information personally.
  - Receive informed consent that defines the procedure and identifies risks and alternatives prior to any procedure.
  - Obtain routine services during hospitalization, including treatment of any chronic conditions.
  - Know appointment times, as well as receive continuity of care.
  - Assessment and treatment of pain.
  - Refuse to participate in research.
  - Transfer facilities pending insurance and clinical status.
  - Receive a medical summary at the end of care.
  - Designate other physicians or organizations, at their request, to receive medical updates.

- Families and patients additionally have the right to determine code status; however, they are unable to demand the continuation of CPR if continuing has been determined to be medically futile per the overseeing provider (also known as "calling" the code).

Patient and Family-Centered Care

- Allow family or friends to visit and stay with the patient if allowed per unit policy and when appropriate.
- Educate the family, as well as the patient, on the situation and any options to consider.
- Establish a family member or friend as a spokesperson who will update the rest of the family of the patient's status.
- Include family in meetings and goals of care discussions.

CARING IN NURSING PRACTICE

Overview

- Theoretical knowledge alone is not enough to function effectively in the nursing profession.
- Caring is the central and most defining concept of nursing. Caring should be patient-centered to ensure the best outcomes for the patient.
- Though caring is not specifically addressed in the nursing code of ethics, it is integrated within each principle of the code.
- Caring in nursing practice promotes patient safety, comfort, and a compassionate, therapeutic, and supportive environment for patients, family, and other staff members. This involves:
  - *Commitment*: ensures that patients' rights and safety are at the forefront of decision-making and care delivery
  - *Communication*: ensures that effective open communication is maintained to place the patients' needs and rights at the forefront of decision-making
  - *Compassion*: ensures patients are treated well and provided with a positive supportive experience
  - *Competence*: ensures that the nurse is held to a high standard of excellence and meets all legal, regulatory, and practice standards to provide quality care
  - *Conscience*: ensures the best moral decision is made even when faced with challenges

 NURSING PEARL

The Nursing Alliance for Quality Care identifies these principles to ensure care is patient-centered:

- Patients should have an active partnership with their families as well as their healthcare providers.
- Patients have the right to make their own healthcare decisions.
- Patients, families, and providers need to share responsibility and accountability.
- Healthcare providers must always respect any privacy boundaries and ensure confidentiality.
- Information sharing and decision-making should be mutual.
- Patient engagement varies from patient to patient and may be influenced by culture or other individual elements.
- Patient advocacy is a critical feature of nursing.
- To fully engage with patients, the nurse needs to identify, appreciate, and acknowledge all cultural, racial, or ethnic backgrounds.
- It is essential to identify and individualize healthcare plans according to the patient and family's educational, language, and literacy needs to ensure full comprehension.

ALERT!

The nurse's engagement with the patient is essential to ensure the safest and highest quality care is being delivered.

Nursing Considerations

- Nursing responsibilities to ensure patient safety include engagement, responsiveness, and vigilance.
- These characteristics promote a therapeutic and supportive environment, as well as promoting compassionate patient care.
  - *Engagement*: the ability of the nurse to empower the patient to be involved in their own care and make informed decisions regarding their own health and healthcare

(continued)

Nursing Considerations (continued)

- *Responsiveness*: the ability of the nurse to provide patient care that is respectful to the patient and addresses all their concerns
- *Vigilance*: the ability of the nurse to identify any potential risks to the patient or signs of clinical deterioration and the ability to act in response to a change in condition

Patient Safety

- Utilize precautions specific to the patient's needs to maintain safety. Examples are as follows:
  - Aspiration precautions
    - ○ Ensure appropriate diet is ordered based on patient's clinical status.
    - ○ Ensure dentures are in place and secure while eating if applicable to patient.
    - ○ Maintain HOB elevated at least 30°.
    - ○ Monitor patient to ensure they are chewing and swallowing adequately.
    - ○ Monitor for coughing and clearance after each bite.
    - ○ Consult speech pathologist for a formal speech evaluation if there is any concern of aspiration.
  - Fall precautions:
    - ○ Place a bed or chair alarm on the patient's surface, as needed.
    - ○ Ensure bed is always locked and in the lowest position.
    - ○ Have a call light within reach of patient at all times.
    - ○ Maintain frequent checks or hourly rounding on patient to ensure safety
    - ○ Use assistive equipment to mobilize patient.
    - ○ Use preventative alerts to signal that patient is a fall alert such as wristband, room flags, grip socks, and so forth.
    - ○ Utilize patient sitter as necessary for high fall risks.
  - Pressure ulcer precautions:
    - ○ Elevate patient's extremities with pillows.
    - ○ Turn patient at least every 2 hr.
    - ○ Use protective barrier cream and lotions to protect the skin.
    - ○ Maintain perineal hygiene as necessary; change pads as soon as soiling is noted.
    - ○ Apply a protective foam/adhesive dressing on bony prominences.
    - ○ Utilize protective boots to prevent breakdown on heels.
    - ○ Request a wound care consult if necessary.
    - ○ Elevate heels off bed or utilize heel protector boots.
    - ○ Place on a pressure redistribution surface, such as a low air loss or pressure relief overlay.
    - ○ Reposition movable devices.
    - ○ Provide support surfaces and special cushions when sitting in the chair.
  - Seizure precautions:
    - ○ Ensure side rails are padded.
    - ○ Have supplemental oxygen and suction equipment readily available at bedside.
    - ○ Maintain low stimulation in room: avoid harsh lighting and loud TV or other noises. Educate visitors to not overstimulate the patient.
  - Suicidal ideation precautions:
    - ○ Ensure patient is wearing hospital attire to signal they are on suicide precautions.
      - ▪ This may include scrubs, a gown of a different color, wristband, or socks.
      - ▪ This may vary across healthcare systems.
    - ○ Follow institutional policy regarding patient personal belongings.
    - ○ Maintain a 1:1 sitter at all times.
    - ○ Minimize visitors as necessary and ensure that visitors do not bring in any objects that the patient may use for harm.

POP QUIZ 12.1

A nurse is caring for a 60-year-old male patient with a history of CHF, CAD, PAD, andT2DM who is requiring surgery for a CABG the next day. The patient has been very anxious since hearing the news that he needs surgery. His wife has stayed with him to help alleviate his anxiety until visiting hr ended. The cardiovascular surgeon has come to obtain consent for the surgery; however, the patient is experiencing increased anxiety that his wife is not here for this conversation. How can the nurse effectively advocate for this patient?

- ○ Remove any objects from room that the patient could potentially use to harm themselves or others.
- ○ Use plastic utensils and paper plates.
- Communicate these precautions to other members of the healthcare team to ensure they are maintaining the safety of the patient, especially if the patient is traveling to other areas of the hospital.
- Explain these precautions to the patient and family to include them in maintaining a safe environment.
- Update the patient's plan of care to reflect these precautions as their condition changes.
  - Some patients may not need these precautions on admission but require them later in their care as their condition changes or vice versa.

Minimize Risk of Medical Errors

- Always use the five rights of medication administration.
  - Right patient
  - Right drug
  - Right dose
  - Right route
  - Right time
- Clarify orders with the physician or pharmacist if unsure or unfamiliar with order.
  - For verbal orders, ask the physician to repeat or spell out the order to ensure it is correct.
  - Limit distractions while taking orders.
- Practice good communication with all members of the healthcare team.
  - Active listening
  - Documentation
  - Verbal communication
- Utilize hospital policies and protocols to ensure accurate patient care.

Engagement

- It is important to build a therapeutic relationship with the patient and family in order to be able to engage with them at the fullest potential.
  - Maintain an active and ongoing partnership with the patient and family by continually looking for social and nonsocial cues and careful assessment of the relationships throughout their care.
  - Maintain an empathetic viewpoint of the patient and be careful to monitor the situation from their perspective.
  - Support the patient as they learn to empower themselves.
  - Offer emotional and mental presence as well as physical presence to build a therapeutic relationship with the patient.
  - Be aware of cultural disparities and integrate cultural differences into practice.
  - Maintain mutuality with the patient, which is essential for shared decision-making.
  - Work with the patient, not just on behalf of the patient.
  - Preserve patient dignity whenever possible.
  - Actively listen to the patient.
  - Be aware of the patient's educational needs and anticipate if resources are needed to assist the patient to fully understand their plan of care.
- Inspire the patient to become engaged in their own treatment once a therapeutic relationship has been established.
- Empower the patient to assume responsibility and accountability for actions that will improve their health and their care.
- Ensure that the patient and family are being heard and engaging in their care.

 ALERT!

Although it is important to build a therapeutic relationship with a patient, remember to maintain and respect privacy boundaries and confidentiality. It is also important for the nurse to take a step back when appropriate.

Responsiveness
Generally, the more responsive the nurse is to a patient, the more engaging the patient will be in their plan of care.
- Use a more flexible and responsive approach that is individualized to the needs of the specific patient population.
- Be available to respond to nonclinical needs or preferences.
- Ensure the patient can easily contact healthcare providers, utilizing new technology or not.
- Adjust care as needed depending on specific groups of patients to fit their needs.
- Show integrity with patients and families.
- Maintain hourly rounding to ensure presence.

Vigilance
- Vigilance begins with a thorough patient physical, psychosocial, and environmental assessment.
- A vigilant assessment includes:
  - Use clinical knowledge to anticipate the patient's physical examination depending on their condition.
  - Compare knowledge of the condition to the patient's presenting symptoms.
  - Anticipate what potential complications could arise with the patient depending on their condition.
  - Identify what these complications would look like clinically, what changes to monitor for, and jump into action if these complications occur.
  - Identify what interventions would be needed for treatment of the condition and any potential complications.
  - Outweigh the risks and benefits of interventions for the patient.
  - Recognize how the patient should respond to interventions.
  - Ensure any potential patient changes are being accurately documented and reported to the healthcare team as necessary.

SYNERGY EXAMPLE

The nurse is providing care to a 24-year-old male patient in the PCU who was admitted for injuries resulting from an MVC. The patient is now paralyzed from L2 down. The patient appears depressed, will not participate in therapy, and does not communicate with staff. The nurse who provides caring practice attempts to build a therapeutic relationship with the patient by addressing him as an individual and not by his injury. The nurse asks the patient about his likes, dislikes, friends, family, what interests him, and so forth., to help build a mutual relationship. Once a relationship has been built, the nurse also helps to identify short-term goals for the patient to help him participate in therapy and utilize his interests to motivate him. As the patient progresses through therapy, the nurse should ensure his safety precautions and goals are addressed as well.

DIVERSITY AND THE NURSING RESPONSE
Overview
- Respecting and valuing all patients is core to the nursing profession.
- Nurses are called on to respond with sensitivity and quality care to all patients, regardless of race, disability, socioeconomic status, religion, age, or sexual orientation.
- Knowledge of diversity and various cultural practices or values is essential to provide patient-centered care and to appropriately advocate and represent patients.
- Diversity in nursing ensures that all patients feel welcome and that they receive the care they deserve.

Nursing Considerations

- The PCU nurse should be familiar with the practices and cultures of the populations in their geographic area.
- Do not assume that the patient and/or family has the same values or beliefs.
  - Get to know the patient on a personal level to identify any differences.
  - Explore these differences with the patient and their family. Ask questions regarding any differences to improve understanding.
  - Accept the information provided by the patient and family and modify the plan of care to fit their needs while still ensuring patient safety.
- Eliminate health disparities that may affect the patient, such as: cultural, racial, and ethnic differences, mental status barriers, and socioeconomic disparities.
- Identify, respect, and address any differences in patients' values, preferences, or needs.

Age

- Use language that is appropriate for the patient's age group.
- Modify nursing care as needed to ensure it is appropriate for the patient.
- Utilize technology as a resource for patient. Take into consideration that the elderly may be less technologically inclined.

Culture

- Ensure the ordered diet meets what the patient needs nutritionally as well as maintains their cultural or religious beliefs.
- Remain open minded and respectful of cultural or religious practices.
  - Allow cultural or religious practices that do not compromise patient or staff wellness or safety.
  - For practices that may compromise patient or staff safety (lighting candles or opening windows), collaborate with patient and family to identify alternative and acceptable solutions.
- Some cultures may use essential oils, lotions, teas, or medicinal herbs for healing purposes. Before allowing the patient or family to use these, ensure they do not have any potential interactions with any current medications.

Education

- Ensure communication to patients and families is at a level everyone can understand and fully comprehend.
- Utilize different techniques to educate patients, as everyone learns differently:
  - Handouts
  - Verbal explanation
  - Videos
  - Demonstration

Ethnicity

- Ask the patient or family if there are any ethnic considerations that need to be considered while they are in the hospital.
- Be aware of certain risk factors and health conditions that may affect specific ethnicities more than others. For example: a disproportionate number of African American males are diagnosed with hypertension when compared to the general population.
- Provide education or resources specific to the patient's and family's ethnic background if necessary.
- Identify any potential language barriers and make necessary accommodations to ensure accurate communication. Utilize medical interpreting services as needed.

Gender

- Respect privacy and boundaries as defined by the patient while still providing competent and safe care.
- Ask transitioning patients what name and pronouns they prefer and inform all essential members of the healthcare team.

Lifestyle
- Lifestyle choices can range from diet and exercise regimen to personal lifestyle choices such as sexual behaviors and use of illegal substances.
- Ask the patient about their lifestyle choices.
- If any poor choice is noted (alcohol, drug, tobacco, obesity, sedentary lifestyle, etc.) provide education and supportive resources to make lasting change.

Spirituality and Religious Beliefs
- Advocate from patient/family perspective, whether similar to or different from personal values.
- Ask the patient about their religion and if there are any special considerations that need to be taken while they are admitted.
- Allow the patient and family time to pray, openly practice their religion, or reflect depending on their religious needs as possible while following institutional guidelines and maintaining patient care.
- Allow religious objects in the room if requested.
- Support visitation with religious leader if requested while abiding by unit and institutional visitor policies.
- Consult chaplain services if requested by the patient or family to perform a prayer, last rites, and so forth.
- Support religious customs throughout patient's hospital stay.

Socioeconomics
- Ensure social work is consulted if necessary to follow up with discharge planning.
- Provide community resources to patients including outpatient exercise or diet programs, community food bank or donation centers, assistance with transportation, and/or securing medical devices or medication.

Values
- Identify what values are important to the patient and integrate them into their hospital care.
- If the patient's values pose a safety concern, collaborate with the patient, providers, and leadership to find an alternative solution that meets both patient needs and maintains safety.

 POP QUIZ 12.2

The nurse is caring for a 72-year-old female of Chinese descent. She is day three post-op, recovering from an MVC where she required surgical repair of her right hip. The family arrives to visit, bringing her favorite foods, pictures from home, and a variety of medicinal healing herbs to assist with her recovery. What should the nurse's response be when the patient asks if she can take the herbal treatments brought from home?

SYNERGY EXAMPLE

The nurse is providing care to a 67-year-old male Muslim patient admitted for a CVA post TPA. The patient is improving and ready for transfer to the step-down unit. The staff is getting ready to transfer the patient at noon; however, the patient is requesting to wait as this is his time for prayer according to the Muslim religion. The nurse appropriately responds to diversity by accepting and accommodating the patient's beliefs, even though the nurse does not practice that same religion, and allows the transfer to wait until the patient has finished his prayers. The nurse communicates this to the other staff and provides the patient with privacy while he is praying.

FACILITATION OF LEARNING

Overview
- A key component of nursing care is the ability to facilitate learning between patients, families, nursing and other healthcare staff, and the community.
- Nurses can facilitate learning by engaging the patient in active learning, identifying any barriers to learning, and incorporating methods to overcome those barriers.

- Barriers to learning for patients may be cognitive, emotional, or psychosocial. These barriers must be identified and addressed before a patient is willing and able to receive new information.
- In addition to patient education, a large component of facilitation of learning applies to nurses educating other nurses in the field. This includes nurse preceptors and nursing educators providing education to new graduate nurses, new hires, or student nurses.

Nursing Considerations

- Facilitation of learning to both patients and new nurses use similar education concepts:
  - Adapt educational programs to fit the needs of the patient and family.
  - Work with the learner to set educational goals.
  - Coach and explain to patients and families at a level they will comprehend.
  - Support the ideas of the new learner and allow them to think of alternatives while offering feedback as needed.
  - Share information for the new learner to make an informed decision, rather than directing them to the answer.
  - Validate the experiences of the patient and/or student nurse.
  - Allow ample time for questions.
  - Identify what is most important to the patient and refocus their attention onto those things if they are overwhelmed.
  - Collaborate with other healthcare providers to incorporate the patient's goals.
  - Use creative ways to integrate education into patient care while providing evidence-based practice.
  - Use the teach-back method to verify learning has occurred:
    - "Please describe the steps for checking blood sugar."
    - "Please repeat back to me what we discussed."
  - Address barriers to learning and ways to overcome obstacles.
  - Engage the learner in various ways:
    - Engage verbally, through discussion.
    - Provide auditory or visual education through recorded audio or videos.
    - Provide written handouts or website resources to investigate.
    - Deliver education formally, but use informal methods as well.
- In addition to the education concepts listed, preceptors should also consider the following when teaching:
  - Share stories: Preceptors can share their experiences and passion for nursing to establish a relationship, as well as discuss how they faced and overcame the same challenges and fears.
  - Assess clinical competency: New nurses may be fearful of making decisions independently. As a preceptor, give them tasks that allow them to develop clinical judgment skills while acting as a resource and standing by to prevent errors.
  - Be an effective communicator.
  - Allow time for reflection at the end of the shift.
  - Be patient and understanding when learning new tasks or procedures.
  - Have clear expectations and provide independent learning experiences. Watching or shadowing cannot replace hands-on experience.

SYNERGY EXAMPLE

The nurse is caring for a patient with a new diagnosis of T2DM and needs to educate him and his wife on how to monitor blood glucose at home. As a competent facilitator of learning, the nurse knows that people learn in different ways. The nurse decides to provide educational pamphlets, videos, and online resources for the patient and his wife. The nurse also demonstrates to the patient and his wife how to use the glucometer to check blood glucose and how to draw up and inject insulin.

To further facilitate his learning, the nurse watches the patient check his blood glucose using his new glucometer while providing feedback. The nurse informs the patient care technician that the patient should be checking his own blood glucose from now on. Collaborate with the assistant to ensure the patient is performing this correctly and asking staff any questions he may have.

COLLABORATION

Overview

- In healthcare, *collaboration* is defined as the ability to work with others toward the same common goal. It is essential in critical care.
  - Collaboration requires all members of the healthcare team to work together, sharing responsibility for problem solving and decision-making.
  - It also requires active listening, effective communication, trust, and a sharing of ideas between all stakeholders (patients, families, and the medical care team).
- Collaboration occurs among all professions and leaders in the healthcare team, patients, and family.
  - Taking care of critically ill patients utilizes staff from all fields, such as physicians, psychologists, pharmacists, respiratory therapists, occupational therapists, physical therapists, registered dieticians, physician assistants, nurse practitioners, and certified technicians.
  - Many critically ill patients have diseases and medical problems that affect multiple body systems. This may require physicians from all levels and specialties, working together to ensure the health and well-being of the patient.
- The nurse is instrumental in promoting collaboration between different members of the healthcare team to eliminate potential knowledge gaps, facilitating information sharing and decision-making, and identifying any barriers to the health and safety of the patient.

Nursing Considerations

- Collaboration cannot effectively take place without open communication between patient, family, and interdisciplinary staff.
  - Effective communication occurs when the healthcare team, who may have different backgrounds, experience, education levels, skill levels, or specialties, can discuss information, ideas, and opinions openly with one another.
  - Participation in daily rounds with the healthcare team promotes collaboration across all skill levels. It also provides focused communication about the patient's treatment plan.
    - ○ Interdisciplinary rounds provide a platform to discuss the patient's clinical status, plan of care, and engage in shared decision-making across all skill levels, making sure the treatment plan is evidence-based, patient-specific, and aligns with the patient's wishes.
    - ○ This allows team members to identify and discuss any potential patient concerns clinically, socially, and psychologically.
    - ○ Daily rounding ensures the whole team is on board with the current plan of care and minimizes back-and-forth miscommunication among members.
    - ○ Additionally, daily rounding provides an opportunity for the patient and family to be involved and listen to the treatment plan.
    - ○ The nurse can prepare for rounds by organizing a basic overview of the patient's status, any concerning findings, and recommendations or suggestions to improve the treatment plan.
- At the core of collaboration is also trust.
  - Trust needs to be evident in the relationships between team-members (how work is done, how words are spoken, and how the results are accounted for). Without trust, collaboration can fall apart quickly.
  - In order to work together to effectively care for the patient, the nurse needs to trust the skills, knowledge, and training of the interdisciplinary team.

 POP QUIZ 12.3

A patient has vocalized feelings of sadness and depression that have worsened throughout their critical illness. Though the patient's clinical status has improved, they still require 35% oxygen via trach collar during the day and ventilator support overnight. Therefore, they are unable to be transferred to the PCU per this hospital's policy. Family and staff have tried engaging to improve the patient's mood, but nothing has made real change. The nurse asks the patient if they would like to go on a "field trip" to see something other than her hospital room and unit. The patient is excited by this and asks when they can go.

Before taking this patient off the unit, what collaborative actions must the nurse take?

- This is especially important in high-stress patient situations, as well as for basic nursing tasks, such as helping with patient bathing or turns, covering for each other during lunch, and answering each other's questions.
- Team learning involves everyone working together toward one common goal and improving patient care using best practice evidence.
- Collaborative leadership allows members of a leadership team to work together to make decisions to keep the unit thriving.
  - This style of leadership among charge nurses, preceptors, assistant nurse managers, and unit managers offers an environment of openness, trust, and comfort, which in turn allows nurses to freely share different perspectives, voices, opinions, and ideas. This is a necessary step for innovation.

SYNERGY EXAMPLE

Interdisciplinary rounding is a good example of collaboration between health disciplines. During interdisciplinary rounding, while each institution may have their own protocol for the flow and order, generally the MD/NP/PA gives a brief overview of the patient's history and physical and then reviews the events of hospital admission. Nursing presents the overnight or daily events and brings up new issues or concerns to the team. Pharmacy reviews medications, dosages, and labs to ensure medications are still appropriate for clinical condition, while the dietitian reviews diet orders, weight gain or loss, and tube feeding composition, if applicable. When new issues arise, they are discussed together, considering all angles and points of view before moving forward with new interventions. This process allows the patient to receive high quality collaborative care.

SYSTEMS THINKING

Overview

- Systems thinking takes into consideration the entire healthcare systems process while providing care for patients.
- It is a holistic approach to advancing healthcare or identifying problems on a global or large system scale. This includes understanding:
  - The patient or whole person within a system
  - Public domain
  - Regional health trends (e.g., increased incidence of diabetes in southern states, regional vaccination rates)
  - National health data (e.g., increased incidence of childhood obesity)
  - World or global health (e.g., increase access to OBGYN or midwifery care in all nations)
- Systems thinking can be applied to providing care for patients, discharge planning, policy creation, and root cause analysis of adverse or sentinel events.

Nursing Considerations

- To be a systems thinker, nurses must:
  - Consider unintended consequences.
  - Fully consider issues taking the systems functioning into consideration.
  - Identify cause and effect relationships within the system.
  - Make meaningful connections between aspects of the system.
  - Observe how aspects of a system changes over time. Note patterns and trends within these changes.
  - Recognize and understand that a systems structure generates behavior.
  - Seek to understand the big picture.

(continued)

Nursing Considerations *(continued)*

- When using systems thinking to identify root cause, the nurse must first:
  - Identify the problem.
  - Identify involved parties.
  - Collect data from charting and/or interviewing.
  - Determine factors which could lead to problem.
  - Identify solutions and/or corrective actions to causative factors.
  - Implement solutions.
  - Identify other areas where this solution could be implemented.

SYNERGY EXAMPLE

A CT scan was completed on a patient over 12 hr after the order was placed, leading to a delay in treatment. A member of the quality control committee performed a root cause analysis to identify the cause of the delay in care. The involved parties include the patient, the family, the assigned nurse, and the providers. After a chart review, additional information was identified. The order was placed at the change of shift, and the oncoming nurse admitted a new patient. Once the order was recognized by the nurse a few hr later, transport was called. However, transportation logs showed over an hr delay. Additionally, CT had to delay this patient's scan because they were overloaded with emergent scans from the emergency department. The investigating nurse identified that a challenging patient assignment, paired with transport delays, and an increased acuity in the emergency department resulted in a delayed scan. A possible solution includes the physician changing the order of the scan from "routine" to "STAT," to prioritize this patient's scan. Also, the CT technician can call the nurse to plan a scheduled time for both the CT scan and transportation.

CLINICAL INQUIRY

Overview

- Clinical inquiry is the process of questioning and evaluating practice to advance evidence-based and informed practice.
- It involves the continual progression of nursing care through questioning and evaluating healthcare practice.
- The nurse can create effective change by practicing evidence-based practice, conducting research, and implementing experiential knowledge.
- The goal is to stay up to date with the most recent professional literature and share this information with others.

Nursing Considerations

The PCU nurse should be familiar with the best practice by engaging in clinical inquiry. This can be performed by doing the following:

- Review and compare research/literature findings to current practice and engage in evidence-based practice or quality improvement projects.
  - This can be done independently or in collaboration with an individual mentor, a like-minded group, or a unit committee.
  - If a research or best practice committee exists within the unit or hospital, consider joining to routinely engage in research or literature findings to identify current best practice.
  - If the unit or hospital does not currently have a research or evidence-based practice committee, speak with unit leadership about possibly starting one.
- Gather knowledge. This can be done by basic internet searches or through rigorous searching of nursing journals or databases.

● Conduct unit specific research. Consider collaborating with unit leadership or a best practice committee to conduct unit specific research to identify possible improvements to policy, procedure, or care process. This can include:

  ● Quality improvement projects involve live monitoring and evaluation of the quality of services provided to patients. Shortcomings and solutions are identified and then tested through additional data collection.

  ● Evidenced-based practice studies are more scholarly experiences focused on literature and research review. Once EBP procedures are identified, they are then implemented into unit practice and procedures and monitored for outcomes.

● Advocate for practice changes to align with research-based practice recommendations.

  ● Be observant of the policies, procedures, or care processes that could be improved or made more efficient.

  ● Identify and discuss findings to unit leadership and/or providers to create meaningful change.

● Share findings with unit leadership, nurse educator, clinical nurse specialist, and staff as appropriate.

  ● Present findings as appropriate through presentations at unit meetings, emails, or hand-outs posted throughout the breakroom or nursing station.

  ● Continue disseminating this information until meaningful and positive change is achieved.

SYNERGY EXAMPLE

During a monthly article review, the nurse learns that chlorhexidine-impregnated dressings can reduce CLABSIs and increase cost effectiveness in the healthcare setting. During the last unit meeting, the nurse educator described the increased rates of patients with CLABSIs in the hospital. The nurse advocates for an increase in the supply of chlorhexidine central line dressings and disinfecting caps for the needleless connectors on the IV tubing. The nurse educates other nurses on the unit to keep the sterile dressing clean, dry, and occlusive, and to change the dressing every 7 days or when soiled.

RESOURCES

Albert, T. (2019). *Why you need to be a systems thinker in health care.* American Medical Association. https://www.ama-assn.org/education/accelerating-change-medical-education/why-you-need-be-systems-thinker-health-care

American Nurses Association. (2015). *Code of ethics for nurses with interpretive statements.* https://www.nursingworld.org/coe-view-only

Chan, T. W., Poon, E., & Hegney, D. (2011). What nurses need to know about Buddhist perspectives of end-of-life care. *Progress in Palliative Care, 19,* 61–65.

Epstein, B., & Turner, M. (2015). The nursing code of ethics: Its value, its history. *Online Journal of Issues in Nursing, 20*(2), 4. https://doi.org/10.3912/OJIN.Vol20No02Man04

Irvin, J. N., Kahn, J. M., Cohen, T. R., & Weingart, L. R. (2018). Teamwork in the intensive care unit. *The American Psychologist, 73*(4), 468–477. https://www.ncbi.nlm.nih.gov/pmc/articles/PMC6662208/

Gaines, K. (2021). What is the nursing code of ethics?. *Nurse.org.* https://nurse.org/education/nursing-code-of-ethics/

Gaylord, N., & Grace, P. (1995). Nursing advocacy: An ethic of practice. *Nursing Ethics, 2*(1), 11–18. https://doi.org/10.1177/096973309500200103

Grace, P. (2018). Enhancing nurse moral agency: The leadership promise of doctor of nursing practice preparation. *OJIN: The Online Journal of Issues in Nursing, 23*(1). https://doi.org/10.3912/OJIN.Vol23No01Man04

Hardin, S. R., & Kaplow, R. (2016). *Synergy for clinical excellence: The AACN synergy model for patient care.* American Association of Critical-Care Nurses.

Institute for Patient- and Family-Centered Care. (n.d.). *Patient- and family-centered care. What is PFCC?* https://www.ipfcc.org/about/pfcc.html

Meyer, G., & Lavin, M. A. (2005). Vigilance: The essence of nursing. *Online Journal of Issues in Nursing, 10*(3), 8. https://pubmed.ncbi.nlm.nih.gov/16225388/

Mick, J. (2017). Funneling evidence into practice. *Nursingcenter.com*. https://www.nursingcenter.com/wkhlrp/Handlers/articleContent.pdf?key=pdf_00006247-201707000-00009

NIH Clinical Center. (n.d.). *Patient bill of rights*. U.S. Department of Health and Human Services, NIH Clinical Center. https://clinicalcenter.nih.gov/participate/patientinfo/legal/bill_of_rights.html

O'Daniel, M. (2008). Professional communication and team collaboration. In R. G. Hughes (Ed.), *Patient safety and quality: An evidence-based handbook for nurses*. Agency for Healthcare Research and Quality. https://www.ncbi.nlm.nih.gov/books/NBK2637/#:~:text=Collaboration%20in%20health%20care%20is,out%20plans%20for%20patient%20care

Six Sigma. (2017, March 10). *Root cause analysis (RCAa) – Important steps*. https://www.6sigma.us/etc/root-cause-analysis-important-steps/

Tarrant, C., Angell, E., Baker, R., Boulton, M., Freeman, G., Wilkie, P., Jackson, P., Wobi, F., and Ketley, D. (2014). Responsiveness of primary care services: Development of a patient-report measure – qualitative study and initial quantitative pilot testing. In *Health services and delivery research*, 2(46). https://www.ncbi.nlm.nih.gov/books/NBK263682/

Welch, J., & Fournier, A. (2018). Patient engagement through informed nurse caring. *International Journal for Human Caring*, 22(1), 1–10. https://doi.org/10.20467/1091-5710.22.1.pg5

POP QUIZ ANSWERS

CHAPTER 2

POP QUIZ 2.1

The nurse's next action would be to increase the patient's oxygen to obtain a saturation >90%. The nurse should then notify the provider of the new ST elevation noted on the EKG and worsening symptoms and vital sign changes.

POP QUIZ 2.2

The nurse's next action should be to auscultate the heart and lungs. Pericarditis after acute chest trauma can quickly progress into a pericardial effusion and/or cardiac tamponade. When auscultating the heart, muffled heart sounds or a pericardial friction rub may present. These assessment findings, in addition to the patient's presentation, are hallmark signs of acute pericarditis.

POP QUIZ 2.3

The nurse should request activity orders and pain relief medication. Activity and movement may elevate BP greater than the 110-mmHg goal. Confirm with the provider what activity orders are appropriate for your patient. Patients with suspected aortic aneurysms should be treated with pain medication and antihypertensives. While this patient's aortic aneurysm was asymptomatic, he did sustain a rib fracture. The pain associated with his acute trauma may contribute to a BP increase and jeopardize the integrity of the aneurysm. Bedside monitoring is also indicated for BP management and sudden vital sign changes in the patient.

POP QUIZ 2.4

This patient has three-vessel disease, which is a contraindication to stent placement or balloon angioplasty. She requires a CABG to treat her CAD and lesions. You should expect cardiothoracic surgery to place orders to urgently prep this patient for surgery.

POP QUIZ 2.5

Notify the provider. This is a surgical emergency, which requires prompt evacuation of the extra fluid from the pericardial sac.

POP QUIZ 2.6

Notify the provider that the patient requires a higher level of care. Vasopressors are not typically administered in the PCU. This patient requires central-line placement, vasopressors, and continuous arterial BP monitoring. Call a rapid response if necessary to gather additional support staff to facilitate quick transfer

POP QUIZ 2.7

Patients with HIV are at risk to develop left ventricular dysfunction, which often progresses to dilated cardiomyopathy and presents with little to no symptoms. If this patient's HIV antibody test comes back positive, then the etiology of his cardiomyopathy has likely been identified. This patient can begin HAART. Prophylaxis for opportunistic infection, which could worsen the clinical condition, can now be administered.

POP QUIZ 2.8

The nurse should notify the provider immediately, call for a rapid response, and prepare for transfer to the ICU.

POP QUIZ 2.9

Patients taking loop diuretics are at risk for developing hypokalemia. If hypokalemia develops in the context of digoxin therapy, patients are at risk for developing digoxin toxicity. Digoxin toxicity manifests with GI symptoms (nausea, vomiting, and anorexia), visual disturbances (blurred vision, photophobia, yellow-tinged vision, and halos), CNS symptoms (fatigue and headache), and dysrhythmia, which can result in cardiac arrest.

POP QUIZ 2.10

Patients with HTN and their family must be educated on the importance of following a low-sodium diet to help achieve BP control. Patients and family may hear that sodium should be avoided; however, many do not understand which foods have high sodium and may need education on what should be avoided. Chinese takeout and fast food has elevated levels of sodium, which can be dangerous for patients with HTN. Advise the wife to bring a breakfast item that adheres to the DASH diet.

POP QUIZ 2.11

Notify the provider immediately and call for necessary support team depending on situation (rapid response, code stroke, code team, etc.). Prepare to transfer to higher level of care.

POP QUIZ 2.12

Patients with mitral valve stenosis and atrial fibrillation are at high risk for embolism development, PE, DVT, or stroke. Anticoagulation or antiplatelet therapy is indicated to prevent these additional complications.

POP QUIZ 2.13

Administer vitamin K as ordered and monitor for excessive bleeding.

CHAPTER 3

POP QUIZ 3.1

Barotrauma occurs from overdistention of the alveoli during mechanical ventilation through increased tidal volumes or high PEEP settings. Barotrauma can lead to pneumothorax, tension pneumothorax, and subcutaneous emphysema.

POP QUIZ 3.2

Intubation and mechanical ventilation is the next step if patient becomes unresponsive to standard treatment.

POP QUIZ 3.3

Patients with no history of smoking or secondhand smoke inhalation should be worked up for alpha 1 antitrypsin deficiency. This is a genetic disorder that can cause COPD.

POP QUIZ 3.4

Respiratory depressants (including opioids, sedatives, alcohol, or other drugs) should be avoided, as they can worsen sleep apnea.

POP QUIZ 3.5

The nurse should clarify the procedure being performed related to the diagnosis with the student. Needle decompression is an appropriate treatment for a tension pneumothorax, but not hemothorax.

POP QUIZ 3.6

Daily oral care with oral cleaning solution.

POP QUIZ 3.7

Lung transplant is considered the last option for treatment of pulmonary HTN. Despite this option, there is the potential for recurrence of pulmonary HTN post lung transplant.

POP QUIZ 3.8

Although the patient wakes up complaining of pain, the respiratory rate is concerning. Providing additional pain medication is contraindicated based on mental status and alertness, oxygen saturation, and respiratory rate. Hold any additional narcotics until the patient's respiratory rate and mental status improve. Consider a reversal agent if the patient continues to be difficult to arouse.

POP QUIZ 3.9

Proning patients who are mechanically ventilated can improve ventilatory status. If no improvement is observed with proning, the patient can be considered a candidate for ECMO.

POP QUIZ 3.10

This is correct. Atelectasis following a thoracic procedure can be an emergency. If chest tube and intubation are indicated and not possible in your current setting, call for immediate transfer to ICU.

CHAPTER 4

POP QUIZ 4.1

Call 911, make sure the patient is in a safe place while waiting for EMS with a patent airway, check the patient's blood sugar, and utilize the emergency glucagon kit.

POP QUIZ 4.2

A fasting blood glucose >125 is concerning for diabetes. While there are other reasons for an elevated fasting blood glucose in the inpatient setting (such as stress or acute illness), the provider should be notified of this finding. Treat as ordered and continue to monitor throughout the course of their PCU admission.

POP QUIZ 4.3

The patient is hypernatremic. Notify the provider and request fluids be exchanged to 0.45% NS.

POP QUIZ 4.4

Untreated hyperglycemia can result in microvascular damage. This most commonly includes neuropathy, retinopathy, and nephropathy. Large vessel damage includes CAD, PVD, and cerebrovascular disease.

POP QUIZ 4.5

Notify the provider, then follow institutional protocol for hypoglycemia. Provide the patient with another 4 oz of juice or bolus of IV dextrose and recheck blood glucose in 15 minutes. Repeat this process until the patient's blood glucose is >70 mg/dL.

CHAPTER 5

POP QUIZ 5.1

The nurse should notify the provider immediately of a suspected GI bleed. Though this patient is receiving IV iron replacement for his iron deficiency anemia, his vital sign changes, abdominal pain, and stool volume, consistency, and distinct odor are consistent with an acute GI bleed. Urgent intervention is needed.

POP QUIZ 5.2

Check the patient's chart to make sure the provider has obtained consent for blood product administration. Verify the patient has an active type and screen prior to administering any blood products. Protocols may vary among institutions, but the patient will most likely need a larger-bore IV to receive his blood products. Insert a large-bore IV or consult the IV therapy team to assist with IV placement. If unsuccessful, the provider may have to place a central line. During an emergency, the blood may be initiated via the 22 gauge IV and switched to larger-bore IV when more access is obtained.

POP QUIZ 5.3

The provider will order the immediate discontinuation of heparin.

CHAPTER 6

POP QUIZ 6.1

Patients with hepatic encephalopathy and elevated ammonia levels should routinely and regularly take lactulose to decrease ammonia level through excretion. It is important to engage in therapeutic communication and reeducate patients on the importance of adhering to these medication orders. If unsuccessful, notify the provider.

POP QUIZ 6.2

The next step is to call for assistance, lay the head of the bed down, and position the patient on their side. The nurse should not insert anything into the patient's mouth during the seizure (tongue blade, suction catheter, etc.). Make sure the patient is free from injury.

POP QUIZ 6.3

Prior to administering their first PO intake/meal, the nurse should confirm that a swallow study has taken place and that the provider diet order allows for the type of food brought in by the family. If a swallow study has not been conducted or the current diet order does not allow for a milkshake, explain this process to the daughter and offer to store the milkshake in the freezer until the swallow study has been completed or the diet order has been appropriately modified based on clinical condition. Consult speech–language pathology to assist with completing the swallow study per hospital protocol.

CHAPTER 7

POP QUIZ 7.1

Large bowel obstruction. Intermittent feculent vomiting with diffuse abdominal pain and constipation are symptoms of large bowel obstruction.

POP QUIZ 7.2

Gastric residuals should be checked by aspirating and measuring gastric contents. If gastric residuals are >250 ml prior to initiating tube feed, the tube feed should be held, and the provider should be notified.

POP QUIZ 7.3

The rigid abdomen with worsening abdominal and back pain, tachycardia, and hypotension indicate that the patient may be bleeding postoperatively. The nurse should call the provider, who will evaluate the need to return to surgery to repair the bleed.

POP QUIZ 7.4

Each hospital and program are different; however, many liver transplant programs do not list patients with history of alcohol abuse unless they have at least 6 months of sobriety. Refer to the transplant coordinator for further questions and explanation.

POP QUIZ 7.5

Minimal fasting before surgery, ambulation soon after surgery, returning to normal eating and drinking within a day of surgery, and multimodal analgesia with appropriate opioid all help decrease the risk of post operative ileus.

POP QUIZ 7.6

Eggs are a good choice because they do not fall under the FODMAP category. Foods that fall under the FODMAP category include dairy, fruit, highly fermentable carbohydrates, onions, sorbitol, certain vegetables, and wheat.

POP QUIZ 7.7

CT angiography is the gold standard for diagnosing bowel ischemia.

CHAPTER 8

POP QUIZ 8.1

This patient needs urgent dialysis to lower the potassium level. Transfer to a higher level of care is indicated to monitor for EKG changes and for initiation of hemodialysis or CRRT (if hemodynamically unstable).

POP QUIZ 8.2

While healthy, these meals are high in potassium. Patients with CKD should limit the amount of potassium in their daily diet. The patient should be educated on the importance of minimizing dietary potassium in addition to adhering to medication therapy.

POP QUIZ 8.3

Patients with hypokalemia may also experience concurrent hypomagnesemia. Hypomagnesemia can exacerbate hypokalemia or make routine supplementation ineffective. Be sure to treat both electrolyte abnormalities to achieve normal values.

CHAPTER 9

POP QUIZ 9.1

Based on this information, the patient displays physical, environmental, and sensory risk factors for falling. Physical risk factors for falls includes a history of diabetes and A-fib. Environmental risk factors include loose rugs and stairs in his house. Sensory risk factors include a history of impaired vision and wearing glasses.

POP QUIZ 9.2

Medication therapy (carbidopa/levodopa), deep brain stimulation, and a combination of exercise programs and cognitive training will help patients improve mobility and stability.

POP QUIZ 9.3

Physical activity helps decrease the risk for developing pneumonia, pressure ulcers, and blood clots.

CHAPTER 10

POP QUIZ 10.1

Although the patient is complaining of pain, she is still experiencing the effects of medications given in the OR/PACU. To provide additional narcotics for a patient with an RR of 8, on 4LNC setting at 92%, responsive only to touch, who is unable to keep eyes open for prolonged periods, may be unsafe and place the patient at risk for further respiratory depression. Consider alternative nonnarcotic medications and nonpharmacological interventions, such as heating pads, ice, or repositioning to manage this patient's pain until she becomes more awake following surgery.

POP QUIZ 10.2

Notify the provider and gather materials to draw stat blood cultures. It is important that two sets of blood cultures be obtained using sterile technique. Each set should include both an anaerobic and aerobic bottle.

POP QUIZ 10.3

If the patient was unresponsive to medical management for hyperkalemia and has decreased urine output, the patient may require dialysis.

CHAPTER 11

POP QUIZ 11.1

The nurse should attempt to de-escalate the situation before the patient becomes more violent by remaining calm and speaking to the patient reassuringly. The nurse should first attempt to engage the patient in conversation and establish a therapeutic relationship. The nurse should incorporate nonverbal communication strategies to appear less threatening. If these techniques are unsuccessful, administer medications or utilize restraints to protect the patient and staff.

POP QUIZ 11.2

Additional medications can be added in combination to address the patient's depression. Once stable, the patient can also undergo psychotherapy or ECT as recommended by the provider.

POP QUIZ 11.3

Be alert for alcohol withdrawal symptoms to develop anywhere between 24 to 72 hr after the patient's last drink.

POP QUIZ 11.4

The nurse could discuss AA or NA, depending on substance abuse disorder. The nurse could also discuss the possibility of inpatient or outpatient rehabilitation programs and the potential for using behavioral health resources like therapists or psychologists to support their recovery.

CHAPTER 12

POP QUIZ 12.1

The nurse should explain to the surgeon that the patient has been anxious all day and to allow the wife to meet with and talk to the surgeon to provide the best patient- and family-centered care. Suggest that the surgeon be on speaker phone with the wife while explaining the surgery to the patient. This would allow the wife to hear about the procedure, as well as ask any questions she may have. This will promote collaboration between the patient, family, and surgeon, as well as ease any anxiety the patient or his wife may have.

POP QUIZ 12.2

Before allowing the patient or family to use any medicinal herbal treatments to assist in her recovery, explain to the family the unit policy for using medicinal herbs. Gather the names and quantities of herbal remedies and consult pharmacy and the provider to determine if there may be any interaction with medications the patient is currently taking. If medicinal herbs are not allowed, collaborate with the family to identify an acceptable alternative solution that allows the patient to practice her cultural beliefs while allowing hospital staff to provide safe care.

POP QUIZ 12.3

The nurse must first discuss and collaborate with the overseeing provider to determine whether her clinical status will allow for this travel. If the provider believes the patient is clinically stable enough for travel, the necessary orders to travel off unit should be obtained. Second, because this patient is trached requiring supplemental 35% oxygen via trach collar, a respiratory therapist should travel with the patient and nurse. If available, a patient care tech may also accompany the patient, nurse, and RT as an additional set of hands. Emergency travel bag/equipment should be taken with the nurse in the event of emergency. Once all orders are obtained and staff is identified, a time and destination for travel should be chosen.

APPENDIX A:
COMMON MEDICATIONS IN THE PCU

Table A.1 Common Antibiotic and Antifungal Medications

General Indications	General Mechanism of Action	General Contraindications, Precautions, and Adverse Effects
Aminoglycosides (e.g., gentamicin, streptomycin, neomycin, etc.)		
Common indications among aminoglycosides: • Bacteremia and sepsis • Bone and joint infections • CAP • Empiric treatment for febrile neutropenia • Infective endocarditis • Intra-abdominal infections • Lower respiratory tract infections • Nosocomial pneumonia • Ophthalmic infections • Surgical infection prophylaxis Specific indications for gentamicin: • Complicated UTIs • Meningitis and ventriculitis • Pelvic inflammatory disease • Pyelonephritis • Skin and skin structure infections Specific indications for streptomycin: • Gram-negative bacillary bacteremia, meningitis or lower respiratory tract infections in combination with other antimicrobials • UTI • Drug susceptible tuberculosis • Specific indications for neomycin: • Adjunctive therapy for hepatic encephalopathy • Infectious diarrhea	• Inhibit bacterial protein synthesis, causing bactericidal effect	• Medication is contraindicated in administration for organisms resistant to aminoglycosides. • Use caution in administering to patients with inflammatory bowel disease, as there is a high likelihood for developing pseudomembranous colitis or *Clostridium difficile*. • Monitor closely for nephrotoxicity or neurotoxicity, including ototoxicity in all aminoglycoside medications. Nephrotoxicity or ototoxicity development requires dose adjustment or discontinuation. • Additional adverse effects include nausea, vomiting, auditory disturbances, headache, skin irritation, rash, anemia, and elevated liver enzymes.

(continued)

Table A.1 Common Antibiotic and Antifungal Medications *(continued)*

General Indications	General Mechanism of Action	General Contraindications, Precautions, and Adverse Effects
Antibiotic, sulfonamide derivative, (TMP-SMX, also known as co-trimoxazol)		
• UTI • Pyelonephritis • Pneumocystic pneumonia • Otitis media • Acute bacterial exacerbations of chronic bronchitis	• Inhibits enzymes in folic acid synthesis pathway, causing bactericidal effects	• Medication is contraindicated in folate deficiency, megaloblastic anemia, G6PD deficiency, severe renal impairment, and hepatic disease. • Use caution in patients with hypothyroidism, colitis or GI disturbances, HIV/AIDS, cardiac disease, and dysrhythmia. • Adverse effects include megaloblastic anemia, aplastic anemia, hemolytic anemia, TTP, angioedema, Stevens-Johnson syndrome, exfoliative dermatitis, anaphylactic reaction, anuria, hyperkalemia, rhabdomyolysis, seizures, hemolysis, leukopenia, QT prolongation, chest pain, dyspnea, nausea, vomiting, itching, fever, and chills.
Antiprotozoals, respiratory (pentamidine)		
• Pneumocystis pneumonia • Leishmaniasis • Oral inhalation antifungal agent used for various fungal infections	• Mechanism of action not clearly known; thought to interfere with fungal DNA and RNA replication	• Use caution if administering rapidly, as it can lead to hypotension. • Use caution in patients with renal, hepatic, or cardiac disease, asthma, or pregnancy. • Adverse effects include dysrhythmia, bronchospasm, elevated AST/ALT, hypoglycemia, tremor, cough, fever, itching, diarrhea, headache, or night sweats.

Azoles (e.g., fluconazole, etc.)

- Cutaneous leishmaniasis
- Cutaneous or lymphocutaneous sporotrichosis
- Skin or skin structure infection caused by *Candida*
- Talaromycosis, coccidioidomycosis, or histoplasmosis prophylaxis in HIV-infected patients
- Primary pulmonary histoplasmosis
- Bacterial vaginosis
- Treatment and prophylaxis treatment for recurrent vulvovaginal candidiasis infections
- Osteomyelitis, bone and joint infection caused by *Candida*
- Infective endocarditis caused by *Candida*
- Infected pacemaker, ICD or VAD caused by *Candida*
- Treatment of meningitis due to *Histoplasma capsulatum* in HIV-infected patients
- CNS infections due to *Coccidioides*, cryptococcus, or *Candida*
- Organ transplant recipients
- Candida prophylaxis in bone marrow transplant or high-risk cancer patients
- Pyelonephritis caused by *Candida*
- UTI caused by *Candida*
- Intra-abdominal infections caused by *Candida*
- Pneumonia caused by *Candida*
- Thrush

- Alter fungal cell membrane to inhibit fungal reproduction and growth through fungistatic action

- Use caution in cardiac, hepatic, or renal conditions.
- Avoid use during pregnancy except in severe, life-threatening emergencies.
- Adverse effects include dizziness, rash, diarrhea, nausea, and headache.

Carbapenems (ertapenem, meropenem, etc.)

Indications for both ertapenem and meropenem:
- Bacterial encephalitis or meningitis
- Intra-abdominal infections
- Complicated skin and skin structure infections

- Inhibit cell wall synthesis by binding to penicillin-binding proteins inside bacterial cell wall, resulting in cell death to prevent organism growth

- Use caution in patients receiving carbapenem treatment who undergo concurrent hematologic testing. A positive Coombs test has been reported in patients taking carbapenems (meropenem).

(continued)

Table A.1 Common Antibiotic and Antifungal Medications *(continued)*

General Indications	General Mechanism of Action	General Contraindications, Precautions, and Adverse Effects
Carbapenems (ertapenem, meropenem, etc.) (continued)		
• Empiric treatment of febrile neutropenia • Bacteremia or sepsis • Pneumonia (CAP or nosocomial) Additional indications for ertapenem: • Complicated UTI and pyelonephritis • Acute pelvic infection • Surgical prophylaxis		• Use caution in patients with cephalosporin, penicillin, or other beta-lactam hypersensitivity, as cross sensitivity is possible. • Use caution in head injury or neurological disease due to risk of seizure associated with carbapenem administration. • Use caution in renal failure, impairment, or dysfunction, as carbapenems are excreted by the kidneys and can result in further damage. • Use caution when administering to patients with inflammatory bowel disease due to high likelihood of developing pseudomembranous colitis and *clostridium difficile*. • Adverse effects include nausea, headache, diarrhea, rash, vomiting, confusion, delirium, hypoglycemia, pseudomembranous colitis, neutropenia, renal failure, and seizure.
Cephalosporins, first generation (cefazolin)		
• First-generation have coverage against most gram-positive cocci as well as gram-negative bacteria, for example, *Escherichia. coli*, *Proteus mirabilis*, and *Klebsiella pneumoniae*. • Upper respiratory tract infections • Skin and skin structure infections • Biliary tract infections • UTI • Infective endocarditis • Surgical infection prophylaxis • Lower respiratory tract infections (pneumococcal pneumonia and CAP) • Bacteremia • Bone and joint infections • Mastitis	• Inhibit cell wall synthesis by binding to penicillin-binding proteins inside bacterial cell wall, resulting in cell death to prevent organism growth causing bactericidal effect	• Do not administer in viral infections or organisms with antimicrobial resistance to cephalosporins. • Use caution in allergy to penicillin, as cross reaction is possible. • Use caution in renal failure, impairment, or dysfunction. Cephalosporins are excreted by the kidneys and can result in further damage. • Adverse effects include headache, diarrhea, nausea, vomiting, maculopapular rash, fever, confusion, bleeding, seizures, azotemia, and renal failure. • Medication is contraindicated in cephalosporin-resistant organisms and viral infection.

Cephalosporins, second generation (cefuroxime)

- Second-generation cephalosporins have coverage against *Haemophilus. influenza, Moraxella catarrhalis,* and *Bacteroides* spp.
- Chronic bronchitis
- Skin and skin structure infections
- UTI
- Treatment of bone and joint infection
- Pharyngitis
- Gonorrhea
- Lyme disease
- Acute otitis media
- Bacteremia
- Meningitis
- Surgical infection prophylaxis
- Tonsillitis
- Sinusitis
- Intra-abdominal infections
- Lower respiratory tract infections
- Pneumonia (CAP and nosocomial)

- Inhibit bacterial cell wall synthesis by binding to specific penicillin-binding proteins within the cell wall, causing bactericidal effect

- Medication is contraindicated in penicillin allergy, viral infections, or bacteria with known drug resistance.
- Use caution in renal failure/impairment, pseudomembranous colitis, and phenylketonuria.
- Adverse effects include nausea, vomiting, flatulence, dyspepsia, dysuria, phlebitis, jaundice, Stevens-Johnson syndrome, and vasculitis.

Cephalosporins, third generation (ceftriaxone)

- Bacteremia and sepsis
- UTI
- Acute bacterial otitis media
- Skin and skin structure infections
- Surgical incision site infections
- Necrotizing infections
- Intra-abdominal infections
- Surgical infection prophylaxis
- Pelvic inflammatory disease
- Bone and joint infections
- Lower respiratory tract infection
- Pneumonia (nosocomial and CAP)

- Inhibit bacterial cell wall synthesis by binding to specific penicillin-binding proteins within the cell wall, causing bactericidal effect

- Medication is contraindicated in penicillin allergy, jaundice, or hyperbilirubinemia in premature neonates, viral infection, or antimicrobial resistance.
- Use caution in GI disease, as it may cause or worsen existing colitis.
- Adverse effects include seizures, bronchospasm, pancreatitis, biliary obstruction, erythema multiforme, acute generalized exanthematous pustulosis, Stevens-Johnson syndrome, renal failure, thrombocytopenia, neutropenia, hypoprothrombinemia, thrombocytopenia, superinfection, edema, nausea, vomiting, headache, jaundice, and itching.

(continued)

Table A.1 Common Antibiotic and Antifungal Medications *(continued)*

General Indications	General Mechanism of Action	General Contraindications, Precautions, and Adverse Effects
Cephalosporins, third generation (ceftriaxone) (continued)		
• Infective endocarditis • Meningitis and vasculitis • Gonorrhea infection • Lyme disease • Congenital syphilis • Bacterial sinusitis • Third-generation cephalosporins: less coverage against most gram-positive organisms, but increase coverage against Enterobacteriaceae, *Neisseria* spp., and *Haemophilus. influenza*	• Inhibit bacterial cell wall synthesis by binding to specific penicillin-binding proteins within the cell wall, causing bactericidal effect	• Medication is contraindicated in penicillin allergy and antimicrobial resistance. • Use caution in colitis, GI disturbances, and renal failure. Cefepime may worsen colitis, other GI issues, and kidney function. • Adverse effects include seizure, anaphylactic shock, Stevens-Johnson syndrome, toxic epidermal necrolysis, erythema multiforme, agranulocytosis, pancytopenia, aplastic anemia, elevated liver enzymes, hypophosphatemia, hypoprothrombinemia, bleeding, colitis, vaginitis, pseudomembranous colitis, hypercalcemia, superinfection, confusion hallucination, rash, vomiting, diarrhea, itching, nausea, headache, and fever.
Cephalosporin, fourth generation (cefepime)		
• Monotherapy for febrile neutropenia • Complicated UTI and pyelonephritis • Intra-abdominal infections • Severe skin and skin structure infections • Pneumonia (CAP and nosocomial) • Bacterial meningitis • Infective endocarditis • Sepsis • Fourth-generation cephalosporins: similar coverage as third-generation cephalosporins but with additional coverage against gram-negative bacteria with antimicrobial resistance, e.g., beta-lactamase		

Cephalosporins, fifth generation (ceftaroline and fosamil)

- Acute bacterial skin and skin structure infections
- CAP
- Sepsis
- Coverage against methicillin-resistant staphylococci and penicillin-resistant pneumococci

- Inhibit bacterial cell wall synthesis by binding to specific penicillin-binding proteins within the cell wall, causing bactericidal effect

- Medication is contraindicated in viral infection and antimicrobial resistance.
- Use caution in patients with colitis, GI disturbances, or renal impairments/failure.
- Adverse effects include hyperkalemia or hypokalemia, bradycardia, seizure, renal failure, agranulocytosis, anaphylaxis, elevated liver enzymes, constipation, hepatitis, hyperglycemia, thrombocytopenia, pseudomembranous colitis, encephalopathy, diarrhea, rash, vomiting, abdominal pain, headache, and dizziness.

Fluoroquinolones (e.g., ciprofloxacin, delafloxacin, levofloxacin, and moxifloxacin)

- UTI, cystitis, and pyelonephritis
- Lower respiratory tract infections, pneumonia (CAP and nosocomial)
- Chronic bronchitis exacerbations
- Skin and skin structure infections
- Animal bite wounds
- Enteric infections
- Mild to moderate acute sinusitis
- Acute prostatitis
- Febrile neutropenia
- Bacterial conjunctivitis
- Ophthalmic infections related to corneal ulcers
- Acute otitis externa
- Bone and joint infections
- Meningococcal infection/prophylaxis
- Intra-abdominal infections
- Peritoneal dialysis infections

- Inhibit DNA synthesis, causing bactericidal effect

- Use caution in patients with cardiac disease or cardiac dysrhythmias, CNS disorders, patients with history of myasthenia gravis, diabetes mellitus, renal impairments, and hepatic dysfunction.
- Adverse effects include hepatotoxicity, phototoxicity, tendon rupture, neurotoxicity, hepatic dysfunction, hyper- or hypoglycemia, exacerbation of myasthenia gravis symptoms, worsening colitis or GI dysfunction, nausea, vomiting, or rash.
- Discontinue immediately with any sign of tendon inflammation or tendon pain. These symptoms often present before tendon rupture.

(continued)

Table A.1 Common Antibiotic and Antifungal Medications *(continued)*

General Indications	General Mechanism of Action	General Contraindications, Precautions, and Adverse Effects
Fluoroquinolones (e.g., ciprofloxacin, delafloxacin, levofloxacin, and moxifloxicin) (continued)		
• Dental infections • Surgical infection prophylaxis • Pulmonary infections in cystic fibrosis • Infective endocarditis • Sepsis • Traveler's diarrhea • Broad spectrum antibiotics useful against gram-negative rods *(Escherichia. coli, Klebsiella* spp., *Proteus* spp., *Pseudomonas* spp., *Pseudomonas aeruginosa, Providencia* spp., and *Serratia marcescens. Streptococcus pneumoniae)*; also effective against *H. influenzae, Moraxella catarrahalis, Legionella* spp., *Mycoplasma* spp., *Chlamydia pneumoniae)* • Effective against gram-positive organisms including *Staphylococcus aureus*, methacillin-resistant *S. aureus* • Effective against anaerobic bacteria, *Mycobacteria, Bacillus anthracis, Francisella tularensis*, and typhoid		
Glycopeptides (vancomycin)		
• Infective endocarditis • Pseudomembranous colitis due to *Clostridium difficile* infection • Enterocolitis • Sepsis and bacteremia • Serious gram-positive infections • Mastitis • Gram-positive lower respiratory infections (CAP and nosocomial pneumonia) • Pleural empyema • Surgical infection prophylaxis • Meningitis and other CNS infections	• Bind to parts of bacterial cell wall, preventing synthesis	• Medication is contraindicated in viral infection and vancomycin-resistant organisms. • Use caution in renal disease, hearing impairment and HF. • Adverse effects include rash, itching, nausea, abdominal pain, fever, diarrhea, and Stevens-Johnson syndrome.

- Bone and joint infections
- Septic arthritis
- Prosthetic joint infections
- Febrile neutropenia
- Intra-abdominal infections
- Peritoneal dialysis related peritonitis
- Used to treat and prevent various bacterial infections caused by gram-positive bacteria, including MRSA
- Effective for streptococci, enterococci, and MSSA infections

Lincosamides (clindamycin)

- Bacteremia
- Lower respiratory tract infections, including CAP and nosocomial pneumonia
- Intra-abdominal infections
- Skin and skin structure infections
- Animal bites
- Diabetic foot ulcer
- Gynecologic infections
- Bacterial vaginosis
- Acne
- Mastitis
- Bone and joint infections
- Bacterial sinusitis
- Acute otitis media
- Surgical infection prophylaxis

- Bind to RNA of bacteria to inhibit protein synthesis

- Medication is contraindicated in patients with a history of enteritis, ulcerative colitis, and pseudomembranous colitis.
- Use caution in patients with diarrhea or hepatic disease.
- Adverse effects include toxic epidermal necrolysis, Stevens-Johnson syndrome, erythema multiforme, exfoliative dermatitis, proteinuria, oliguria, superinfection, fungal overgrowth, pseudomembranous colitis, edema, leukopenia, thrombocytopenia, elevated hepatic enzyme, fever, fatigue, dizziness, vomiting, nausea, headache, and itching.

(continued)

Table A.1 Common Antibiotic and Antifungal Medications *(continued)*

General Indications	General Mechanism of Action	General Contraindications, Precautions, and Adverse Effects
Macrolides (azithromycin)		
• Mild to moderate bacterial exacerbations of chronic bronchitis in patients with COPD • Acute otitis media • Bacterial conjunctivitis • CAP • Skin and skin structure infections • Pelvic inflammatory disease • Gonorrhea • *Mycobacterium* infection • Acute bacterial sinusitis • Bacterial endocarditis prophylaxis	• Inhibit protein synthesis in bacterial cells, causing bacteriostatic effect • Bactericidal in high concentrations	• Medication is contraindicated in patients with a history of jaundice or hepatic dysfunction prior to macrolide use, viral infection, and drug-resistant bacteria. • Use caution in renal impairment, cardiovascular disease, colitis, or GI disease, and in patients with a history of myasthenia gravis. • Adverse effects include photosensitivity, dysrhythmia and QT prolongation, renal failure, hyperkalemia, bronchospasm, seizures, elevated liver enzymes, hyperbilirubinemia, constipation, jaundice, superinfection, anemia, dermatitis, and hypo- or hyperglycemia.
Oxazolidinones (linezolid)		
• Lower respiratory tract infections • CAP and nosocomial pneumonia • Skin and skin structure infections • Sepsis and bacteremia caused by vancomycin-resistant enterococcus • MRSA bacteremia • MRSA-associated bone and joint infection • Septic arthritis • Prosthetic joint infections • Meningitis and other CNS infections • Febrile neutropenia • Intra-abdominal infections • Peritonitis	• Inhibit bacterial protein synthesis by preventing translation and protein production thus preventing bacterial growth	• Medication is contraindicated in concurrent use of metrizamide or iohexol during procedures requiring radiographic contrast administration. • Use caution in uncontrolled hypertension, concurrent use with MAOIs, diarrhea, pseudomembranous colitis, history of seizures, and diabetes (may cause hypoglycemia). • Adverse effects include myelosuppression, short-term decreased fertility in males, hypoglycemia, pancytopenia, optic neuritis, seizures, anaphylaxis, angioedema, anemia, thrombocytopenia, elevated hepatic enzymes, hypertension, hypoglycemia, pseudomembranous colitis, diarrhea, vomiting, abdominal pain, rash, itching, and tooth discoloration.

Penicillins (ampicillin)

- Severe infections including bacteremia
- Infective endocarditis
- Respiratory tract infections
- Skin and skin structure infections
- Genitourinary infections
- UTI
- GI infection

- Inhibit cell wall synthesis to produce a bactericidal effect, preventing organism growth

- Medication is contraindicated in penicillin-resistant organisms.
- Use caution in renal impairments, cephalosporin and carbapenem hypersensitivity, colitis and other GI disturbances, and mononucleosis.
- Adverse effects include antibiotic-associated colitis, anaphylaxis, exfoliative dermatitis, seizures, rash, nausea, vomiting, leukopenia, thrombocytopenia, platelet dysfunction, anemia, elevated hepatic enzymes, pseudomembranous colitis, superinfection, or diarrhea.

Tetracyclines (doxycycline)

- Necrotizing ulcerative gingivitis
- Treatment when penicillins are contraindicated
- Uncomplicated gonorrhea
- Chlamydia
- Psittacosis
- Respiratory tract infections
- Skin and skin structure infection
- Severe acne
- Rocky mountain spotted fever
- Cholera

- Bind to ribosomes of susceptible bacteria and inhibit protein synthesis
- Bacteriostatic, bactericidal in high concentrations

- There are no direct contraindications.
- Use caution in renal impairment/failure, hepatic disease, colitis, and GI disease.
- Adverse effects include photosensitivity, exfoliative dermatitis, enterocolitis, hepatic failure, pericarditis, anaphylaxis, hemolytic anemia, azotemia, blurred vision, dysphagia, erythema, thrombocytopenia, neutropenia, nail discoloration, headache, vomiting, diarrhea, nausea, rash, and tooth discoloration.

Note: All agents are contraindicated in the presence of hypersensitivity to the medication or one of its components.

RESOURCES

Hooper, D., Calderwood, S., & Bogorodskaya, M. (n.d.). Fluroquinolones. *UpToDate.* https://www.uptodate.com/contents/fluoroquinolones
Prescribers' Digital Reference. (n.d.). *Amikacin sulfate* [Drug information]. PDR Search. https://www.pdr.net/drug-summary/Amikacin-Sulfate-amikacin-sulfate-676
Prescribers' Digital Reference. (n.d.). *Ampicillin* [Drug information]. PDR Search. https://www.pdr.net/drug-summary/Ampicillin-for-Injection-ampicillin-677
Prescribers' Digital Reference. (n.d.). *Azithromycin* [Drug information]. PDR Search. https://www.pdr.net/drug-summary/Azithromycin-azithromycin-24249
Prescribers' Digital Reference. (n.d.). *Bactrim* [Drug information]. PDR Search. https://www.pdr.net/drug-summary/
    Bactrim-Bactrim-DS-sulfamethoxazole-trimethoprim-686
Prescribers' Digital Reference. (n.d.). *Cefazolin* [Drug information]. PDR Search. https://www.pdr.net/drug-summary/Cefazolin-Sodium-cefazolin-sodium-1193

Prescribers' Digital Reference. (n.d.). *Cefepime (Maxipime)* [Drug information]. PDR Search. https://www.pdr.net/drug-summary/Maxipime-cefepime-hydrochloride-3215.5755

Prescribers' Digital Reference. (n.d.). *Ceftriaxone* [Drug information]. PDR Search. https://www.pdr.net/drug-summary/Ceftriaxone-ceftriaxone-1723

Prescribers' Digital Reference. (n.d.). *Cefuroxime* [Drug information]. PDR Search. https://www.pdr.net/drug-summary/Zinacef-cefuroxime-242

Prescribers' Digital Reference. (n.d.). *Ciprofloxacin* [Drug information]. PDR Search. https://www.pdr.net/drug-summary/Ciprofloxacin-Injection-ciprofloxacin-3255

Prescribers' Digital Reference. (n.d.). *Clindamycin* [Drug information]. PDR Search. https://www.pdr.net/drug-summary/Cleocin-Phosphate-Injection-clindamycin-1865

Prescribers' Digital Reference. (n.d.). *Doxycycline* [Drug information]. PDR Search. https://www.pdr.net/drug-summary/Doxycycline-doxycycline-24308

Prescribers' Digital Reference. (n.d.). *Ertapenem* [Drug information]. PDR Search. https://www.pdr.net/drug-summary/Invanz-ertapenem-359

Prescribers' Digital Reference. (n.d.). *Fluconazole* [Drug information]. PDR Search. https://www.pdr.net/drug-summary/Diflucan-fluconazole-1847

Prescribers' Digital Reference. (n.d.). *Gentamicin sulfate* [Drug information]. PDR Search. https://www.pdr.net/drug-summary/Gentamicin-Injection-40-mg-mL-gentamicin-sulfate-3299

Prescribers' Digital Reference. (n.d.). *Merrem* [Drug information]. PDR Search. https://www.pdr.net/drug-summary/Merrem-meropenem-2055

Prescribers' Digital Reference. (n.d.). *Neomycin* [Drug information]. PDR Search. https://www.pdr.net/drug-summary/Neomycin-Sulfate-neomycin-sulfate-819

Prescribers' Digital Reference. (n.d.). *Pentamidine* [Drug information]. PDR Search. https://www.pdr.net/drug-summary/NebuPent-pentamidine-isethionate-1408

Prescribers' Digital Reference. (n.d.). *Streptomycin* [Drug information]. PDR Search. https://www.pdr.net/drug-summary/Streptomycin-streptomycin-1600

Prescribers' Digital Reference. (n.d.). *Teflaro (ceftaroline fosamil)* [Drug information]. PDR Search. https://www.pdr.net/drug-summary/Teflaro-ceftaroline-fosamil-158

Prescribers' Digital Reference. (n.d.). *Tobramycin* [Drug information]. PDR Search. https://www.pdr.net/drug-summary/Tobramycin-tobramycin-916

Prescribers' Digital Reference. (n.d.). *Vancomycin* [Drug information]. PDR Search. https://www.pdr.net/drug-summary/Vancocin-vancomycin-hydrochloride-802

Prescribers' Digital Reference. (n.d.). *Zyvox (Linezolid)* [Drug information]. PDR Search. https://www.pdr.net/drug-summary/Zyvox-linezolid-2341

Table A.2 Common Pain and Sedation Medications

General Indications	General Mechanism of Action	General Contraindications, Precautions, and Adverse Effects
Analgesics with antipyretic activity: acetaminophen		
• Fever • Mild pain or temporary relief of headache, myalgia, back pain, musculoskeletal pain, dental pain, dysmenorrhea, arthralgia and minor aches, and pains with the common cold or flu. • Moderate to severe pain with adjunctive opioid analgesics • Osteoarthritis pain • Acute migraine	• Increase pain threshold by inhibiting prostaglandin synthesis through the COX pathway	• Medication is contraindicated in severe hepatic impairment or severe active hepatic disease. • Use caution in renal disease or patients with G6PD • Adverse effects include elevated hepatic enzymes, rash, jaundice, hypoprothrombinemia, neutropenia, angioedema, hemolytic anemia, and rhabdomyolysis.
Barbiturates (phenobarbital)		
• Status epilepticus • Maintenance of all types of seizures • Short-term treatment of insomnia • Procedural sedation • Relief of preoperative anxiety • Sedation maintenance • Relieves anxiety, tension, and apprehension	• Nonselective CNS depressant with sedative hypnotic actions	• Medication is contraindicated in pulmonary disease in which obstruction or dyspnea is present, hepatic disease or hepatic encephalopathy, pregnancy, and porphyria. • Use caution in acute pain, as paradoxical reactions can occur. • Use caution during rapid IV administration, as this can cause bronchospasm. • Do not abruptly discontinue medication, as withdrawal can occur. • Adverse effects include suicidal ideation, megaloblastic anemia, bradycardia, depression, tolerance, impaired cognition, respiratory depression, confusion, elevated liver enzymes, hepatitis, jaundice, neutropenia, dependence, emotional lability, rash, nausea, vomiting, fatigue, decreased libido, and ptosis.

(continued)

Table A.2 Common Pain and Sedation Medications *(continued)*

General Indications	General Mechanism of Action	General Contraindications, Precautions, and Adverse Effects
Gabapentinoids (gabapentin)		
• Adjunct treatment of partial seizures • Neuropathic pain • Moderate to severe restless leg syndrome • ALS • Tremor • Nystagmus • Spasticity due to MS • Pruritis • Fibromyalgia • Dysautonomia following severe TBI • Alcohol dependence	• Exact mechanism of action with GABA receptors unknown • Show a high affinity for binding sites throughout the brain correspondent to the presence of the voltage-gated calcium channels, especially alpha-2-delta-1, which seems to inhibit release of excitatory neurotransmitters in presynaptic area which participate in epileptogenesis	• There are no contraindications to use. • Use caution in renal failure and pulmonary disease. Gabapentin is excreted in the kidneys; dose adjustments may be required for patients in renal failure or with renal impairments. • Do not abruptly discontinue, as withdrawal symptoms can occur. • Adverse effects include hyperglycemia, tolerance, depression, confusion and memory impairments, dehydration, jaundice, respiratory depression, dizziness, headache, fatigue, nausea and vomiting, tremor, decreased libido, back pain, emotional lability, skin irritation, diarrhea, and irritability.
General anesthetics: etomidate		
• General anesthesia induction • Sedation during rapid sequence intubation • Procedural sedation	• Increase GABA transmission by increasing the number of GABA receptors available through displacement of natural binding of GABA inhibitors	• There are no true contraindications. • Avoid use, if possible, with sepsis or septic shock. • Use caution in geriatric patients, as it can cause cardiac depression. • Use caution in hepatic disease, as etomidate is metabolized in the liver. • Adverse effects include apnea, laryngospasm, bradycardia, dysrhythmia, anaphylaxis, respiratory depression, hypoventilation, hypo/hypertension, sinus tachycardia, nausea, and vomiting.

General anesthetics: ketamine

- General anesthesia induction/maintenance
- Preanesthetic sedation
- Treatment of refractory bronchospasm in status asthmaticus
- Treatment-resistant depression in adults
- Moderate to severe pain
- Induction agent during rapid sequence intubation
- ICU sedation

- Interrupt pathways in the brain prior to producing somesthetic sensory blockade and selectively depress the thalamo-neocortical system

- Medication is contraindicated in which additional blood pressure increase would be hazardous, including hypertension, hypertensive crisis, stroke, head trauma, intercranial mass, or intracranial bleeding.
- Use caution in glaucoma or patients with increased ICP, alcoholism, substance abuse, and thyrotoxicosis.
- Adverse effects include bradycardia, diabetes insipidus, dysrhythmia, laryngospasm, apnea, ocular hypertension, increased ICP, hallucinations, delirium, hypertension, respiratory depression, confusion, withdrawal, psychosis, dysphoria, urinary incontinence, nightmares, nausea, vomiting, anxiety, and insomnia.

General anesthetics: propofol

- General anesthesia
- ICU sedation
- Conscious sedation
- Refractory status epilepticus
- Refractory migraine
- Postoperative nausea and vomiting prophylaxis
- Agitation associated with alcohol withdrawal

- Inhibit NMDA receptors through channel gating modulation with agonistic activity at the GABA receptor

- Propofol is contraindicated when general anesthesia or sedation is contraindicated.
- Use caution in cardiac disease, sepsis, and hypovolemia, as these patients will be more susceptible to propofol-induced hypotension.
- Use caution in pancreatitis and hyperlipidemia, due to high lipid content, propofol can exacerbate or worsen these conditions.
- Adverse effects include bradycardia, dysrhythmia, laryngospasm, bronchospasm, hyperkalemia, ileus, hypotension, edema, hypoventilation, euphoria, wheezing, elevated hepatic enzymes, respiratory depression, hypertriglyceridemia, hepatomegaly, and drowsiness.

(continued)

Table A.2 Common Pain and Sedation Medications *(continued)*

General Indications	General Mechanism of Action	General Contraindications, Precautions, and Adverse Effects
Opioids: fentanyl		
• Control of moderate to severe pain • Intraoperative or procedural management of severe pain • Postoperative pain management • Management of chronic severe pain in opioid-tolerant patients requiring around the clock long-term opioid treatment • Management of severe breakthrough cancer pain in opioid tolerant patients • Short-term management of acute postoperative pain • Adjunctive management of general anesthesia maintenance • Major surgery • Analgesia/sedation in mechanically ventilated patients • Sedation and analgesia prior to rapid sequence intubation • Management of dyspnea in patients with end stage cancer or lung disease • Procedural sedation	• Bind to pain receptors in the body to decrease pain pathways and alleviate pain	• Transdermal fentanyl patches are contraindicated in patients with known or suspected paralytic ileus or GI obstruction. • Nonparenteral fentanyl is contraindicated in status asthmaticus or severe respiratory depression. • Do not stop taking medication abruptly, as it may cause withdrawal symptoms. • Use caution in patients with history of alcoholism or substance abuse, as there is a high risk for psychological dependence. • Use with caution in patients with respiratory disorders, as it may cause respiratory depression. • Use caution in head trauma and neurological disorder, as it may increase drowsiness and decrease respirations. • Adverse effects include GI obstruction, bradycardia, laryngospasm, respiratory depression, pneumothorax, apnea, chest wall rigidity, ileus, dysrhythmia, constipation, hypokalemia, hypoventilation, dyspnea, confusion, hallucinations, dysphoria, blurred vision, psychological and physiological dependance, withdrawal, rash, vomiting, abnormal dreams, drowsiness, fatigue, paranoia, anxiety, agitation, emotional lability, and nausea.

Opioids: hydrocodone

- Treatment of chronic severe pain requiring around the clock long term opioid treatment
- Treatment of refractory restless leg syndrome

- Agonistic activity at the mu receptors resulting in changes in the perception of pain at the spinal cord and into the CNS

- Medication is contraindicated in patients with significant respiratory depression, acute or severe asthma, known or suspected GI obstruction, or paralytic ileus.
- Use caution in substance abuse, depression, geriatric populations, CNS depression and/or head trauma, increased ICP, psychosis, opioid naive patients, seizures, cardiac disease, adrenal insufficiency, hypothyroidism, or myxedema.
- Long-term use may increase risk of infertility.
- Adverse reactions include GI obstructions, seizures, apnea, SIADH, respiratory arrest, constipation, depression, dyspnea, confusion, withdrawal if abruptly discontinued, respiratory depression, hypoxia, hypotension, psychological and physiological dependence, infertility, nausea, tremor, anxiety, dizziness, and drowsiness.

Opioids: hydromorphone

- Relief of moderate to severe pain
- Management of chronic severe pain in opioid-tolerant patients requiring around the clock long-term opioid treatment
- Analgesia and/or sedation in mechanically ventilated patients

- Acts at the mu receptor causing changes in perception to pain at the spinal cord and into the CNS

- Medication is contraindicated in patients with respiratory depression, status asthmaticus (immediate release tablets), paralytic ileus (extended-release tablets), and sulfite hypersensitivity.
- Use caution in substance abuse, opioid naïve patients, head trauma or CNS depression, cardiac disease, geriatric populations, adrenal insufficiency, hypothyroidism, and myxedema.

(continued)

Table A.2 Common Pain and Sedation Medications *(continued)*

General Indications	General Mechanism of Action	General Contraindications, Precautions, and Adverse Effects
Opioids: hydromorphone (continued)		
		• Adverse reactions include bronchospasm, GI obstruction, bradycardia, anaphylaxis, laryngospasm, apnea, respiratory arrest, ileus, constipation, depression, dysphoria, hallucinations, confusion, euphoria, withdrawal if abruptly discontinued, urinary retention, nausea, drowsiness, vomiting, fatigue, dizziness, diarrhea, anxiety, tremor, paranoia, and lethargy.
Opioids: morphine		
• Acute and chronic moderate to severe pain	• Act at the mu receptor, causing changes in perception to pain at the spinal cord and into the CNS	• Medication is contraindicated in significant respiratory depression in unmonitored settings, acute or severe bronchial asthma (oral solutions), respiratory depression or hypoxia, upper airway obstruction, acute alcoholism, or delirium tremens (rectal route), known or suspected GI obstruction or paralytic ileus, hypovolemia, circulatory shock, cardiac dysrhythmia or HF secondary to chronic lung disease, and concurrent use with MAOI therapy.
• Management of chronic severe pain in patients who require daily around the clock long-term opioid treatment		
• Dyspnea in patients with end stage cancer or pulmonary disease		
• Procedural sedation		
• Painful diabetic neuropathy		• Use caution in substance abuse, alcoholism, opioid naïve patients, CNS depression, head trauma, seizures or increased ICP, cardiac disease, adrenal insufficiency, hypothyroidism, and myxedema.
• Refractory restless leg syndrome		

Opioids: oxycodone

- Treatment of severe pain
- Management of chronic severe pain in patients requiring daily around the clock long-term opioid management
- Painful diabetic neuropathy
- Restless leg syndrome

- Mu receptor agonist that changes pain perceptions at the spinal cord and into the CNS

- Do not abruptly discontinue, as withdrawal symptoms can occur.
- Adverse effects include ileus, bradycardia, dysrhythmia, increased ICP, bronchospasm, GI obstruction, laryngospasm, depression, confusion, hypoxia, edema, euphoria, delirium, dysphagia, hallucinations, psychosis, physiological dependence, adrenocortical insufficiency, drowsiness, diarrhea, constipation, headache, fever, nausea, restlessness, and vomiting.

- Medication is contraindicated in patients with significant respiratory depression, patients with hypercarbia, GI obstruction, and paralytic ileus.
- Use caution in opioid naïve patients, with abrupt discontinuation, CNS depression, head trauma, psychosis and increased ICP, cardiovascular disease, seizures, adrenal insufficiency, hypothyroidism, and myxedema.
- Adverse effects include laryngospasm, seizure, ileus, bradycardia, GI obstruction, constipation, euphoria, dysphoria, confusion, blurred vision, dysuria, dyspnea, hypotension, hallucinations, nausea, drowsiness, vomiting, diarrhea, abdominal pain, or fatigue.

(continued)

Table A.2 Common Pain and Sedation Medications (*continued*)

General Indications	General Mechanism of Action	General Contraindications, Precautions, and Adverse Effects
Opioids: tramadol		
• Moderate to moderately severe acute pain • Moderate chronic pain or moderately severe chronic pain in patients requiring continuous around the clock treatment for an extended period of time • Adjunctive treatment of osteoarthritis • Diabetic neuropathy • Postherpetic neuralgia • Postoperative shivering	• Agonistic activity at the central opiate receptor	• There are no direct contraindications. • Use caution in polysorbate 80 hypersensitivity, CNS depression, head trauma, seizure and increased ICP, severe pulmonary disease, biliary disease, GI obstruction or GI disease, substance abuse, renal or hepatic impairments, geriatric population, adrenal insufficiency, hypothyroidism, and myxedema. • Adverse effects include hepatic failure, pancreatitis, bradycardia, seizures, pulmonary edema, dysrhythmia, bronchospasm, constipation, hallucinations, hypertension, hypertonia, dyspnea, urinary retention, peripheral edema, blurred vision, withdrawal with abrupt discontinuation, hepatitis, amnesia, confusion, nausea, dizziness, headache, vomiting, drowsiness, agitation, and pruritus.
Sedatives: benzodiazepines (midazolam)		
• Procedural sedation • Amnesia induction • Control of preoperative anxiety • General anesthesia induction and maintenance • Seizures • Sedation maintenance in mechanically ventilated patients • Relief of agitation and/or anxiety • Treatment of status epilepticus refractory to standard therapy • Sedation during RSI • Treatment of alcohol withdrawal including delirium tremens	• Act on the hypothalamic, thalamic, and limbic regions to produce CNS depression	• Medication is contraindicated in sleep apnea or severe respiratory insufficiency/failure that is not mechanically ventilated, acute closed angle glaucoma. • Use caution in geriatric populations, psychiatric conditions including bipolar, depression, mania, psychosis or suicidal ideation, CNS depression, hepatic disease, substance use/abuse, and dementia. • Adverse effects include coma, seizure, apnea, pneumothorax, dysrhythmia, bradycardia, delirium, confusion, hypotension, hallucinations, memory impairment, constipation, respiratory depression, tolerance, psychological dependance,

Sedatives: dexmedetomidine

• Sedation induction and maintenance of mechanically ventilated ICU patients • Procedural sedation of nonintubated patients undergoing surgical procedure • Preanesthetic sedation	• Centrally act as agonist to alpha2-adrenoceptors, resulting in sedation and analgesia without significant ventilatory effects	• There are no direct contraindications. • Use caution in patients with hypovolemia, diabetes, bradycardia, hypotension, uncontrolled hypertension, hepatic disease, and renal failure. • Adverse effects include hypotension and bradycardia (may require decreased dose or discontinuation), dysrhythmia, hyperkalemia, renal failure, apnea, respiratory depression, hypoxia, hypovolemia, anemia, nausea, anxiety, fever, vomiting, diaphoresis, dizziness, headache, and diarrhea.

RESOURCES

Prescribers' Digital Reference. (n.d.). *Acetaminophen* [Drug information]. PDR Search. https://www.pdr.net/drug-summary/Ofirmev-acetaminophen-1346
Prescribers' Digital Reference. (n.d.). *Amidate (etomidate)* [Drug information]. PDR Search. https://www.pdr.net/drug-summary/Amidate-etomidate-675
Prescribers' Digital Reference. (n.d.). *Ativan* [Drug information]. PDR Search. https://www.pdr.net/drug-summary/Ativan-Injection-lorazepam-996
Prescribers' Digital Reference. (n.d.). *Ativan* [Drug information]. PDR Search. https://www.pdr.net/drug-summary/Precedex-dexmedetomidine-hydrochloride-1271
Prescribers' Digital Reference. (n.d.). *Dilaudid* [Drug information]. PDR Search. https://www.pdr.net/drug-summary/
    Dilaudid-Injection-and-HP-Injection-hydromorphone-hydromorphone-hydrochloride-490
Prescribers' Digital Reference. (n.d.). *Diprovan* [Drug information]. PDR Search. https://www.pdr.net/drug-summary/Diprivan-propofol-1719
Prescribers' Digital Reference. (n.d.). *Fentanyl* [Drug information]. PDR Search. https://www.pdr.net/drug-summary/Fentanyl-Citrate-fentanyl-citrate-2474
Prescribers' Digital Reference. (n.d.). *Ketamine* [Drug information]. PDR Search. https://www.pdr.net/drug-summary/Ketalar-ketamine-hydrochloride-1999#10
Prescribers' Digital Reference. (n.d.). *Morphine* [Drug information]. PDR Search. https://www.pdr.net/drug-summary/Morphine-Sulfate-Tablets-morphine-sulfate-1520
Prescribers' Digital Reference. (n.d.). *Neurontin* [Drug information]. PDR Search. https://www.pdr.net/drug-summary/Neurontin-gabapentin-2477.4218
Prescribers' Digital Reference. (n.d.). *Oxycodone* [Drug information]. PDR Search. https://www.pdr.net/drug-summary/Oxycodone-HCl-oxycodone-hydrochloride-24333
Prescribers' Digital Reference. (n.d.). *Phenobarbital* [Drug information]. PDR Search. https://www.pdr.net/drug-summary/Phenobarbital-Elixir-phenobarbital-2669#10
Prescribers' Digital Reference. (n.d.). *Zohydro-ER (hydrocodone)* [Drug information]. PDR Search. https://www.pdr.net/drug-summary/
    Zohydro-ER-hydrocodone-bitartrate-3389

Table A.3 Common Intravenous Fluids

General Indications	General Mechanism of Action	General Contraindications, Precautions, and Adverse Effects
D5NS		
• Parenteral (IV) treatment for hypoglycemia and hyperkalemia • Nutritional and parenteral nutrition	• Replace and supplement glucose, supplies energy to cells	• Medication is contraindicated in hyperglycemia and severe dehydration. Dextrose solutions can worsen the patient's hyperosmolar state. • Use caution in hypernatremia, hyperchloremia, metabolic acidosis, infection, diabetes, hepatic disease, in HF with fluid overload, and electrolyte imbalance. • Adverse effects include hyperglycemia.
D5W		
• Parenteral (IV) treatment for hypoglycemia and hyperkalemia • Nutritional and parenteral nutrition • Oral glucose tolerance test	• Replace and supplement glucose • Supply energy to cells	• Medication is contraindicated in hyperglycemia and severe dehydration. Dextrose solutions can worsen the patient's hyperosmolar state. • Use caution in infection, diabetes, hepatic disease, heart failure with fluid overload, and electrolyte imbalance. • Adverse effects include hyperglycemia.
Normal saline (sodium chloride, 3%, 0.9%, 0.45%)		
• Dehydration or hypovolemia, including during diabetic ketoacidosis and shock • Hyponatremia • Mucolysis and sputum induction in patients with cystic fibrosis • Treatment of nasal congestion and dryness • Nutritional supplementation • Temporary relief of corneal edema • Treatment of increased ICP (3% hypertonic solution) • Inpatient management of viral bronchiolitis	• Regulate membrane potential of cells to help maintain water/sodium balance and homeostatic function	• There are no direct contraindications. • Use caution in hypernatremia, hyperchloremia, HF with fluid overload, and metabolic acidosis. • Adverse effects include HF, encephalopathy, hypernatremia, and sodium retention.

Lactated Ringer's solution

- Any condition requiring volume repletion or electrolyte supplementation
- Hypotension
- Any condition requiring an increase of pH level

- Regulate homeostasis by supplementing water and electrolyte balance

- There are no true contraindications.
- Use caution in alkalosis, diabetes, metabolic disturbances (hypokalemia, hypercalcemia, or metabolic acidosis), dysrhythmia, hypoxemia, and pulmonary, cardiovascular and hepatic disease.
- Adverse effects include change in taste, weight gain, vomiting, stomach pain, seizures, nausea, dizziness, faintness, nervousness, confusion, blurred vision, or edema.

RESOURCES

Mayo Foundation for Medical Education and Research. (2021, February 1). *Lactated ringer's (INTRAVENOUS route) side effects*. https://www.mayoclinic.org/drugs-supplements/lactated-ringers-intravenous-route/side-effects/drg-20489612?p=1

Prescribers' Digital Reference. (n.d.). *Dextrose monohydrate* [Drug information]. PDR Search. https://www.pdr.net/drug-summary/5--Dextrose-dextrose-monohydrate-24283

Prescribers' Digital Reference. (n.d.). *Sodium chloride* [Drug information]. PDR Search. https://www.pdr.net/drug-summary/Sodium-Chloride-sodium-chloride-24245

Table A.4 Common Steroid Medications

General Indications	General Mechanism of Action	General Contraindications, Precautions, and Adverse Effects
Corticosteroids (prednisone, dexamethasone, methylprednisolone)		
• Maintenance therapy of primary or secondary adrenocortical insufficiency • Congenital adrenal hyperplasia • Kidney transplant rejection prophylaxis • Chronic graft versus host disease • Acute lymphocytic leukemia • Chronic lymphocytic leukemia • Short-term treatment of hypercalcemia secondary disease • Inflammatory bowel disease • Crohn's disease • Ulcerative colitis • Rheumatic conditions • Systemic autoimmune conditions • Hemolytic anemia • Asthma exacerbation • Thrombocytopenia or ITP • Myasthenia gravis • Psoriatic arthritis • Proteinuria in nephrotic syndrome • Severe erythema multiforme or Stevens-Johnson syndrome • Treatment of ACE-inhibitor-induced angioedema • Allergic disorders including anaphylaxis • ARDS • Pneumonia • Hodgkin lymphoma • Multiple myeloma • Duchenne muscular dystrophy	• Inhibit steps in the inflammatory pathway to prevent systemic infection and inflammation of the lungs and to reduce mucus production	• Patients receiving corticosteroids for an extended time or in high doses are at increased risk of immunosuppression, making them more prone to infection. • Avoid in patients with Cushing's syndrome. • Use caution in untreated infection, diabetes, glaucoma, immunosuppression, and liver disease. • Adverse effects include growth inhibition, osteoporosis, osteopenia, impaired wound healing, immunosuppression, candidiasis, fluid retention, hypernatremia, euphoria, hallucinations, hyperglycemia, nausea, weight gain, fluid retention, emotional lability, headache, hoarseness, diaphoresis, and bronchospasm. • Medication may reduce glucose tolerance, causing hyperglycemia in diabetic patients.

- Carpal tunnel syndrome
- Autoimmune hepatitis
- Primary amyloidosis
- Exacerbation of COPD
- Idiopathic or viral pericarditis
- Interstitial nephritis
- Bell's palsy
- Transplant rejection
- Guillain-Barré Syndrome

RESOURCES

Prescribers' Digital Reference. (n.d.). *Prednisone* [Drug information]. PDR Search. https://www.pdr.net/drug-summary/Prednisone-Prednisone-Intensol-prednisone-2575

AA	Alcoholics Anonymous
AACN	American Association of Critical-Care Nurses
ABG	arterial blood gas
ABI	ankle-brachial index
ACE	angiotensin-converting enzyme
ACEI	angiotensin-converting enzyme inhibitor
ACHS	before meals and at bedtime
ACLS	advanced cardiovascular life support
ACS	acute coronary syndrome
ACT	activated clotting time
ADA	American Diabetes Association
A-fib	atrial fibrillation
AIDS	acquired immunodeficiency syndrome
AKI	acute kidney injury
ALS	amyotrophic lateral sclerosis
AMS	altered mental status
ANA	American Nurses Association
ARB	angiotensin receptor blocker
ARDS	acute respiratory distress syndrome
ASI	alcohol severity index
AST	aspartate aminotransferase
ATP	adenosine triphosphate
AV	atrioventricular
AVF	arteriovenous fistula
BiPAP	bilevel positive airway pressure
BM	bowel movement
BMP	basic metabolic panel
BNP	B-type natriuretic peptide
BP	blood pressure
BUN	blood urea nitrogen
CABG	coronary artery bypass graft
CAD	coronary artery disease
CAP	community-acquired pneumonia
CAUTI	catheter-associated urinary tract infection
CBC	complete blood count
CDE	certified diabetes educator
CERP	continuing education recognition points
CHF	congestive heart failure
CIWA	clinical institute withdrawal assessment
CK	creatine kinase
CKD	chronic kidney disease
CK-MB	creatine kinase-MB

CLABSI	central-line-associated bloodstream infection
CMP	comprehensive metabolic panel
CNS	central nervous system
COPD	chronic obstructive pulmonary disease
COWS	clinical opiate withdrawal scale
COX	cyclooxygenase-1
CPAP	continuous positive airway pressure therapy
CPK	creatine phosphokinase
Cr	creatinine
CRP	C-reactive protein
CRRT	continuous renal replacement therapy
CV	cardiovascular
DASH	dietary approaches to stop hypertension
DI	diabetes insipidus
DIC	disseminated intravascular coagulation
DM	diabetes mellitus
DNR	do not resuscitate
DNI	do not intubate
DKA	diabetic ketoacidosis
DVT	deep vein thrombosis
E. coli	*Escherichia coli*
EBV	Epstein-Barr virus
EBP	evidence-based practice
ECMO	extracorporeal membrane oxygenation
EGD	esophagogastroduodenoscopy (upper GI endoscopy)
eGFR	estimated glomerular filtration rate
ELISA	enzyme-linked immunosorbent assay
EMS	emergency medical services
ERCP	endoscopic retrograde cholangiopancreatography
ESR	erythrocyte sedimentation rate
ESRD	end-stage renal disease
ETOH	ethanol
EVAR	endovascular repair
FODMAP	fermentable oligosaccharides, disaccharides, monosaccharides, and polyols
G6PD	glucose-6-phosphate dehydrogenase
GABA	gamma-aminobutyric acid
GAD	generalized anxiety disorder
GCS	Glasgow Coma Scale
GERD	gastroesophageal reflux disease
GFR	glomerular filtration rate
GI	gastrointestinal
H/H	hemoglobin and hematocrit
HAART	highly active antiretroviral therapy
HbA1c	glycosylated hemoglobin
HF	heart failure
HHS	hyperosmolar hyperglycemic syndrome
H. influenza	*Haemophilus influenza*
HIT	heparin-induced thrombocytopenia
HOB	head of bed
HR	heart rate
HSV	herpes simplex virus
HTN	hypertension
IABP	intraaortic baloon pump

I/O	intake/output
IBS	irritable bowel syndrome
ICD	implantable cardioverter defibrillator
ICH	intracerebral hemorrhage
ICP	intracranial pressure
IgE	immunoglobulin E
IgM	immunoglobulin M
IM	intramuscular
INR	international normalized ratio
ITP	immune thrombocytopenic purpura
IV	intravenous
IVF	intravenous fluid
IVIG	intravenous immunoglobulin
JVD	jugular vein distention
KUB	kidney, ureter, and bladder x-ray
LAD	left anterior descending artery
LDH	lactic acid dehydrogenase
LFT	liver function test
LV	left ventricle
LVAD	left ventricular assist device
MAO	monoamine oxidase
MAOI	monoamine oxidase inhibitor
MAP	mean arterial pressure
MDRO	multidrug-resistant organism
MI	myocardial infarction
MODS	multiple organ dysfunction syndrome
MONA-B	morphine, oxygen, nitroglycerin, aspirin, beta blocker
MRA	magnetic resonance angiography
MRSA	methicillin-resistant *Staphylococcus aureus*
MS	multiple sclerosis
MSSA	methicillin-susceptible *Staphylococcus aureus*
NA	Narcotics Anonymous
NASH	non alcoholic steatohepatitis
NCCA	National Commission of Certifying Agencies
NG	nasogastric
NIHSS	National Institutes of Health Stroke Scale (NIH Stroke Scale)
NIPPV	nasal intermittent positive pressure ventilation
NMDA	N-methyl-D-aspartate
NPO	nothing by mouth
NS	normal saline
NSAID	nonsteroidal anti-inflammatory drug
NSR	normal sinus rhythm
NSTEMI	non-ST-elevation myocardial infarction
OB	obstetrics
OBGYN	obstetric–gynecologic
OG	orogastric
OR	operating room
OSA	obstructive sleep apnea
OT	occupational therapy
OTC	over the counter
PAC	premature atrial contraction
PACU	post-anesthesia care unit
PAD	peripheral arterial disease

PCA	patient-controlled analgesia
PCC	prothrombin complex concentrate
PCCN	progressive care certified nurse
PCI	percutaneous coronary intervention
PCR	polymerase chain reaction
PCU	progressive care unit
PDE-5	phosphodiesterase-5
PE	pulmonary embolism
PEEP	positive end-expiratory pressure
PEFR	peak expiratory flow rate
PICC	peripherally inserted central catheter
PIV	peripheral intravenous line
PKU	phenylketonuria
PMI	point of maximal impulse
PO	mouth per os (by mouth)
PPE	personal protective equipment
PRN	as needed
PT	physical therapy; prothrombin time
PTT	partial thromboplastin time
PVC	premature ventricular contractions
PVD	peripheral vascular disease
Q2H	every 2 hr
RBC	red blood cell
RCA	right coronary artery
RPR	rapid plasma reagin
RRT	renal replacement therapy
RSI	rapid sequence intubation
RVC	remature ventricular contractions
RVR	rapid ventricular response
SA	sinoatrial
SBP	spontaneous bacterial peritonitis
SCD	sequential compression device
ScvO2	central venous oxygen saturation
SIADH	syndrome of inappropriate secretion of antidiuretic hormone
SNRI	serotonin–norepinephrine reuptake inhibitor
SSI	surgical site infection
SSRI	selective serotonin reuptake inhibitor
STAT	for urgent or rush
STEMI	ST-elevation myocardial infarction
SVR	sustained virologic response
SVT	supraventricular tachycardia
TBI	traumatic brain injury
T2DM	type 2 diabetes
TEE	transesophageal echocardiogram
TEG	thromboelastography
TIA	transient ischemic attack
TIPS	transjugular intrahepatic portosystemic shunt
TMP-SMX	trimethoprim-sulfamethoxazole
TPA	tissue plasminogen activator
TPN	total parenteral nutrition
TSH	thyroid-stimulating hormone
TTE	transthoracic echocardiogram

TV	television
UNOS	United Network for Organ Sharing
UTI	urinary tract infection
VAC	vacuum-assisted closure
VAD	vascular access device
VATS	video-assisted thoracoscopic surgery
VBG	venous blood gas
VS	vital signs
VT	ventricular tachycardia
WBC	white blood count

INDEX

Printed in the United States
by Baker & Taylor Publisher Services